Pathology

Notice

Medicine is an ever-changing science. As new research and clinical experience broaden our knowledge, changes in treatment and drug therapy are required. The editor and the publisher of this work have checked with sources believed to be reliable in their efforts to provide information that is complete and generally in accord with the standards accepted at the time of publication. However, in view of the possibility of human error or changes in medical sciences, neither the editors nor the publisher nor any other party who has been involved in the preparation or publication of this work warrants that the information contained herein is in every respect accurate or complete, and they are not responsible for any errors or omissions or for the results obtained from use of such information. Readers are encouraged to confirm the information contained herein with other sources. For example and in particular, readers are advised to check the product information sheet included in the package of each drug they plan to administer to be certain that the information contained in this book is accurate and that changes have not been made in the recommended dose or in the contraindications for administration. This recommendation is of particular importance in connection with new or infrequently used drugs.

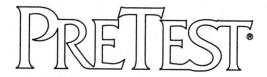

Pathology

PreTest®
Self-Assessment
and Review

Eighth Edition

Edited by
Earl J. Brown, M.D.
Associate Professor
Department of Pathology
Quillen College of Medicine
Johnson City, Tennessee

Chief of Hematopathology
Department of Pathology
VA Medical Center
Mountain Home, Tennessee

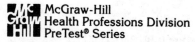 McGraw-Hill
Health Professions Division
PreTest® Series

New York   St. Louis   San Francisco   Auckland
Bogotá   Caracas   Lisbon   London   Madrid
Mexico City   Milan   Montreal   New Delhi
San Juan   Singapore   Sydney   Tokyo   Toronto

Pathology : PreTest® Self-Assessment and Review, 8/e
International Editions 1996

Exclusive rights by McGraw-Hill Book Co.–Singapore for manufacture and export.
This book cannot be re-exported from the country to which it is consigned by
McGraw-Hill.

1 2 3 4 5 6 7 8 9 0 CWP FC 9 8 7 6 5

The editors were Gail Gavert and Bruce MacGregor.
The production supervisor was Gyl A. Favours.
This book was set in Times Roman by Compset, Inc.

Library of Congress Cataloging-in-Publication Data

Pathology : PreTest self-assessment and review / edited by
    Earl Brown. – 8th ed.
      p.   cm.
    Includes bibliogrpahical references.
    ISBN 0-07-052086-0 (pbk.)
    1. Pathology – Examinations, questions, etc.   I. Brown, Earl,
    1956 –   .   II. Series.
      [DNLM: 1. Pathology–examination questions.   QZ 18.2 P297 1996]
    RB31.P325   1996
    616.07'076–dc20
    DNLM/DLC
    for Library of Congress   95-5740

When ordering this title, use ISBN 0-07-113617-7

Printed in Singapore

Contents

Preface

The study of pathology, a science so basic to clinical medicine, has been abbreviated sadly in many medical schools in recent years, and this at a time when explosive growth is occurring in the science. Recent advances in immunopathology, diagnosis of bacterial and viral diseases including AIDS, and detection of infectious agents such as papillomavirus in cervical dysplasia are proceeding at a tremendous rate. The eighth edition of *Pathology: PreTest® Self-Assessment and Review* includes such new subject areas as predictive values in the interpretation of laboratory data, importance of cytokines, the molecular basis of genetic and other disease processes, and molecular biology techniques as these apply to lymphoproliferative disorders and other tumors.

The medical student must feel submerged at times in the flood of information — occasionally instructors may have similar feelings. This edition is not intended to cover all new knowledge in addition to including older anatomic and clinical pathology. It is, rather, a serious attempt to present important facts about many disease processes in hopes that the student will read much further in major textbooks and journals and will receive some assistance in passing medical school, licensure, or board examinations.

Introduction

Each *PreTest® Self-Assessment and Review* allows medical students to comprehensively and conveniently assess and review their knowledge of a particular basic science, in this instance Pathology. The 500 questions parallel the format and degree of difficulty of the questions found in the United States Medical Licensing Examination (USMLE) Step 1. Practicing physicians who want to hone their skills before USMLE Step 3 or recertification may find this to be a good beginning in their review process.

Each question is accompanied by an answer, a paragraph explanation, and a specific page reference to an appropriate textbook or journal article. A bibliography listing sources can be found following the last chapter of this text.

An effective way to use this PreTest is to allow yourself one minute to answer each question in a given chapter. As you proceed, indicate your answer beside each question. By following this suggestion, you approximate the time limits imposed by the Step.

After you finish going through the questions in the section, spend as much time as you need verifying your answers and carefully reading the explanations provided. Pay special attention to the explanations for the questions you answered incorrectly—but read *every* explanation. The authors of this material have designed the explanations to reinforce and supplement the information tested by the questions. If you feel you need further information about the material covered, consult and study the references indicated.

PreTest®

Pathology

General Pathology

DIRECTIONS: Each question below contains five suggested responses. Select the **one best** response to each question.

1. A 49-year-old man suffers an acute myocardial infarction because of the sudden occlusion of the left anterior descending coronary artery. The areas within the ventricle of myocardial necrosis can best be described as

(A) coagulative necrosis
(B) liquefactive necrosis
(C) fat necrosis
(D) caseous necrosis
(E) fibrinoid necrosis

2. Which group of factors is most important in the cellular pathogenesis of acute ischemia?

(A) Mitochondrial hyperplasia, lysozyme release, membrane injury
(B) Reduced ATP, increased calcium influx, membrane injury
(C) Lipid deposition, reduced protein synthesis, nuclear damage
(D) Ribosome detachment, glycolysis, nuclear damage
(E) Mitochondrial condensation, glycolysis, sodium cell loss

3. The involution of the thymus that occurs with aging is an example of the process of programmed cell death that is best described as

(A) apoptosis
(B) pyknosis
(C) karyorrhexis
(D) karyolysis
(E) pinocytosis

4. An understanding of complex disorders like hereditary spherocytosis, Chédiak-Higashi syndrome, and alcoholic liver disease has improved with molecular discoveries in

(A) lysosomal release
(B) recombinant DNA
(C) cytoskeletal makeup
(D) membrane phospholipids
(E) lipid accumulation

5. The irregular eosinophilic hyaline inclusions within the hepatocytoplasm shown below are

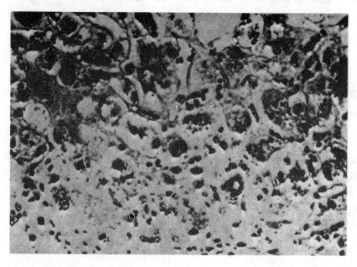

(A) Russell bodies
(B) parasites
(C) characteristic of chronic alcoholism
(D) characteristic of viral hepatitis
(E) characteristic of carbon tetrachloride poisoning

6. As visualized by the electron microscope, all the following are cell organelles EXCEPT

(A) lysosomes
(B) the Golgi complex
(C) the endoplasmic reticulum
(D) desmosomes
(E) microbodies

7. Which of the following provides an example of concomitant hyperplasia and hypertrophy?

(A) Uterine growth during pregnancy
(B) Left ventricular cardiac hypertrophy
(C) Enlargement of skeletal muscle in athletes
(D) Breast enlargement at puberty
(E) Cystic hyperplasia of the endometrium

8. Early during the acute inflammatory process neutrophils marginate to the periphery of blood vessels. An important adhesive surface protein found on these neutrophils, but absent in patients with leukocyte adhesion deficiency type 1, is

(A) E-selectin
(B) L-selectin
(C) leukocyte function antigen 1 (LFA-1)
(D) intracellular adhesion molecule 1 (ICAM-1)
(E) vascular adhesion molecule 1 (VCAM-1)

9. Defects in chemotaxis resulting in increased susceptibility to infection are associated with all the following EXCEPT

(A) diabetes mellitus, juvenile type
(B) chronic granulomatous disease of childhood
(C) chronic renal failure
(D) Chédiak-Higashi syndrome
(E) thermal injury

10. A very important mediator of the systemic effects of inflammation is

(A) gamma interferon (γ-IFN)
(B) beta tumor necrosis factor (β-TNF)
(C) interleukin 1 (IL-1)
(D) interleukin 2 (IL-2)
(E) interleukin 3 (IL-3)

11. The chemical mediators of inflammation listed below often proceed in a cascade after activation EXCEPT

(A) complement
(B) kinin
(C) arachidonic acid
(D) fibrinopeptides
(E) neutral proteases

12. Leukotrienes differ from prostaglandins in the mediation of inflammation by more potent actions in all the following EXCEPT

(A) chemotaxis
(B) vasoconstriction
(C) bronchoconstriction
(D) pain
(E) vascular permeability

13. The cells of the mononuclear phagocyte system originate from the

(A) spleen
(B) liver
(C) lymph node
(D) bone marrow
(E) thymus

14. Infectious diseases associated with a granulomatous response include all the following EXCEPT

(A) tuberculosis
(B) coccidioidomycosis
(C) schistosomiasis
(D) sarcoidosis
(E) cat-scratch disease

15. In an evaluation of an 8-year-old boy who had had recurrent infections since the first year of life, findings included enlargement of the liver and spleen, lymph node inflammation, and a superficial dermatitis resembling eczema. Microscopic examination of a series of peripheral blood smears taken during the course of a staphylococcal infection indicated that the bactericidal capacity of the boy's neutrophils was impaired or absent. Which of the following is the most probable diagnosis?

(A) Chronic granulomatous disease
(B) Congenital agammaglobulinemia
(C) Hereditary thymic dysplasia
(D) Chédiak-Higashi syndrome
(E) Wiskott-Aldrich syndrome

16. Normal levels of C-reactive protein (CRP) are most often observed in

(A) acute viral illness
(B) pneumococcal pneumonia
(C) active rheumatoid arthritis
(D) active pulmonary tuberculosis
(E) acute myocardial infarction

17. Type I collagen is found in all the following EXCEPT

(A) tendon
(B) dermis
(C) cartilage
(D) fascia
(E) bone

18. An exudate is the result of

(A) increased venous pressure
(B) sodium retention
(C) decreased plasma oncotic pressure
(D) increased capillary permeability
(E) lymphatic obstruction

19. "Heart failure cells" are present within the alveoli as a result of

(A) petechial hemorrhage
(B) ecchymoses
(C) purpura
(D) active hyperemia
(E) passive hyperemia

20. Procoagulant factors produced by endothelial cells include

(A) thrombomodulin
(B) prostacyclin
(C) von Willebrand factor
(D) thromboxane A_2
(E) fibrinogen

21. The action of streptokinase involves the formation of

(A) antithrombin III
(B) protein C
(C) plasmin
(D) thrombin
(E) C'1 inactivator

22. A patient hospitalized for fractures of the long bones who develops mental dysfunction, increasing respiratory insufficiency, and renal failure should be suspected of having

(A) fat embolism syndrome
(B) disseminated intravascular coagulopathy
(C) myocardial infarction
(D) aortic valve disease
(E) respiratory distress syndrome

23. Which of the following statements regarding transmural intestinal infarction is true?

(A) Thromboemboli usually originate in the ileofemoral veins
(B) The colon is more commonly affected than the small intestine
(C) Colonic infarction classically affects the hepatic flexure
(D) Arterial occlusion results in pallor of the affected segment
(E) Up to 25 percent of cases are due to nonocclusive hypoperfusion

24. Endotoxic shock is commonly caused by all the following organisms EXCEPT

(A) *Pseudomonas aeruginosa*
(B) *Escherichia coli*
(C) *Proteus* species
(D) *Corynebacterium diphtheriae*
(E) *Klebsiella pneumoniae*

25. All the following cytologic and membrane alterations can generally be found in neoplastic cells EXCEPT

(A) changes in pseudopodia and microvilli
(B) changes in the cytoskeleton
(C) acquisition of surface-associated glycoproteins
(D) increased lectin agglutinability
(E) decreased membrane transport

26. The gross texture and resilience of a given tumor are largely influenced by which of the following?

(A) Presence or absence of connective tissue stroma
(B) Degree of malignancy
(C) Interface between normal tissue and tumor
(D) Type of epithelium present
(E) Relative blood supply

27. An increased incidence of neoplasia has been observed in all the following EXCEPT

(A) primary (genetic) immunodeficient states
(B) immunosuppressed recipients of transplants
(C) acquired immunodeficiency syndrome (AIDS)
(D) therapy with radiation and radiomimetic drugs
(E) sarcoidosis

28. The incidences of all the following malignancies are higher in China or Japan when compared with those in the United States EXCEPT

(A) nasopharyngeal carcinoma
(B) liver carcinoma
(C) gastric carcinoma
(D) choriocarcinoma
(E) prostatic carcinoma

29. Oncogene activation has been implicated in the development of all the following malignancies EXCEPT

(A) carcinoma of the urinary bladder
(B) neuroblastoma
(C) chronic myelocytic leukemia
(D) Burkitt's lymphoma
(E) retinoblastoma

30. An example of a cancer suppressor gene is

(A) c-*abl*
(B) *bcr*
(C) c-*myc*
(D) p53
(E) *ras*

31. Hypertrophic osteoarthropathy is most often associated with

(A) bronchiectasis
(B) infective endocarditis
(C) bronchogenic carcinoma
(D) mesothelioma
(E) inflammatory bowel disease

32. An African boy with a rapidly expanding mass in the region of the jaw and cheek is thought to have Burkitt's lymphoma. These cells are growing rapidly because of

(A) their permanent nature
(B) shortening of the cell cycle
(C) nonsequencing of the EBV genome
(D) fewer G_0 cells entering the cycle
(E) delayed progression from G_2 to mitosis

33. Environmental and industrial pollutants are becoming increasingly relevant in human oncogenesis. Which of the following combinations is most closely allied with human neoplasia?

(A) Asbestos, silica, arsenicals
(B) Diethylstilbestrol, radioactive ducts, cyanide
(C) Aflatoxin, beryllium vapor, benzidine
(D) Polyvinyl chloride, nickel, chromium
(E) Carbon tetrachloride, lead, chloroform

34. While many factors affect a tumor's behavior, which of the following can be expected to influence the biology of a given tumor the *most*?

(A) Lack of a peripheral capsule
(B) Histologic differentiation
(C) Presence of inflammation
(D) Size of the tumor
(E) Nuclear cytoplasmic ratio

35. All the following are correct associations of special histologic stains of tumor markers with the appropriate tumors EXCEPT

(A) human chorionic gonadotropin (hCG) and trophoblastic tumors
(B) alpha-fetoprotein (AFP) and liver cell cancer
(C) prostate-specific antigen (PSA) and prostate cancer
(D) carcinoembryonic antigen (CEA) and colon cancer
(E) chloroacetate esterase (CAE) and stomach cancer

36. Characteristics of granular cell tumors commonly include all the following EXCEPT

(A) location in the tongue
(B) PAS-positive, diastase-resistant granules
(C) association with pseudoepitheliomatous hyperplasia
(D) frequent malignant change
(E) origin from Schwann cell precursors

---

37. The photomicrograph below shows a labeling phenomenon of dark cytoplasmic granules within select cells. This staining technique has all the following characteristics EXCEPT

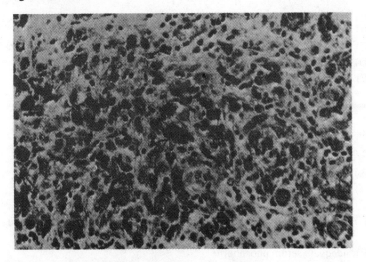

(A) it relies on neutral polysaccharides for a positive reaction
(B) it relies on antigen-antibody binding
(C) it may be used to identify proteins
(D) it may be used to identify tumor cell markers
(E) it may be used to identify viruses and other microorganisms

38. The histologic pattern of the lymph node section shown below is likely to support a diagnosis of

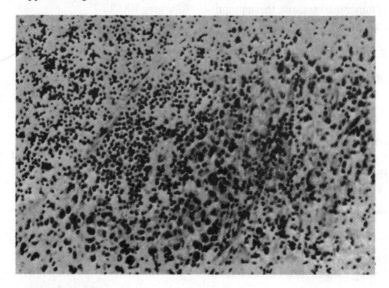

(A) sickle cell anemia
(B) carcinoma
(C) leukemia
(D) infectious mononucleosis
(E) rheumatoid arthritis

---

39. A significant deficiency in vitamin D might be expected to lead to

(A) hyperostosis
(B) relative excess of osteoid tissue
(C) increased absorption of calcium
(D) decreased production of bone matrix
(E) adequate serum phosphorus

40. A deficiency of vitamin E would most likely result in

(A) night blindness
(B) rickets
(C) a bleeding diathesis
(D) spinocerebellar degeneration
(E) megaloblastic anemia

41. The specimen shown in the photomicrograph below is from a mass removed from the thigh of a 58-year-old man. Using the current nomenclature, this lesion is compatible with

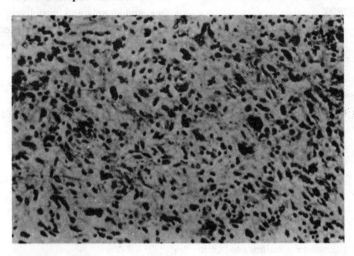

(A) nodular fasciitis
(B) rhabdomyosarcoma
(C) myositis ossificans
(D) osteogenic sarcoma
(E) malignant fibrous histiocytoma

---

42. All the following characteristics are true of liposarcoma EXCEPT that it

(A) presents varied histology
(B) is commonly found in the retroperitoneum
(C) frequently gives rise to embolization in lymphatics
(D) is the most common soft tissue sarcoma
(E) arises very rarely in subcutaneous tissue

43. Vitmain K is required for the synthesis of all the following EXCEPT

(A) prothrombin
(B) clotting factor VII
(C) clotting factor VIII
(D) clotting factor IX
(E) clotting factor X

44. Fibrosarcoma, shown in the photomicrograph below, may be characterized by all the following EXCEPT

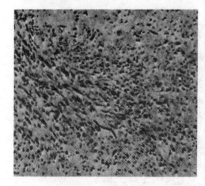

(A) interlacing bundles of anaplastic spindle cells
(B) occasional similarity to "cellular fibroma"
(C) fibroblastic or myofibroblastic differentiation
(D) relative infrequency of occurrence
(E) prominent arborizing vascularization

45. Which of the following drugs may cause bronchospasm?

(A) Bleomycin
(B) Methotrexate
(C) Nitrofurantoin
(D) Aspirin
(E) Amiodarone

46. An apathetic male infant in an underdeveloped country is found to have peripheral edema, a "moon" face, and an enlarged, fatty liver. Which of the following is one mechanism involved in the pathogenesis of this child's abnormalities?

(A) Decreased protein intake leading to decreased lipoproteins
(B) Decreased caloric intake leading to hypoalbuminemia
(C) Decreased carbohydrate intake leading to hypoglycemia
(D) Decreased fluid intake leading to hypernatremia
(E) Decreased fat absorption leading to hypovitaminosis

47. A woman taking oral contraceptives during the reproductive years increases, even if only minimally, her risk of developing the following EXCEPT

(A) pulmonary infarction
(B) myocardial infarction
(C) vaginal adenosis
(D) venous thrombus
(E) liver cell adenoma

48. Alcohol may be the most significant cause of public health problems in the United States. All the following entities are correlated with alcohol abuse EXCEPT

(A) subdural hematoma
(B) esophageal carcinoma
(C) elevated creatine phosphokinase
(D) primary biliary cirrhosis
(E) portal vein thrombosis

49. δ-Aminolevulinic acid is excreted in increased amounts in the urine of patients with

(A) lead poisoning
(B) carcinoma of the pancreas
(C) chronic pyelonephritis
(D) vitamin C intoxication
(E) ulcerative colitis

50. Effects of radiation exposure on tissue include all the following EXCEPT

(A) double-stranded chromosomal breaks
(B) formation of free radicals
(C) abnormal mitotic figures
(D) endothelial swelling
(E) epidermal hyperplasia

51. An industrial foundry worker who has been chronically exposed to heavy metal vapors has developed a radiographic pattern of pulmonary "honeycombing." Which of the following heavy metals is most likely responsible?

(A) Cobalt
(B) Lead
(C) Cadmium
(D) Mercury
(E) Arsenic

52. A comatose 27-year-old woman is brought to the emergency room by paramedics, and the strong odor of bitter almonds is present. The differential diagnosis must include the possibility of poisoning by

(A) ethylene glycol
(B) carbon monoxide
(C) mercury
(D) cyanide
(E) methanol

53. If a mutant gene is not expressed phenotypically in a person, this is said to represent

(A) variable expressivity
(B) reduced penetrance
(C) codominance
(D) genetic heterogeneity
(E) nondisjunction

54. A chromosomal aberration that results in a disturbance in the normal gene balance is termed

(A) nondisjunction
(B) euploidy
(C) aneuploidy
(D) breakage
(E) variance

55. All the following genetic disorders are autosomal recessive (AR) EXCEPT

(A) alkaptonuria
(B) familial hypercholesterolemia
(C) phenylketonuria (PKU)
(D) myeloperoxidase deficiency
(E) cystic fibrosis (CF)

56. A 45-year-old man presents with severe pain in both knee joints. At the time of surgery, his cartilage is found to have a dark blue-black color. Further evaluation revealed that this patient's urine darkened rapidly with time. The most likely diagnosis for this abnormality is

(A) hyperphenylalaninemia
(B) tyrosinemia
(C) tyrosinase-positive oculocutaneous albinism
(D) alcaptonuria
(E) maple syrup urine disease

57. In tissues affected by the predominant form of Niemann-Pick disease, which of the following is found at abnormally high levels?

(A) Sphingomyelin
(B) Sphingomyelinase
(C) Kerasin
(D) Acetyl coenzyme A
(E) Ganglioside

58. The abnormality most compatible with a diagnosis of von Gierke's disease is a deficiency of

(A) glucose-6-phosphatase
(B) glucose-6-phosphate dehydrogenase
(C) branching enzyme
(D) muscle phosphorylase
(E) lysosomal glucosidase

59. Mechanisms responsible for Down's syndrome include all the following EXCEPT

(A) nondisjunction during first meiotic division
(B) mosaicism
(C) translocation
(D) centric fusion (Robertsonian translocation)
(E) formation of isochromosomes

60. A 2-month-old girl presents with a soft, high-pitched, mewing cry and is found to have several congenital heart defects. The most likely chromosomal abnormality producing these symptoms is

(A) 5p−
(B) 11p−
(C) 13q−
(D) 21q−
(E) 22q−

61. All the following symptoms are associated with Klinefelter's syndrome EXCEPT

(A) large, soft testes
(B) gynecomastia
(C) eunuchoidism
(D) azospermia
(E) elevated urinary gonadotropins

62. A young woman of average intelligence and short stature who has never menstruated is under clinical investigation for Turner's syndrome. However, a buccal smear shows some cells with one Barr body. Which of the following best explains this finding?

(A) Laboratory error
(B) The patient is a male
(C) Classic XO pattern
(D) Turner's mosaic pattern
(E) Klinefelter's syndrome

63. A 15-year-old phenotypically female patient presents for workup of primary amenorrhea and is found to have an XY karyotype. The most likely diagnosis is

(A) Turner's syndrome
(B) mixed gonadal dysgenesis
(C) true hermaphroditism
(D) male pseudohermaphroditism
(E) female pseudohermaphroditism

64. An 8-year-old boy is found to have progressive corneal vascularization, deafness, notched incisors, and a flattened nose. The most likely cause of these changes is congenital infection by

(A) toxoplasma
(B) rubella
(C) cytomegalovirus
(D) herpes simplex virus
(E) *Treponema pallidum*

65. Which one of the following abnormalities of the eye is a markedly premature infant most at risk for developing soon after birth?

(A) Presbyopia
(B) Pinguecula
(C) Pterygium
(D) Macular degeneration
(E) Retrolental fibroplasia

66. In hemolytic disease of the newborn, all the following statements are correct EXCEPT

(A) erythroblastosis fetalis develops because of prior maternal sensitization
(B) anemia and hepatosplenomegaly are characteristic
(C) anti-D immunoglobulin should be given to a sensitized mother before delivery
(D) both ABO and Rh antigens cause hemolytic disease of the newborn
(E) there is transplacental transmission of maternal antibody

67. Rearrangement of immunoglobulin chains is seen in

(A) T lymphocytes
(B) B lymphocytes
(C) macrophages
(D) Langerhans' cells
(E) natural killer cells

68. The cells seen in the following photomicrograph were stained by ABC technique using OKT1 (Leu-1), OKT3 (Leu-4), and OTK11 (Leu-5) cluster designation CD5, CD3, and CD2. The result indicates that the cells are of what origin?

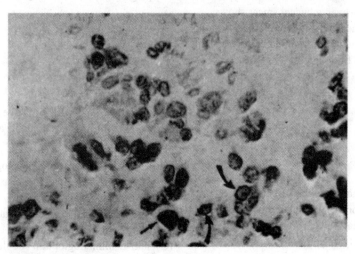

(A) T lymphocytes
(B) Oat cells
(C) Mesothelial cells
(D) EAC rosettes
(E) Melanoma cells

---

69. Characteristically, B lymphocytes do all the following EXCEPT

(A) constitute 10 to 15 percent of peripheral blood lymphocytes
(B) occur in lymphoid follicles and the superficial cortex of lymph nodes
(C) express surface immunoglobulins IgM and IgD
(D) express cluster differentiation antigen CD8
(E) possess complement component (C3) receptors

70. The mixed lymphocyte reaction is used to define which one of the following?

(A) HLA-A
(B) HLA-DQ
(C) Complement components
(D) Tumor necrosis factor alpha (TNFα)
(E) Beta$_2$ microglobulin

71. In antigen recognition by cytotoxic T lymphocytes, the T-cell receptor recognizes antigens bound to

(A) class I antigens
(B) class II antigens
(C) class III antigens
(D) C3b
(E) Fc portion of IgG

72. There is a strong association between ankylosing spondylitis and

(A) HLA-B27
(B) HLA-DR3
(C) HLA-DR4
(D) HLA-A3
(E) HLA-BW47

73. After receiving incompatible blood, a patient develops a transfusion reaction in the form of back pain, fever, shortness of breath, and hematuria. This type of immunologic reaction is classified as a

(A) systemic anaphylactic reaction
(B) systemic immune complex reaction
(C) delayed-type hypersensitivity reaction
(D) complement-mediated cytotoxicity
(E) T-cell–mediated cytotoxicity

74. Delayed-type hypersensitivity reactions of the tuberculin skin test type

(A) appear within 1 or 2 h
(B) require an intact T-lymphocyte population
(C) show dermal infiltrates of granulocytes
(D) are associated uniquely with small antigens
(E) do not require previous exposure to the antigen

75. An allograft is a graft between

(A) a human and an animal
(B) two individuals of different species
(C) two individuals of the same species
(D) two individuals of the same inbred strain
(E) identical twins

76. True statements concerning diagnostic specificity include all the following EXCEPT

(A) Scl-70 antibody is specific for diffuse systemic sclerosis
(B) antibodies to nucleolar RNA are specific for diffuse systemic sclerosis
(C) antibodies to double-stranded DNA are specific for systemic lupus erythematosus (SLE)
(D) antibodies to antinuclear antibody (ANA) are specific for SLE
(E) anti-Sm antibodies are specific for SLE

77. A patient with severe diabetic renal disease receives a donor cadaver kidney, following which a progressive rise in the serum creatinine occurs over a period lasting 5 months. In the photomicrograph below, what single finding is most characteristic for chronic rejection?

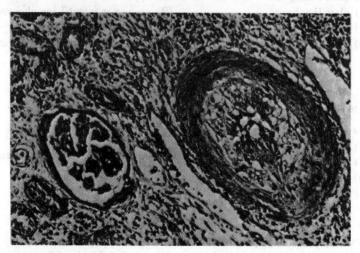

(A) Damaged glomeruli
(B) Interstitial fibrosis
(C) Interstitial inflammation
(D) Tubular atrophy
(E) Vascular changes

---

78. A 32-year-old woman sees her physician because of "stiffness" and intolerance to cold temperatures in her fingers. Her face has a "mask-like" quality. It would be appropriate in the systems review to ask about

(A) headaches and dizziness
(B) swallowing difficulties
(C) sun hypersensitivity
(D) thyroid trouble
(E) family history

79. The most feared clinical complication of a patient with an isolated IgA deficiency is

(A) tetany
(B) anaphylaxis
(C) angioedema
(D) thrombocytopenia
(E) lymphoma

80. Systemic lupus erythematosus (SLE), a multisystem disease of autoimmune origin, is characterized by all the following statements EXCEPT

(A) polyclonal B-cell activation is essential to the pathogenesis
(B) cardiac involvement is the most common cause of death
(C) visceral lesions are mediated by type III hypersensitivity
(D) joint involvement (arthritis) is common clinically
(E) hypergammaglobulinemia is usual

81. All the following statements regarding primary Sjögren's syndrome are true EXCEPT

(A) xerostomia is a major symptom
(B) anti-SSB antibodies are major markers
(C) renal glomerular lesions are common
(D) rheumatoid factor is often present
(E) there is increased frequency of HLA-DR3

82. Which of the following conditions is most likely to be associated with cancer?

(A) Systemic lupus erythematosus
(B) Hypertension
(C) Polymyositis
(D) Autoimmune thyroiditis
(E) Arteriosclerosis

83. Patients with common variable immunodeficiency (CVI) have

(A) no B lymphocytes in peripheral blood
(B) hypergammaglobulinemia
(C) thymic aplasia
(D) increased incidence of autoimmune diseases
(E) deficiency of adenosine deaminase

84. A 23-year-old man with full-blown AIDS is noted to be severely neutropenic. Which of the following abnormalities is most likely to be seen on further investigation?

(A) Macrocytic anemia
(B) Normal CD4 lymphocyte count
(C) Thrombocytopenia
(D) Lymphocytosis
(E) Hypocellular bone marrow

85. Current knowledge concerning AIDS (acquired immunodeficiency syndrome) includes all the following EXCEPT

(A) the causative agent is HIV
(B) the causative agent belongs to the retrovirus group
(C) T lymphocytes of the helper/inducer subset are infected
(D) cytotoxic/suppressor T cells are markedly increased
(E) the incidence of non-Hodgkin's lymphomas is increased in AIDS

86. Which of the following diseases is caused by a togavirus?

(A) Epidemic keratoconjunctivitis
(B) Dengue fever
(C) Eastern encephalitis
(D) Yellow fever
(E) St. Louis encephalitis

87. All the following diseases are associated with herpesviruses EXCEPT

(A) shingles
(B) chickenpox (varicella)
(C) influenza
(D) cytomegalic inclusion disease
(E) mononucleosis

88. A 19-year-old man living in New Mexico presents to a local clinic after a one-day history of fever, myalgia, chills, headache, and malaise. He complains of vomiting, diarrhea, abdominal pain, tachypnea, and a productive cough. His white cell count was elevated with an increase in the number of bands. Atypical lymphocytes were also found in the peripheral blood. He was treated with antibiotics, but the next day he developed acute respiratory failure with cardiopulmonary arrest and died. Postmortem examination of the lungs revealed intraalveolar edema, rare hyaline membranes, and a few interstitial lymphoid aggregates. The feature that most clearly separates this disease from hemorrhagic fever with renal syndrome caused by *Hantavirus* is

(A) increased capillary permeability
(B) noncardiogenic pulmonary edema
(C) peripheral leukocytosis
(D) atypical lymphocytosis
(E) abdominal pain

89. Pathogenic pneumococci typically exhibit all the following EXCEPT

(A) inhibition of growth by ethylhydrocupreine (Optochin)
(B) M protein in their cell walls
(C) bile solubility
(D) positive Neufeld quellung reactions
(E) detection of capsular polysaccharides by counterimmunoelectrophoresis (CIE)

90. The cells in the photomicrograph shown below are from a drop of cerebrospinal fluid. The most likely diagnosis is

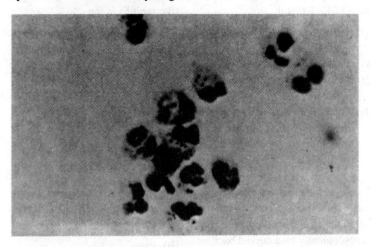

(A) subarachnoid hemorrhage
(B) viral meningitis
(C) tuberculous meningitis
(D) bacterial meningitis
(E) leukemic meningitis

91. A 6-year-old boy developed a facial rash that had the appearance of a slap to the face. The rash, which was composed of small red spots, subsequently involved the upper and lower extremities. The patient also complained of arthralgia and suddenly developed a life-threatening aplastic crisis of the bone marrow. The most likely infectious agent causing these symptoms is

(A) rhinovirus
(B) parainfluenza virus
(C) parvovirus
(D) measles virus
(E) rubella virus

92. Lobar pneumonia is caused predominantly by

(A) *Klebsiella pneumoniae*
(B) *Staphylococcus pyogenes*
(C) *Haemophilus influenzae*
(D) *Streptococcus pneumoniae*
(E) *Legionella pneumophila*

93. Which of the following organisms produces signs and symptoms that mimic acute appendicitis?

(A) Enteropathic *Escherichia coli*
(B) *Enterobius vermicularis*
(C) *Trichomonas hominis*
(D) *Yersinia enterocolitica*
(E) *Bacillus anthracis*

94. All the following statements about *Listeria monocytogenes* are true EXCEPT that it

(A) causes neonatal and adult meningitis
(B) causes food-borne outbreaks
(C) causes frequent epithelioid granulomas
(D) is an opportunistic agent in the immunosuppressed or pregnant
(E) is a gram-positive intracellular bacillus

95. Organisms that can cause outbreaks around coastal areas of the United States and are characterized microscopically by a curved bacillus include

(A) *Mycobacterium avium*
(B) *Mycobacterium bovis*
(C) *Mycobacterium marinum*
(D) *Vibrio cholerae*
(E) *Mycobacterium kansasii*

96. An adult patient in the summer months suffers a rash on one of the extremities followed several weeks later by arthritis of the knee. In addition to viral and bacterial disorders and rheumatoid joint disease, which of the following should also be considered in the differential diagnosis?

(A) Hemarthrosis
(B) Reiter's disease
(C) Lyme disease
(D) Charcot's joint
(E) Baker's cyst

97. The most specific of the commonly used tests for diagnosing active syphilis is the

(A) rapid plasma reagin (RPR) test
(B) *Treponema pallidum* immobilization (TPI) test
(C) fluorescent treponemal antibody-absorption (FTA-ABS) test
(D) Veneral Disease Research Laboratory (VDRL) test
(E) Kolmer test

98. Spirochetal infections include all the following EXCEPT

(A) bejel
(B) yaws
(C) relapsing fever
(D) Weil's disease
(E) lymphogranuloma venereum

99. The organism *Mycoplasma pneumoniae* exhibits all the following characteristics EXCEPT which one?

(A) It is enclosed by a membrane but lacks cell walls
(B) It causes 50 percent of pneumonias in college students
(C) It is often accompanied by the presence of cold agglutinins in serum
(D) It is beyond resolution of light microscopy
(E) It causes granuloma formation

100. An adult migrant farm worker in the San Joaquin Valley of California has been hospitalized for 2 weeks with progressive lassitude, fever of unknown origin, and skin nodules on the lower extremities. A biopsy of one of the deep dermal nodules shown in the photomicrograph below reveals the presence of

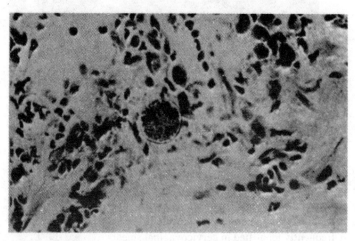

(A) Russell bodies
(B) malignant lymphoma
(C) coccidioides spherule
(D) lymphomatoid granulomatosis
(E) erythema nodosum

---

101. Characteristic features of lepromatous leprosy include all the following EXCEPT

(A) nerve involvement
(B) numerous bacilli in histiocytes
(C) frequent polyclonal hypergammaglobulinemia
(D) association with erythema nodosum
(E) encroachment of infiltrate on basal epidermis

102. Unusual characteristics of mycobacteria, such as resistance to toxic agents, environmental viability, and unusual stain reactions, can be attributed to their

(A) acid fastness
(B) aerobic requirements
(C) high lipid content
(D) peptidoglycan content
(E) plasma membrane

103. The photomicrograph below of a duodenal aspiration smear shows an organism that

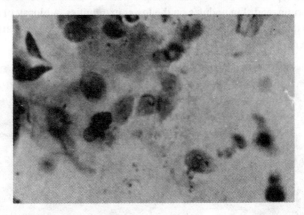

(A) is often numerous in lymph nodes
(B) infects principally the large intestine
(C) is transmitted by the genus *Triatoma*
(D) is the most common intestinal parasite in the U.S.
(E) is frequently identified in cervicovaginal smears

104. The photomicrograph below was prepared after a distal colonic biopsy was performed. The most likely diagnosis is

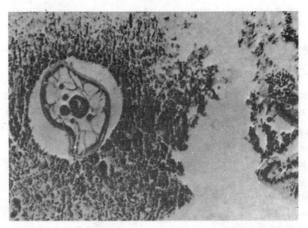

(A) clonorchiasis
(B) enterobiasis
(C) filariasis
(D) strongyloidiasis
(E) schistosomiasis

105. All the following statements about *Mycobacterium tuberculosis* are true EXCEPT

(A) it has a long doubling time
(B) its cell wall contains large amounts of lipid
(C) it frequently infects silica miners
(D) it is prone to drug-resistant mutation
(E) it is a facultative anaerobe

106. Sections of tissue infected with blastomyces would be expected to show organisms with

(A) nonbranching pseudohyphae and blastocysts
(B) acute-angle branching, septate hyphae
(C) wide-angle branching, nonseptate hyphae
(D) broad-based budding
(E) large spheres with external budding

107. As a result of active world travel, parasitic infestations are far from being considered exotic diseases in the United States today. A pulmonary phase is part of the development of all the following helminths EXCEPT

(A) *Necator americanus*
(B) *Strongyloides stercoralis*
(C) *Ascaris lumbricoides*
(D) *Wuchereria bancrofti*
(E) *Toxocara*

108. Parathyroid hormone, by its action on target organs, is known to cause all the following EXCEPT

(A) increased intestinal calcium absorption
(B) increased renal tubular reabsorption of calcium
(C) increased serum phosphate levels
(D) mobilization of calcium from bone
(E) decreased renal tubular reabsorption of phosphate

109. The enzyme activity curve labeled II, shown below, best represents the pattern for which of the following serum enzymes after an uncomplicated acute myocardial infarction?

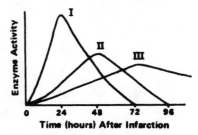

(A) Aspartate aminotransferase
(B) Creatine phosphokinase
(C) Lactic dehydrogenase
(D) Alkaline phosphatase
(E) 5′-Nucleotidase

110. Elevated levels of serum amylase may be found in all the following conditions EXCEPT

(A) acute pancreatitis
(B) biliary tract disease
(C) mumps
(D) renal insufficiency
(E) congestive heart failure

111. Elevated levels of serum alkaline phosphatase are expected findings in each of the following conditions EXCEPT

(A) obstructive jaundice
(B) cirrhosis
(C) hepatitis
(D) polycythemia vera
(E) pregnancy (last trimester)

112. Hyperuricemia often occurs secondary to all the following disorders EXCEPT

(A) leukemias
(B) lymphomas
(C) chondrocalcinosis (pseudogout)
(D) Lesch-Nyhan syndrome
(E) chronic renal disease

113. The table below shows the normal serum values for the five isoenzymes of lactic dehydrogenase (LDH) and the values obtained for one patient. The diagnosis most compatible with the patient's values is

Isoenzyme	Normal % activity	Patient's % activity
LDH_1	20–35	18
LDH_2	30–40	24
LDH_3	20–30	13
LDH_4	5–15	26
LDH_5	1–15	19

(A) acute hepatitis
(B) pernicious anemia
(C) pulmonary infarct
(D) myocardial infarct
(E) cerebrovascular accident

DIRECTIONS: Each group of questions below consists of lettered headings followed by a set of numbered items. For each numbered item select the **one** lettered heading with which it is **most** closely associated. Each lettered heading may be used **once, more than once, or not at all.**

Questions 114–115

For each of the disorders listed, choose the most appropriate feature.

(A) Mental retardation and self-mutilation
(B) Deficiency of α-galactosidase A
(C) Second most common cause of genetic mental retardation
(D) Situs inversus
(E) Deficiency of hexosaminidase A

114. Fabry's disease

115. Tay-Sachs disease

Questions 116–119

Match each vitamin deficiency with the disorder with which it is most likely to be associated.

(A) Microcytic anemia
(B) Perifollicular petechiae
(C) Wernicke-Korsakoff syndrome
(D) Macrocytic anemia
(E) Night blindness

116. Pyridoxine deficiency

117. Ascorbic acid deficiency

118. Folate deficiency

119. Thiamine deficiency

Questions 120–123

Match the following characteristics and diseases

(A) Tick-borne disease
(B) Granulomatous inflammation
(C) Meningitis
(D) Mosquito-borne disease
(E) Endotoxins in cell walls

120. Histoplasmosis

121. Cryptococcosis

122. Rocky Mountain spotted fever

123. Yellow fever

Questions 124–127

For each disease that causes blindness, select the characteristic with which it is most likely to be associated.

(A) Silver-wire arterioles
(B) Variable modes of inheritance
(C) Microaneurysms
(D) Bitot's spots
(E) Pannus formation

124. Diabetic retinopathy

125. Keratomalacia

126. Trachoma

127. Retinitis pigmentosa

Questions 128–131

Match each disorder or description with the immunoglobulin with which it is most likely to be associated.

(A) IgA
(B) IgD
(C) IgE
(D) IgM
(E) IgG

128. Anaphylaxis

129. The major circulating immunoglobulin

130. Berger's disease

131. Waldenström's macroglobulinemia

Questions 132–135

For each of the proteins listed, choose the disease with which it is most likely to be associated.

(A) Rheumatoid arthritis
(B) Senile cardiac amyloidosis
(C) Nodular lymphoma
(D) Alzheimer's disease
(E) Medullary carcinoma of the thyroid
(F) Long-term hemodialysis

132. Amyloid light chain (AL) protein

133. Amyloid-associated (AA) protein

134. Beta$_2$ amyloid protein

135. Transthyretin

General Pathology
Answers

1. The answer is A. *(Robbins, 5/e, pp 5–17.)* The cause of cell injury and death may sometimes be inferred from the type of necrosis present. Coagulative necrosis, characterized by loss of the cell nucleus, acidophilic change of the cytoplasm, and preservation of the outline of the cell, is seen in sudden, severe ischemia of many organs. It is not present, however, in acute ischemic necrosis of the brain. Myocardial infarction resulting from the sudden occlusion of the coronary artery is a classic example of coagulative necrosis. In liquefactive necrosis, the dead cells are completely dissolved by hydrolytic enzymes. This type of necrosis can be seen in ischemic necrosis of the brain and in acute bacterial infections. Fat necrosis, seen with acute pancreatic necrosis, is fat cell death caused by lipases. Fibrinoid necrosis is an abnormality seen sometimes in injured blood vessels where plasma proteins abnormally accumulate within the walls of blood vessels. Caseous necrosis is a combination of coagulative and liquefactive necrosis, but the necrotic cells are not totally dissolved and remain as amorphic, coarsely granular, eosinophilic debris. This type of necrosis grossly has the appearance of clumped cheese. It is classically seen in tuberculous infections. Gangrenous necrosis of extremities is also a combination of coagulative and liquefactive necrosis. In dry gangrene the coagulative pattern is predominate, while in wet gangrene the liquefactive pattern is predominate.

2. The answer is B. *(Robbins, 5/e, pp 4–11.)* Injury to the cell membrane, the loss of cell ATP, and the influx of Ca^{2+} into the mitochondria are thought to be the most critical of multiple cellular events after experimental ischemia in animals. A major detriment following reduction of cell oxygen tension is the cessation or reduction in ATP because of falling oxidative phosphorylation; this occurs early in hypoxia. While increasing anaerobic glycolysis subsequently occurs, the pivotal step is loss of the energy-producing ATP, which leads to cell Na^+ accumulation, K^+ efflux, and Ca^{2+} influx, by reduced effectiveness of the active transport Na^+ pump. Cells greatly enlarge as a consequence of isoosmotic water accumulation. These changes are still reversible if oxygen tension is restored. Continuing hypoxia results in mitochondrial damage (vacuole formation), which is irreversible. Cell death will occur when lysosomes break down and release proteases, RNA and DNAases, and cathepsins. Central nervous system cells are most susceptible to ischemia (survival of 5 min or less); liver and kidney cells survive up to 2 h; and epidermal cells tolerate several hours of hypoxia.

3. The answer is A. *(Robbins, 5/e, pp 17–21. Rubin, 2/e, pp 23–25.)* As cells die, the nuclear chromatin clumps and then aggregates along the nuclear membrane. As this clumping of chromatin continues, the nucleus becomes smaller and stains deeply basophilic (blue). This cellular process is called *pyknosis.* The nucleus may then break up into many clumps (*karyorrhexis*) or there may be decreased staining of chromatin (*karyolysis*). *Apoptosis* is a distinctive pattern of cell death that usually involves single cells. There is typically no inflammatory response. Apoptotic cells appear histologically as intensely eosinophilic (red) bodies with or without dense, fragmented nuclear material. Apoptosis is described as a programmed suicide process of cells that occurs by the stimulation of endogenous endonucleases. It is the type of cell death seen during embryonic development or hormone-induced atrophy of tissue; an example is the involution of the thymus that occurs with aging. Apoptosis may result from some bacterial toxins or viral infections, an example of which are Councilman bodies, which are found in the liver of some patients with viral hepatitis. Abnormalities of the genes involved in apoptosis may contribute to the formation of some malignancies. A different process is *pinocytosis,* which is the uptake of small, soluble macromolecules into the cytoplasm of phagocytic cells.

4. The answer is C. *(Robbins, 5/e, pp 23–24, 589–591. Rubin, 2/e, p 17.)* Cytoskeletal filament proteins compose the framework of cells involved in cell functions, such as pinocytosis, structural stability, contractility, organelle movement, and cell motility. The cytoskeleton is seen ultrastructurally as microtubules (25 nm diameter) of tubulin protein; intermediate filaments (8 to 10 nm) of keratins, desmin, vimentin, glial and neurofilaments; thin filaments of actin (6 to 8 nm); and thick filaments (15 nm) of myosin. Every cell has tubulin and actin, while most have some myosin. Epithelial cells have any of the many types of cytokeratins, with a few having the mesenchymal filament vimentin. Muscle cells and fibroblasts have desmin. Glial cells and neurons contain glial and neurofilament protein, respectively. Phagocytosis is impaired in the Chédiak-Higashi syndrome because of a defect in the polymerization of microtubules. Alcoholic "hyaline" (Mallory's bodies) in alcoholic liver disease appears to be composed of prekeratins. Red cells have a membrane skeleton made up of spectrin, ankyrin, actin, and protein 4.1. In hereditary spherocytosis a genetic defect is responsible for abnormal spectrin that is unable to bind protein 4.1 required for the stability of the red cell membrane.

5. The answer is C. *(Robbins, 5/e, pp 31–32, 858.)* Hyaline inclusions, as shown in the illustration, may appear in liver cells injured by chronic alcoholism and have been shown by ultrastructure studies to result from the close packing of fibrils. The appearance of these inclusions is not a morphologic expression of cell injury. Alcoholic hyaline inclusions (Mallory's bodies) are nonspecific and occur in Wilson's disease, Indian childhood cirrhosis, bypass operations for morbid obesity, and alcoholic hepatitis. They react with antibodies to cytokeratins, which suggests they are related to the intermediate filament keratin.

6. The answer is D. *(Anderson, 9/e, pp 2–3.)* The cytoplasmic matrix contains numerous organelles with highly specialized functions. Whereas mitochondria are the "power" units of the cell involved with the Krebs cycle and anaerobic metabolism, the endoplasmic reticulum is a complex network of rodlike tubules containing ribosomes and is involved in protein synthesis (rough endoplasmic reticulum). Lysosomes are round bodies containing enzymes involved in inflammation. These include the sulfatases, desoxyribonucleases, hydrolases, and acid phosphatases. The Golgi apparatus (complex) is made up of tiny vesicles, membranes, and vacuoles and is also involved in protein synthesis, as it receives the synthesized proteins from the endoplasmic reticulum. The Golgi complex appears to collect, segregate, and export protein. Microbodies are membrane-bound spheres that contain catalase and oxidases. Epithelial cells, especially surface-lining cells, are held together by connections referred to as *intercellular junctions.* Desmosomes (squamous cells), tight junctions (zonula occludens), and gap junctions (nexuses) are examples of such membrane connectors.

7. The answer is A. *(Robbins, 5/e, pp 44–47. Rubin, 2/e, pp 7–9.)* In uterine growth during pregnancy, both cell proliferation involving the endometrial glands and muscle enlargement of the uterine wall occur. These processes offer models of both hyperplasia and hypertrophy. When both are present, DNA synthesis is markedly accelerated. Hyperplasia is an increase in the number of cells, whereas hypertrophy is an increase in cell size, as in cardiac muscle hypertrophy in response to volume overload or peripheral vascular hypertension. Enlargement of breast tissue resulting from hormonal influences is due solely to an increase in cell numbers.

8. The answer is C. *(Robbins, 5/e, pp 57–59. Rubin, 2/e, pp 49–52.)* Adhesion molecules are important in cell-to-cell interactions, such as leukocyte adhesion to endothelial cells during acute inflammation. These adhesion molecules consist of three families: integrins, selectins, and immunoglobulins. Integrins are transmembrane glycoproteins composed of alpha and beta sub-units. Beta-1-integrins are found on lymphocytes, monocytes, basophils, and eosinophils, while beta-2-integrins are found on all leukocytes. The beta-2-integrins (also called CD11/CD18 molecules) consist of MO-1, leukocyte function antigen 1 (LFA-1), and gp 150,95. Activation of phagocytic cells early during inflammation increases the expression of integrins on their surface. The genetic disease leukocyte adhesion deficiency type 1 is characterized by recurrent bacterial infections and impaired leukocyte adhesion. Patients have a deficiency of the beta chains of LFA-1 and Mac-1 integrins. The selectins, in contrast, consist of E-selectin, found on endothelial cells, P-selectin, found on endothelial cells and platelets, and L-selectin, found on most leukocytes. The immunoglobulin family includes two endothelial adhesion molecules: ICAM-1 (intracellular adhesion molecule 1) and VCAM-1 (vascular adhesion molecule 1).

9.   The answer is B. *(Robbins, 5/e, p 64. Rubin, 2/e, pp 60, 1031–1032.)* The enzymatic defect that exists in chronic granulomatous disease of childhood does not impair chemotaxis or the cell's ability to engulf bacteria but rather involves a failure to produce hydrogen peroxide after engulfment. Chemotactic defects resulting in inhibition of the capacity of leukocytes to infiltrate an area of infection or injury may be due to intracellular defects, as found in Chédiak-Higashi syndrome, in other genetic defects, and in diabetes mellitus. Chronic renal failure and cirrhosis may be associated with factors in the circulation that impair chemotaxis. Thermal injuries are also associated with acquired defects in leukocyte chemotaxis.

10.   The answer is C. *(Robbins, 5/e, pp 70–71, 73–74, 84–85.)* Two of the major systemic effects of inflammation (acute-phase reactions) are fever and leukocytosis. Both of these reactions are largely under the control of the cytokines IL-1 or α-TNF (cachectin) or both. These two cytokines have many similar functions, including induction of fever, release of ACTH, leukocytosis, and other systemic acute-phase responses. IL-1 initiates fever by inducing synthesis of prostaglandin $E_2(PGE_2)$ in the anterior hypothalamus, followed by transmission via the posterior hypothalamus, vasomotor center, and sympathetic nerves to cause skin vasoconstriction. Leukocytosis occurs initially because of rapid release of cells from the postmitotic reserve pool of the bone marrow, which is caused by IL-1 and α-TNF and associated with a "shift to the left" of immature cells. β-TNF, another cytokine, has no major role in acute-phase reactions. It takes part in T-cell cytotoxicity and its release may injure cell membranes directly in T-cell–mediated lysis.

11. The answer is E. *(Robbins, 5/e, pp 21–22, 66–70.)* Lysosomes contain many substances involved in inflammation including alkaline and acid phosphatase, collagenases, lysozymes, lactoferrin, myeloperoxidase, cationic proteins, and acid proteases. Of these, the neutral proteases (elastase, collagenase, cathepsin G) function in stages of inflammatory confinement and wound healing by degrading tissue matrix like collagen, fibrin, cartilage, elastin, and basement membranes. The other mediators cascade as follows: complement cascade starts classically by an antigen-antibody complex or alternately by nonimmunologic stimuli. C5a leads to chemotaxis while the complement complex C5b-9 leads to cell lysis. The kinins are activated by Hageman factor (XIIA), via prekallikrein, into bradykinin. The fibrinopeptides of the clotting system can also be activated by Hageman factor or by extrinsic tissue thromboplastin to result in a polymerized fibrin clot. The important cascades of arachidonic acid metabolites (cyclooxygenase, lipoxygenase), leading to functioning vasodilators (prostaglandins) and membrane permeability factors (leukotrienes), are the most complex of all, beginning with the actions of phospholipase.

12. The answer is D. *(Robbins, 5/e, pp 68–70, 73–74.)* Leukocytes, including basophils, are involved with the production of derivatives of a very important polyunsaturated fatty acid, arachidonic acid. By a complex two-path cascade system, the metabolites of arachidonic acid eventually yield prostaglandins (vasodilators) and leukotrienes (vasoconstrictors). The biosynthesis begins by activation of plasma membrane phospholipase A_2 and proceeds either by the action of fatty acid cyclooxygenase on arachidonic acid to form prostaglandins, or by the action of lipoxygenase to yield leukotrienes (hydroperoxyeicosatetraenoic acid in platelets, mast cells, and leukocytes). While many substances can be chemotactic, few are known to be as potent as several of the leukotrienes. Leukotriene B_4 as a chemotactic agent is involved in neutrophil aggregation, while leukotrienes C_4, D_4, and E_4 are involved with increased vascular permeability, bronchoconstriction, and vasoconstriction. Prostaglandin E and prostacyclin probably account for most vasodilatation seen in inflammation. The prostaglandins are involved in producing both pain and fever in inflammation.

13. The answer is D. *(Robbins, 5/e, pp 76–78. Henry, 18/e, pp 799–800.)* There is evidence that most, if not all, macrophages originate from a committed bone marrow stem cell, which differentiates into a monoblast and then a promonocyte, which in turn matures into a monocyte in the circulating peripheral blood. When called upon, the circulating monocyte can enter into an organ or tissue bed as a tissue macrophage (previously called a *histiocyte*).

Examples of tissue macrophages are Kupffer cells (liver), alveolar macrophages (lung), osteoclasts (bone), Langerhans cells (skin), microglial cells (central nervous system), and possibly the dendritic immunocytes of the dermis, spleen, and lymph nodes. The entire system, including the peripheral blood monocytes, constitutes the mononuclear phagocyte system.

14. The answer is D. *(Robbins, 5/e, pp 80–82.)* Granulomatous inflammation is characterized by the presence of granulomas, consisting of 1- to 2-mm foci of modified macrophages (epithelioid cells) surrounded by mononuclear cells, mainly lymphocytes. It is a chronic inflammation initiated by a variety of infectious and noninfectious agents. Indigestible organisms or particles, or T-cell–mediated immunity to the inciting agent, or both, appear essential for formation of granulomas. Although tuberculosis is the classic infectious granulomatous disease, several other infectious disorders are characterized by formation of granulomas, including deep fungal infections (coccidioidomycosis and histoplasmosis), schistosomiasis, syphilis, brucellosis, lymphogranuloma venereum, and cat-scratch disease. In sarcoidosis, a disease of unknown cause, the granulomas are noncaseating, which may assist in histologic differentiation from tuberculosis. No organisms are found in lesions of sarcoidosis.

15. The answer is A. *(Robbins, 5/e, pp 218–219. Rubin, 2/e, pp 1031–1032.)* The classic form of chronic granulomatous disease usually afflicts boys and causes their death before they reach the age of 10 years. Key findings in chronic granulomatous disease include lymphadenitis, hepatosplenomegaly, eczematoid dermatitis, pulmonary infiltrates that are associated with hypergammaglobulinemia, and defective ability of neutrophils to kill bacteria. The last finding is thought to be caused by a delay in the release of neutrophilic lysosomal enzymes responsible for intracellular bactericidal action. Although defective neutrophilic bactericidal action also is associated with Chédiak-Higashi syndrome, this syndrome is distinguished by photophobia and oculocutaenous albinism. Thrombocytopenia is a feature of Wiskott-Aldrich syndrome.

16. The answer is A. *(Henry, 18/e, pp 224–225. Robbins, 5/e, p 84.)* C-reactive protein (CRP) elevations, as well as elevations in the erythrocyte sedimentation rate, are nonspecific markers of inflammatory conditions. The CRP rises faster and returns to normal earlier than the erythrocyte sedimentation rate in most inflammatory diseases. Most bacterial infections, rheumatoid arthritis, rheumatic fever, and diseases leading to necrosis and tissue damage will elevate the CRP. CRP elevations do not occur in most viral illnesses.

17. The answer is C. *(Robbins, 5/e, pp 87–89, 132–133. Rubin, 2/e, pp 70–74, 226–227.)* Type I collagen is found in skin, tendon, bone, dentin, and fascia; type II collagen is found only in cartilage; type III collagen (reticulin) appears in skin, blood vessels, uterus, and embryonic dermis. Type IV collagen, a component of basement laminae of epithelial and endothelial cells, does not have the typical 67-nm banding of types I, II, and III. Synthesis of collagen includes lysine oxidation, resulting in alpha-chain cross-linkages with structural stability of collagen. Decreased formation of cross-linkages in collagen and elastin occurs in Marfan's syndrome, an autosomal dominant disorder of connective tissues, with skeletal abnormalities including arachnodactyly, lens subluxation, and cystic medionecrosis of aorta with aneurysm and sometimes rupture.

18. The answer is D. *(Robbins, 5/e, pp 53–57, 93–97.)* Edema is the accumulation of excess fluid in the interstitial tissue or body cavities. It may be caused by inflammation (inflammatory edema) or may be due to abnormalities involving the Starling forces acting at the capillary level (noninflammatory edema or hemodynamic edema). Inflammatory edema is caused by increased capillary permeability, which is the result of vasoactive mediators of acute inflammation. An exudate is inflammatory edema fluid resulting from increased capillary permeability. It is characterized by a high protein content, much cellular debris, and a specific gravity greater than 1.020. Pus is an inflammatory exudate having numerous leukocytes and cellular debris. In contrast, transudates result from either increased intravascular hydrostatic pressure or from decreased osmotic pressure. They are characterized by a low protein content and a specific gravity of <1.012. Noninflammatory edema is the result of abnormalities of the hemodynamic (Starling) forces acting at the level of the capillaries. Increased hydrostatic pressure may be caused by arteriolar dilatation, hypervolemia, or increased venous pressure. Hypervolemia may be caused by sodium retention seen in renal disease, and increased venous pressure can be seen in venous thrombosis, congestive heart failure, or cirrhosis. Decreased plasma oncotic pressure is caused by decreased plasma protein, the majority of which is albumin. Decreased albumin levels may be caused by loss of albumin in the urine, which occurs in the nephrotic syndrome, or by reduced synthesis, which occurs in chronic liver disease. Lymphatic obstruction may be caused by tumors, surgical resection, or infections, for example, infection with filarial worms and consequent elephantiasis.

19. The answer is E. *(Robbins, 5/e, pp 97–99.)* Hemorrhage is the leakage of blood from a blood vessel. Blood may escape into the tissue, producing a hematoma, or it may escape into spaces, producing a hemothorax, hemopericardium, or hemarthrosis. Superficial hemorrhages into the skin or mucosa are classified as petechiae (small, pinpoint capillary hemorrhages), purpura (diffuse, multiple, superficial hemorrhages), or ecchymoses (larger, confluent areas of hemorrhages). Hyperemia is an excess amount of blood within an organ. It may be caused by increased arterial supply (active hyperemia) or impaired venous drainage (passive hyperemia). Examples of active hyperemia include the increased blood flow during exercise, blushing, or inflammation. Examples of passive hyperemia, or congestion, include the changes produced by chronic heart failure. These changes include chronic passive congestion of the lung or the liver. The lung changes are characterized by intraalveolar, hemosiderin-laden macrophages, called "heart failure cells." The congestion in the liver is characterized by centrilobular congestion, which is seen grossly as a "nutmeg" appearance of the liver.

20. The answer is C. *(Robbins, 5/e, pp 68–70, 100–103.)* The three main components of hemostasis include endothelial cells, platelets, and the coagulation system. Endothelial cells exhibit both procoagulant and anticoagulant properties. Their procoagulant activities involve activation of the extrinsic coagulation cascade by their production of tissue factor (thromboplastin) and stimulation of platelet aggregation by their production of von Willebrand's factor and platelet-activating factor. Their anticoagulant activities involve the production of prostacyclin (PGI_2), thrombomodulin, and plasminogen activator. The contrasting actions of the arachidonic acid metabolites prostacyclin and thromboxane $A_2(TxA_2)$ produce a fine-tuned balance for the regulation of clotting. TxA_2, a product of the cyclooxygenase pathway of arachidonic acid metabolism, is synthesized in platelets and is a powerful platelet aggregator and vasoconstrictor. The prostaglandin PGI_2, also a product of the cyclooxygenase pathway but produced by endothelial cells, inhibits platelet aggregation and causes vasodilation. Aspirin, a cyclooxygenase inhibitor, blocks the synthesis of both TxA_2 and PGI_2 and is used in the treatment of coronary artery disease. Fibrinogen, which is produced by the liver, is cleaved by thrombin to form fibrin.

21. The answer is C. *(Henry, 18/e, pp 738–742. Robbins, 5/e, pp 103–106.)* The most important control of the coagulation cascade is the fibrinolytic system, the main component of which is plasmin. Plasminogen is converted into plasmin by either factor XII or a plasminogen activator (PA). Examples of PA's include tissue plasminogen activator (tPA), urokinase plasminogen activator, and streptokinase. Once formed, plasmin splits fibrin and also degrades both fibrinogen and coagulation factors VIII and V. Also important in the control of the coagulation cascade are plasma protease inhibitors, which include antithrombin III, protein C, and C′1 inactivator. Antithrombin

III in the presence of heparin inhibits thrombin, XIIa, XIa, Xa, and IXa, while protein C in the presence of heparin inhibits thrombin, XIIa, XIa, Xa, and IXa. C'1 inactivator inhibits XIa, XIIa, and kallikrein. The significance of these control mechanisms is illustrated by patients with deficiencies of antithrombin III or protein C who develop recurrent thromboemboli. Thrombin acts differently in the coagulation cascade by converting fibrinogen to fibrin.

22. The answer is A. *(Robbins, 5/e, pp 113–114. Rubin, 2/e, pp 272–273.)* Fat embolism syndrome can supervene as a complication within 3 days following severe trauma to the long bones. However, the pathogenesis must be regarded as unknown because simple entrance of microglobular fat into the circulation as a result of damage to small vessels in marrow tissue occurs in over 90 percent of patients with trauma and bone fracture, yet the syndrome occurs in only a minority of such patients. Laboratory and clinical findings can simulate those of intravascular coagulopathy, which may be a component of fat embolism syndrome, with a major difference of split products of fibrin seen mainly in intravascular coagulopathy. Plasma levels of free fatty acids are elevated in fat embolism and may contribute to pulmonary vascular alterations. At autopsy fat material can be demonstrated in fat stains of frozen sections of lung, brain, and kidney in patients who had the syndrome.

23. The answer is E. *(Robbins, 5/e, pp 114–116, 787–789.)* Transmural intestinal infarction is that part of the spectrum of mesenteric ischemia in which there is ischemic necrosis of the full thickness of the intestinal wall. Fifty percent of cases involve the small intestine only and are a result of thrombotic or embolic occlusion of the superior mesenteric artery. Thromboemboli arise from intracardiac mural thrombi, prostheses or valvular vegetations, or from complicated atherosclerotic plaques in the aorta. Arterial thrombi usually occur over atherosclerotic plaques. Twenty-five percent of cases result from nonocclusive hypoperfusion of the small or large intestine.

Arterial and venous occlusion both lead to hemorrhagic infarction with intense congestion and discoloration of the affected bowel segment. The area of the colon most often affected is the splenic flexure, which represents the watershed region of supply between the superior and inferior mesenteric arteries.

24. The answer is D. *(Robbins, 5/e, pp 117–119)* Septic shock is caused by the gram-negative, endotoxin-producing aerobic rods mentioned in the question. It results from pooling of blood in the peripheral circulation. A common cause of sepsis in burn wounds is *Pseudomonas aeruginosa*. The major target in severe shock is the kidneys, which suffer acute ischemic tubular necrosis, affecting proximal and distal nephrons in septic shock. Gram-negative endotoxic shock has a 70 percent mortality.

25. The answer is E. *(Robbins, 5/e, pp 245–248. Rubin, 2/e, pp 148–151.)* Generally tumor cells, by virtue of their transformation, exhibit ultrastructural alterations as visualized by electron microscopy as well as physiologic changes. Membrane projections (microvilli, filopodia, pseudopodia) may become blunted, or lost altogether. Neoplastic transformation may be associated with formation of projections in some cells, but the loss of attenuation of surface projections is more characteristic of neoplastic cells. Cytoskeletal microfilaments and tubules become disorganized, while intermediate filaments (keratins, desmin, vimentin) may increase. In addition to formation of membrane-associated glycoproteins (tumor antigens), there is increased "shedding" and loss of surface antigens. Fibronectin, for instance, is lost from tumor cell surfaces and may be measured in the patient's plasma as cold-insoluble globulin. Surface glycolipids (many are receptor sites) are diminished or lost in some neoplastic cells, theoretically enabling tumor cells to escape the growth inhibitory effects of chalones. Plant lectins can agglutinate cells because their property of divalency cross-links sugars on neighboring cells. This lectin agglutinability is increased in many malignant cells. Fundamental to the biologic behavior of neoplastic cells is the increased demand for cell nutrients, which is aided by an observed increase in membrane transport in neoplastic cells.

26. The answer is A. *(Robbins, 5/e, pp 242, 248–250.)* All tumors whether benign or malignant have a supporting stroma composed of varying amounts of connective tissue and blood supply. The cellularity can range from that of a highly cellular lesion, such as oat cell carcinoma of the lung or Burkitt's lymphoma, to that of a relatively hypocellular lesion, such as a hyalinized neurilemmoma, but the cellularity of the tumor per se does not usually influence the texture. Firmness and even hardness of tumors are a function of the amount of collagenous stroma present. The term *desmoplasia* refers to a collagenized and fibroblastic stroma; an example is carcinoma of the breast, which has the texture of a water chestnut because of the concurrent proliferation of the fibrous stroma with the carcinoma. Tumors that lack a collagenized fibrous stroma tend to be softer regardless of the tumor cellularity per se. Malignant tumors of mesenchyme have a fleshy character because of very little connective tissue stroma; examples include fibrosarcoma, liposarcoma, and leiomyosarcoma. There are a few exceptions to the desmoplastic rule, and an obvious example is a tumor of cartilage in which the hyaline cartilage matrix accounts for the firmness; some chondrosarcomas, however, may be soft and friable.

27. The answer is E. *(Robbins, 5/e, pp 215–219, 228–231, 283–286, 293, 712–714.)* Immunodeficiency states often predispose to the development of neoplasia. The primary immunodeficiencies most clearly associated with an increased incidence of malignancy are common variable immunodeficiency, severe combined immunodeficiency, Wiskott-Aldrich syndrome, and ataxia-telangiectasia (in which defective repair of DNA may also play a role). The neoplasms in these genetic immunodeficiencies are predominantly non-Hodgkin's lymphomas, often immunoblastic, and often extranodal. Secondary immunodeficiency states occur in patients immunosuppressed for organ transplantation and tumors that develop are mainly high-grade, non-Hodgkin's lymphomas, frequently extranodal, especially in the CNS. Transplant patients also show an increased incidence of Kaposi's sarcoma, and a slight increase of squamous cell carcinoma in skin and oral tissues has been reported. The significant increase in neoplasia due to irradiation and radiomimetic drugs—primarily an increase in acute nonlymphoid leukemia—appears to be largely independent of immunosuppression. AIDS, a major devastating example of secondary immunodeficiency, was first recognized in 1981 through the increased incidence of Kaposi's sarcoma in young homosexual men. Subsequent studies established a considerable increase of high-grade, non-Hodgkin's lymphomas in patients infected with human immunodeficiency virus (HIV). Such lymphomas include small noncleaved cell, immunoblastic, and diffuse large cell lymphomas. There also may be an increase in Hodgkin's disease of aggressive type in HIV infection. Sarcoidosis is not associated with an increased incidence of malignancy.

28. The answer is E. *(Robbins, 5/e, pp 253–254. Rubin, 2/e, pp 192–197.)* There are marked differences in the incidence of various types of cancer in different parts of the world. Nasopharyngeal carcinoma, associated with the Epstein-Barr virus, is rare in most parts of the world, except for parts of the Far East, especially China. Liver cancer is associated with both hepatitis B infection and high levels of aflatoxin B1. It is endemic in large parts of Africa and Asia. The highest rates for gastric carcinoma are found in Japan. Trophoblastic diseases, including choriocarcinoma, have high rates of disease in the Pacific rim areas of Asia. In contrast, Asian populations have a very low incidence of prostate cancer. American blacks have a high incidence, while the rate in American and European whites is in between.

29. The answer is E. *(Robbins, 5/e, pp 259–270. Rubin, 2/e, pp 173–183.)* Proto-oncogenes are genes that code for proteins involved in normal growth and development. These normal cellular genes may become oncogenic by being incorporated into a viral genome by a process called *retroviral transduction*, which forms viral oncogenes (v-oncs). They can also be activated by other processes, such as mutations, that form cellular oncogenes (c-oncs). These oncogenes, which are associated with certain malignancies, can be classified into different classes based on various postulated mechanisms of cellular activation. The *abl* oncogene, which is associated with chronic myeloid leukemia, acts through a tyrosine-like kinase, which is a protein involved in signal transduction. The *ras* family of oncogenes, associated with neuroblastoma and urinary bladder cancer, code for a protein, *p21*, which is similar to GTP-binding proteins (G proteins). The product of some oncogenes, such as *myc,* which is associated with Burkitt's lymphoma, are found only in the nucleus and are classified as nuclear regulatory proteins. Some genes, rather than being associated with the formation of cancer, are associated with the suppression of cancer. A classic example of these "anti-oncogenes" involves the formation of retinoblastoma. Both normal alleles, the "anti-oncogenes," which are located at the retinoblastoma (Rb) locus on chromosome 13, must be inactivated for the development of retinoblastoma. This is the basis of the famous "two-hit" hypothesis developed by Knudson. There is also a higher incidence of other cancers in these patients, especially osteogenic sarcoma.

30. The answer is D. *(Robbins, 5/e, pp 259–263, 265–270.)* Most proto-oncogenes are genes that encode for proteins that promote cell growth, but cancer suppressor genes encode proteins that suppress cellular proliferation. Examples of tumor suppressor genes are Rb (associated with retinoblastoma), p53, APC, NF1, DCC, and WT1. The p53 gene, located on chromosome 17, is the single most common target for genetic alterations in human cancers. It is found in many cases of colon, breast, and lung cancers. Mutations in the APC (adenomatous polyposis coli) gene lead to the development of tumors that may progress to adenocarcinomas of the colon, while mutations in the NF1 (neurofibromatosis type 1) gene lead to the development of neurofibromas, some of which may progress to neurofibrosarcomas. DCC (deleted in colon carcinoma) is a tumor suppressor gene located on chromosome 18, which is related to the formation of carcinomas of the colon and stomach. Deletion of WT1, located on chromosome 11, is associated with the development of Wilms' tumor, a childhood neoplasm of the kidney. Genes c-*abl,* located on chromosome 9, and *bcr,* located on chromosome 22, are translocated in cases of chronic myelocytic leukemia. The gene c-*myc,* located on chromsome 8, is translocated in cases of Burkitt's lymphoma. The *ras* oncogene is involved in the genesis of many human cancers. It is not a normal suppressor gene.

31. The answer is C. *(Robbins, 5/e, pp 296–297.)* Hypertrophic osteoarthropathy is a syndrome consisting of periosteal new bone formation with or without digital clubbing and joint effusion. It is seen usually in an adult who complains of aching bone pain, especially in distal extremities. While it is most common in association with lung carcinoma (up to 10 percent of cases), it also occurs with pleural mesothelioma, chronic lung disease such as bronchiectasis or lung abscess, infective endocarditis, and less commonly, with cirrhosis or inflammatory bowel disease (ulcerative colitis). It may occur with congenital heart, lung, or liver disease in children and in familial and idiopathic forms. Radiographs show periosteal thickening with new bone formation on diaphyseal ends of long bones. Treatment is that of the associated disorder; the arthropathy is reversible with surgical resection or medical correction of the underlying disease.

32. The answer is B. *(Robbins, 5/e, pp 264–265, 273–275, 641–642.)* Burkitt's lymphoma is one of the most rapidly growing tumors known to oncologists. Most tumors grow without inhibition by means of a decrease in the time spent within the cell growth cycle itself, a reduction in the total numbers of cells dying, or many more stable cells leaving G_0 to enter the cycle at G_1. One or all of these mechanisms may be in effect, along with a lack of inhibition of cell growth. Such inhibition is not completely understood, but cells are known to be delayed in progressing to mitosis from G_2. Permanent cells are essentially nondividing and usually die. In African Burkitt's lymphoma, but not necessarily in American Burkitt's lymphoma, high titers of serum antibody to Epstein-Barr viral capsid antigen have been described, along with incorporation of the viral genome. A translocation occurs between chromosome 8 (site of proto-oncogene c-*myc*) and chromosome 14, which carries the heavy-chain Ig gene, t (8;14).

33. The answer is D. *(Robbins, 5/e, pp 283–284.)* The association of the chemical and physical environment (with its implied hazards of toxic wastes, mainly from industrial pollution) with the development of tumors in humans is becoming a specialized field in itself. Major legislation and public health efforts are just beginning to place emphasis on these hazards. A major clue to the implication of environmental factors lies in the clustering of rare tumor types in populations in which such an incidence is unexpected. For example, cases of angiosarcoma of the liver (a relatively rare tumor) were identified in employees of a rubber company and in a few residents living near the plant where the monomer vinyl chloride was present in the atmosphere. Exposure to asbestos in shipyard, roofing, and insulation workers has led to the development of not only pleural and peritoneal malignant mesotheliomas, but solid malignant tumors of the lung and viscera as well. Although it increases the risk of tuberculosis, silicosis has not, by itself, increased the risk of developing cancer. Similarly, beryllium vapor (from the manufacture of alloys, ceramics, high-technology electronics, and fluorescent light bulbs) causes marked granulomatous disease but has not been identified as a carcinogen. Cyanide is lethal if ingested. Carbon tetrachloride and chloroform may cause hepatic necrosis and are potentially lethal, but neither is implicated in tumorigenesis. Foundry workers are at risk of developing pulmonary and nasal sinus cancers when they are regularly exposed to nickel or chromium compounds.

34. The answer is B. *(Robbins, 5/e, pp 245–248, 297.)* As all medical oncologists and students of oncology are painfully aware, tumors do not read textbooks and cannot be expected to follow predicted courses in every clinical circumstance. Thus, many exceptions and deviations from the expected occur. An important predictor of a given tumor's behavior, however, is the differentiation, which is a histologic parameter that gives some index as to the degree of resemblance of the tumor to the cell of origin; that is, differentiation states to what degree the tumor resembles its parent cell or tissues. Well-differentiated tumors resemble their cells of origin to a great extent, while poorly differentiated tumors do not resemble their origins to an appreciable extent. With some exceptions tumors may be expected to behave according to their differentiation. Furthermore, the growth rate of tumors appears to correlate with their level of differentiation, with the less-differentiated tumors growing faster than well-differentiated ones. The term *grade* implies differentiation and in some cases may be synonymous; for example, grade I tumors are well differentiated, while grade III tumors are poorly differentiated. Higher grade tumors tend to have more mitoses, which generally correlate with aggressiveness and poorer outcome.

35. The answer is E. *(Henry, 18/e, pp 692–695. Robbins, 5/e, pp 300–301.)* Tumor markers are a diverse group of biochemical substances associated with the presence of some tumors and include hormones, oncofetal antigens, isozymes, proteins, mucins, and glycoproteins. Human chorionic gonadotropin (hCG) is a hormone associated with trophoblastic tumors, especially choriocarcinoma. Alpha-fetoprotein (AFP) is a glycoprotein synthesized by the yolk sac and the fetal liver and is associated with yolk sac tumors of the testes and liver cell carcinomas. Prostate-specific antigen (PSA) and prostatic acid phosphatase (PAP) are associated with cancer of the prostate. Carcinoembryonic antigen (CEA) is a glycoprotein associated with many cancers including adenocarcinomas of the colon, pancreas, lung, stomach, and breast. It may also be increased in some benign disorders. Chloroacetate esterase (CAE) (not to be confused with CEA) is a histochemical stain used in the differentiation of acute leukemias.

36. The answer is D. *(Silverberg, 2/e, pp 291, 882–883.)* Granular cell tumors (formerly known as *granular cell myoblastomas*) are benign neoplasms that frequently contain S-100 protein. They may originate from Schwann-cell precursors. The most frequent locations are the tongue and subepidermal and subcutaneous tissues of the trunk (breast and many other sites). The eosinophilic cytoplasmic granules are phagolysosomes. These tumors are rarely malignant, though poorly encapsulated, and they frequently cause pseudoepitheliomatous hyperplasia of overlying epithelium, which is difficult to differentiate from squamous cell carcinoma.

37. The answer is A. *(Robbins, 5/e, p 299. Silverberg, 2/e, pp 103–116.)* The photomicrograph in the question shows an immunoperoxidase reaction, a technique fostered by Sternberger in the early 1970s to identify antigens within cells by the use of an antibody specific for the antigen sought. Following incubation with a specific antibody directed against the target antigen (primary antibody incubation), a secondary antibody incubation is conducted using heterologous immune sera directed against the first antibody. For example, the primary antibody may be rabbit antihuman IgG. If human IgG is present on or within a given cell, binding occurs. Secondary antibody could then be goat antirabbit, which now binds to the rabbit IgG. Then horseradish peroxidase-antiperoxidase conjugate is applied, which links to the antibody complexes. The last step is a chromogen substrate, in this case rust-brown diaminobenzidine. Rust-brown granules indicate a positive reaction. This useful technique (or a modification of it, such as the use of highly specific and sensitive monoclonal antibodies with avidin-biotin conjugate rather than peroxidase-antiperoxidase) is used to identify tumor-associated antigens, viruses, and other microorganisms, proteins, and hormones.

38. The answer is B. *(Anderson, 9/e, p 1474.)* The lymph-node section shown in the photomicrograph contains metastatic carcinoma cells and was probably excised from a patient who has carcinoma. The tumor cells are clustered in small nests within the node and are separated by stromal tissue. The cellular clustering is characteristic of carcinomas that have metastasized to lymph nodes.

39. The answer is B. *(Robbins, 5/e, pp 414–418.)* Vitamin D is essential for maintenance of normal bone remodeling in the adult; therefore, a significant deficiency in adults leads to poorly mineralized bone, or osteomalacia. Deficiency also results in decreased intestinal absorption of calcium, inadequate serum calcium and phosphorus, and, therefore, impaired mineralization of osteoid. Defective mineralization of osteoid causes formation of soft, easily deformed bones. Since there is no decreased production of osteoid matrix, a relative excess of woven bone or osteoid with wide osteoid seams results.

40. The answer is D. *(Robbins, 5/e, pp 411–419, 603–608.)* Vitamin E functions primarily as an antioxidant. Deficiencies of vitamin E may produce spinocerebellar degeneration and skeletal muscle abnormalities. Manifestations of these changes include decreased tendon reflexes, ataxia, and loss of pain, position, and vibration sense. Night blindness is one manifestation of vitamin A deficiency. Other symptoms of vitamin A deficiency include dry eyes (xerophthalmia), squamous metaplasia of mucous membranes, and vulnerability to infections. Vitamin D deficiency results in an excess of unmineralized matrix in the bone. In children this results in rickets, and in adults it results in osteomalacia. Megaloblastic anemia, characterized by macrocytic erythrocytes, is the result of a deficiency of either vitamin B_{12} or folate.

41. The answer is E. *(Anderson, 9/e, pp 1853–1860. Robbins, 5/e, p 1267.)* *Malignant fibrous histiocytoma (MFH)* is the current term used to designate sarcomatous growths of the deep soft tissues. This is principally a disease of the lower extremity and thigh in middle- to advanced-aged patients of both sexes, but it has also been reported as occurring in far-removed areas, such as the adventitia of the thoracic aorta and the ocular orbit. It has also occurred with some frequency years after irradiation. The tumor is composed of a background of spindle cells with varying amounts of collagen (hence, fibrous) and scattered, giant, bizarre, xanthomatous and myoblastic-like cells (hence, histiocytic). In the past, many of these tumors were undoubtedly labeled as "pleomorphic liposarcomas" and "pleomorphic adult rhabdomyosarcomas," both of which must be differentiated from MFH. This does not imply, of course, that pleomorphic liposarcomas and adult rhabdomyosarcomas do not exist simply because a new term has been introduced, but rather that strict histologic criteria should be adhered to in order to exclude MFH—namely, that malignant myoblasts with cytoplasmic striations (rhabdomyosarcoma) and lipoblasts (liposarcoma) must be unequivocally demonstrated. The prognosis is poor for MFH.

42. The answer is C. *(Robbins, 5/e, pp 1262–1263.)* Liposarcomas are the most common soft tissue sarcoma of adults, arise deeply in the thigh or retroperitoneum, and are liable to metastasize by embolization in blood vessels (nonmyxoid types). Histology is varied—well-differentiated, myxoid, round cell, or pleomorphic—depending on tumor type. Myxoid liposarcoma is the most common variant. The pleomorphic type is undifferentiated and easily confused with other poorly differentiated mesenchymal sarcomas. The clinical picture is also varied. Well-differentiated and myxoid types are locally invasive and recurrent, if they are not completely excised, but they are rarely metastatic. Round-cell and pleomorphic types are often aggressive with widespread metastases, local recurrence, and poor 5-year survival.

43. The answer is C. *(Lee, 9/e, pp 570–572.)* Vitamin K is not required for the biosynthesis of coagulation factor VIII, which has an uncertain participation as a trace protein in the intrinsic coagulation pathway and is also known as the antihemophilic factor. Vitamin K, although its biochemical mode of action remains unclear, is required for the biosynthesis and maintenance of normal concentrations of coagulation factors II (prothrombin), VII, IX, and X.

44. The answer is E. *(Robbins, 5/e, pp 1262–1263, 1265–1266.)* Fibrosarcomas are most frequent in the retroperitoneum, followed by the superficial or deep tissues of the extremities and especially around the knee. They form one of the less common tumors of soft tissue since many previously diagnosed as fibrosarcoma have been reclassified as malignant fibrous histiocytoma or aggressive fibromatosis (desmoid). Slowly growing, well-differentiated fibrosarcomas may be difficult to differentiate from "cellular fibromas." Histologically they may form interlacing bundles of malignant spindle cells, which is called a "herringbone" pattern. Hypoglycemia may be associated with fibrosarcoma. A prominent arborizing vascular proliferation forming a "chicken-wire" pattern is characteristic of liposarcomas.

45. The answer is D. *(Robbins, 5/e, p 719.)* Drug-induced respiratory changes include bronchospasm, pulmonary edema, hypersensitivity pneumonitis, and chronic pneumonitis with fibrosis. Amiodarone, given for ventricular tachycardia, is concentrated in the lung and causes pneumonitis, with resultant fibrosis in 5 to 15 percent of patients. The cytotoxic drug bleomycin, used in cancer chemotherapy, also causes pneumonitis and fibrosis because of direct drug toxicity and stimulation of inflammatory cells to infiltrate alveoli. Methotrexate, another cytotoxic anticancer agent that inhibits synthesis of DNA, and nitrofurantoin both may cause hypersensitivity pneumonitis. Very small doses of aspirin may cause asthmatic attacks and urticaria in patients with rhinitis and nasal polyps. In these patients, aspirin probably inhibits the cyclooxygenase pathway of arachidonic acid metabolism with no effect on the lipoxygenase pathway, so that decreased prostaglandins, increased bronchoconstrictor leukotrienes, and asthma result. In acute salicylate poisoning, the initial event is respiratory stimulation with loss of carbon dioxide.

46. The answer is A. *(Anderson, 9/e, pp 548–550. Robbins, 5/e, pp 327–328.)* Protein-calorie malnutrition in underdeveloped countries leads to a spectrum of symptoms from kwashiorkor at one end to marasmus at the other. Marasmus, caused by a lack of caloric intake (i.e., starvation), leads to generalized wasting, stunted growth, atrophy of muscles, and loss of subcutaneous fat. There is no edema or hepatic enlargement. These children are alert, not apathetic, and are ravenous. In contrast, children with kwashiorkor, which is characterized by a lack of protein despite adequate caloric intake, have peripheral edema, a "moon" face, and an enlarged, fatty liver. The peripheral edema is caused by decreased albumin and sodium retention, while the fatty liver is caused by decreased synthesis of the lipoproteins necessary for the normal mobilization of lipids from liver cells. Additionally these children have "flaky paint" areas of skin and abnormal pigmented streaks in their hair ("flag sign"). In children with marasmus, the skin is inelastic due to loss of subcutaneous fat. In either severe kwashiorkor or marasmus, thymic atrophy may result in the reduction in number and function of circulating T cells. B-cell function (i.e., immunoglobulin production) is also depressed, so that these children are highly vulnerable to infections.

47. The answer is C. *(Robbins, 5/e, pp 385–387, 1044–1045.)* Despite current controversy, most researchers agree that women taking oral contraceptives are at risk, however small, of developing myocardial infarction, especially if the woman is a cigarette smoker, and vascular thrombi that may lead to strokes and pulmonary embolism and infarction. Also very minimal in terms of numbers of cases are hepatic adenomas, which have been recorded in patients taking oral estrogens over a protracted period of time. Conflicting evidence is found concerning the risk of developing endometrial carcinoma. Some researchers have shown a definite risk of developing uterine cancer, but not all series have demonstrated a positive correlation. The same problem exists in estimation of the risk of developing breast cancer. Vaginal adenosis develops not in the women taking estrogens themselves, but rather in the female offspring of mothers who received diethylstilbestrol (DES) while pregnant. Some of these daughters have also developed clear cell carcinoma of the cervix, an adenocarcinoma that carries a rather poor prognosis. DES binds to cell nuclear DNA and hence may act as a cocarcinogen rather than as a mere promoter.

48. The answer is D. *(Robbins, 5/e, pp 388–390, 868–869.)* The seemingly innumerable deleterious effects of alcohol abuse are recognized as constituting a major public health problem even in non-Western locations, such as Africa and Asia. The effects may be socioeconomic (divorce, absenteeism, and high insurance rates due to automobile accidents), political, moral, or organic. Indeed, it is difficult to think of an organ or organ system that does not develop a physical dysfunction, either reversible or irreversible, in response to excessive intake of ethanol. Subdural hematomas are commonly seen in alcoholics. Portal vein thrombosis is rarely seen in the absence of nutritional or Laënnec's cirrhosis. Levels of the muscle and cardiac enzyme creatine phosphokinase may be elevated in states of alcoholic myocardiosis, cardiomyopathy, alcoholic rhabdomyolysis, or trauma to skeletal muscles while the patient is in an alcoholic toxic state. Primary biliary cirrhosis occurs predominantly in middle-aged women and its etiology is unknown, although marked immunologic factors have been described, as well as marked copper deposition in the liver with normal serum ceruloplasmin.

49. The answer is A. *(Robbins, 5/e, pp 390–392.)* Increased amounts of δ-aminolevulinic acid (ALA) and coproporphyrin are found in the urine of patients who have ingested lead. Lead interferes with erythropoiesis by inhibiting the activity of several enzymes, including δ-ALA synthetase and ALA dehydrase. Thus the various degrees of anemia that are usually associated with lead poisoning are likely to be mediated by interference with erythropoietic-dependent enzymes, causing a microcytic, hypochromic anemia with basophilic stippling of the erythrocytes. Additional clinical findings include abdominal colic and a wristdrop and footdrop caused by a peripheral demyelinating neuropathy.

50. The answer is E. *(Robbins, 5/e, pp 402–408.)* Ionizing radiation, which is used in clinical diagnosis and therapy, induces changes in many different organ systems of the body. Its effects may be direct or indirect. Direct effects on target tissues produce single- or double-stranded chromosomal breaks in DNA. Indirect effects result in the formation of free radicals. Radiation also causes bizarre nuclear morphology along with abnormal mitotic figures. Changes induced in blood vessels include swelling and vacuolation of endothelial cells along with secondary thromboses and hemorrhages. The skin shows epidermal atrophy, not hyperplasia, and hyalinization and fibrosis of the dermis. There is atrophy of skin appendages and dilatation of the blood vessels. Effects on the blood include lymphopenia and granulocytopenia. Sterility is an effect on the gonads in both males and females, and the gastrointestinal tract is frequently damaged, leading to nausea and vomiting.

51. The answer is C. *(Anderson, 9/e, pp 209–213.)* Heavy metal poisoning may occur via the respiratory route owing to contaminated inhalant and vapors. Such poisoning is usually industrially related, as with mercury (calomel workers), arsenic (pesticides), and lead (batteries and paints). Cadmium has been implicated in producing not only an acute form of pneumonia, but, with chronic exposure to small concentrations of cadmium vapors, diffuse interstitial pulmonary fibrosis and an increased incidence of emphysema as well. The "honeycomb" radiologic pattern is indicative of an interstitial fibrotic process and may be the result of repeated pneumonitis and bronchitis. Cadmium can also be found in tobacco smoke. Cobalt poisoning leads to myocardiopathy, mercury poisoning leads to renal tubular damage, and lead poisoning leads to liver necrosis and cerebral edema. Arsenic poisoning, in addition to carrying an increased risk of lung and skin cancer, may cause death by inhibition of respiratory enzymes and cardiac subendocardial hemorrhages complicated by gastroenteritis with shock.

52. The answer is D. *(Robbins, 5/e, p 397. Rubin, 2/e, pp 308–313.)* Many environmental chemicals are potential causes of quite serious human diseases. Cyanide causes cellular damage by binding to cytochrome oxidase and inhibiting cellular respiration. It is a component of amygdalin, which is found in the pits of several fruits, such as apricots and peaches. Cyanide poisoning is betrayed by the presence of the odor of bitter almonds. Ethylene glycol, commonly used as an antifreeze, is toxic to humans. It causes acute tubular necrosis in the kidney. Carbon monoxide replaces oxygen in hemoglobin and causes the formation of carboxyhemoglobin and anoxia. Despite the extreme cyanosis, it produces a characteristic cherry-red color to the skin. Mercury toxicity damages both the kidney (proximal tubular necrosis) and the brain. The neurologic symptoms include mental changes and a tremor. Mercury was used in the hat industry, and the symptoms of toxicity resulted in the expression "mad as a hatter." Methanol, originally called "wood alcohol," is metabolized in the body to formaldehyde and formic acid. These metabolites cause necrosis of retinal ganglion cells, which produces blindness.

53. The answer is B. *(Robbins, 5/e, pp 127–129, 152–154.)* Mendel's laws deal with single-gene mutations that may be inherited or acquired de novo, with expression of the abnormality highly variable. In autosomal dominant inheritances, if a mutant gene is unexpressed, this is called *reduced penetrance* and it may vary by a percentage that reflects the degree of expression. *Variable expressivity* refers to expression of the trait in all who harbor the mutant gene, but with different expressions of the abnormality. *Nondisjunction* refers to a failure of disjoining of a homologous pair of chromosomes during meiosis (may result in aneuploidy). *Codominance* refers to the full expression of both alleles of a gene pair. *Genetic heterogeneity* applies to multiple-loci mutations (each in a different location, reflecting multiple different mutations), which can result in the same or similar expressed abnormality.

54. The answer is C. *(Robbins, 5/e, pp 152–153.)* Any deviation from the normal number of chromosomes, from their normal structure, or a combination of the two is an aberration that, if unbalanced, is termed *aneuploidy.* If the alterations remain balanced (balanced translocations), the condition is termed *euploidy.* Aneuploidy can result from the addition of a single chromosome to a pair (trisomy) or from translocations, inversions, duplications, and deletions.

55. The answer is B. *(Robbins, 5/e, pp 28, 63–64, 135–137, 449–454. Rubin, 2/e, pp 230–234, 240–244.)* Familial hypercholesterolemia (FH) is a common autosomal dominant (AD) disorder caused by mutation in the low-density lipoprotein (LDL) receptor gene located on chromosome 19. These gene mutations impair LDL transport and catabolism, with accumulation of LDL cholesterol in plasma. Elevated cholesterol levels result in skin xanthomas, early atherosclerosis, and increased risk of myocardial infarction. There is absent or deficient LDL receptor activity in homozygotes and one-half normal receptor activity in heterozygotes. CF is a fairly common AR disorder in whites (1:2500). Exocrine glands produce viscous mucus and sweat with high sodium and chloride concentration. The mutant gene product is unknown but the CF gene is localized on the long arm of chromosome 7. CF is manifest clinically only in homozygotes; parents are asymptomatic heterozygous carriers of the trait. PKU is an AR disorder of amino acid metabolism due to mutation in the gene coding for phenylalanine hydroxylase. Chromosome location is 12 and six different mutations are known. Myeloperoxidase deficiency has a frequency of 1:2000; slow bacterial killing is the major problem. Alkaptonuria is rare, the mutant gene product is homogentisic acid oxidase, and abnormal pigmentation of connective tissue (ochronosis) will result.

56. The answer is D. *(Robbins, 5/e, pp 132, 147–148, 449–450. Rubin, 2/e, pp 240–244.)* Several autosomal recessive disorders involve inborn errors of amino acid metabolism. Alkaptonuria (ochronosis) is caused by the excess accumulation of homogentisic acid. This results from a block in the metabolism of the phenylalanine-tyrosine pathway, which is caused by a deficiency of homogentisic oxidase. Excess homogentisic acid causes the urine to turn dark upon standing after a period of time. It also causes a dark coloration of the sclera, tendons, and cartilage. After years, many patients will develop a degenerative arthritis. Phenylketonuria (PKU), also called *hyperphenylalaninemia*, results from a deficiency of phenylalanine hydroxylase, an enzyme that oxidizes phenylalanine to tyrosine in the liver. Infants are normal at birth, but rising phenylalanine levels (hyperphenylalaninemia) results in irreversible brain damage. The excess phenylacetic acid in the urine results in a "mousy" odor. A lack of the enzyme fumarylacetoacetate hydrolase results in increased levels of tyrosine (tyrosinemia). Chronic forms of the disease are associated with cirrhosis of the liver, kidney dysfunction, and a high risk of developing hepatocellular carcinoma. Maple syrup urine disease is associated with an enzyme defect that causes the accumulation of branched-chain α-keto acid derivatives of isoleucine, leucine, and valine. *Albinism* refers to a group of disorders characterized by an abnormality of the synthesis of melanin. Two forms of oculocutaneous albinism are classified by the presence or absence of tyrosinase, which is the first enzyme in the conversion of tyrosine to melanin. Albinos are at a greatly increased risk for the development of squamous cell carcinomas in sun-exposed skin.

57. The answer is A. *(Robbins, 5/e, pp 142–143.)* Sphingomyelin, a lipid composed of phosphocholine and a ceramide, characteristically is found in abnormally high concentrations throughout the body tissues of patients who have any one of the forms of Niemann-Pick disease. Division of this disease into five categories is generally accepted; type A, the acute neuronopathic form, is the one that has the highest incidence. The lack of sphingomyelinase in type A is the metabolic defect that prevents the hydrolytic cleavage of sphingomyelin, which then accumulates in the brain. Patients who have the type A form usually show hepatosplenomegaly at 6 months of age, progressively lose motor functions and mental capabilities, and die during the third year of life.

58. The answer is A. *(Robbins, 5/e, pp 146–147. Rubin, 2/e, pp 240–241.)* The glycogen storage diseases are due to defective metabolism of glycogen, and at least eleven syndromes from genetic defects in the responsible enzymes have been described. Most of these glycogenoses are inherited as autosomal recessive disorders. Von Gierke's disease (type I) results from deficiency of glucose-6-phosphatase, the hepatic enzyme needed for conversion of G6P to glucose, with glycogen accumulation particularly in the enlarged liver and kidney and hypoglycemia. Diagnosis requires biopsy demonstration of excess liver glycogen plus either absent or low liver G6P activity, or a diabetic glucose tolerance curve, or hyperuricemia. Von Gierke's disease is the major hepatic or hepatorenal type of glycogenosis. Lysosomal glucosidase deficiency causes Pompe's disease (type II). Glycogen storage is widespread but most prominent in the heart (cardiomegaly). In brancher glycogenosis (type IV) there is accumulation of amylopectin or abnormal glycogen in liver, heart, skeletal muscle, and brain. The major myopathic form, McArdle's disease (type V), is due to lack of muscle phosphorylase. Glucose-6-phosphate dehydrogenase (G6PD) deficiency may cause oxidant-induced hemolytic anemia. The gene is X-linked recessive. One variant is present in about 10 percent of American blacks.

59. The answer is E. *(Robbins, 5/e, pp 152–156. Rubin, 2/e, pp 216–220.)* Nondisjunction is the failure of paired chromosomes or chromatids to separate during anaphase, either during mitosis or meiosis. Nondisjunction during the first meiotic division is responsible for trisomy 21 in about 93 percent of patients with Down's syndrome. Nondisjunction during mitosis of a somatic cell early during embryogenesis results in mosaicism in about 2 percent of patients with Down's syndrome. Translocation of an extra long arm of chromosome 21 causes about 5 percent of Down's syndrome cases. An important type of translocation, the Robertsonian translocation (centric fusion), involves two nonhomologous acrocentric chromosomes with the resultant formation of one large metacentric chromosome and one small chromosomal fragment, which is usually lost. Carriers of this type of translocation may produce children with Down's syndrome. Isochromosomes result from abnormal division of the centromere in a transverse plane. They are important in the pathogenesis of Turner's syndrome, not Down's syndrome.

60. The answer is A. *(Robbins, 5/e, p 156. Rubin, 2/e, p 220.)* Several genetic diseases are characterized by a deletion of part of an autosomal chromosome. The 5p−syndrome is also called the *cri du chat syndrome* as affected infants characteristically have a high-pitched cry similar to that of a kitten. Additional findings in this disorder include severe mental retardation, microcephaly, and congenital heart disease. The 11p−syndrome is characterized by the congenital absence of the iris (aniridia) and is often accompanied by Wilms tumor of the kidney. The 13q−syndrome is associated with the loss of the Rb suppressor gene and the development of retinoblastoma. Signs and symptoms of patients with either 21q− or 22q− are similar to those of Down's syndrome.

61. The answer is A. *(Anderson, 9/e, p 874.)* The findings of small, firm testes, eunuchoidism, gynecomastia, and mental retardation constitute the classic manifestations of Klinefelter's syndrome, a type of hypogonadism. The seminiferous tubules may be sclerosed and hyalinized. Urinary levels of gonadotropin are usually elevated; the elevation is thought to result from the absence of controlling testicular hormones, not from pituitary dysfunction.

62. The answer is D. *(Robbins, 5/e, pp 158–159.)* The Barr body represents a sex chromatin clump attached to the nuclear membrane that originates from an entire X chromosome and can easily be seen by using light microscopy to examine scrapings of the epithelium of the inside buccal mucosa. According to the formula M = n − 1, the total number of X chromatin masses equals the number of cellular X chromatin masses seen in the nucleus minus 1. Hence, normal males are 0 = 1 −1 (no Barr body), and normal females are 1 = 2 − 1 (one Barr body). In classic Turner's syndrome (XO), the expected buccal smear would be 0 = 1 − 1 (no Barr bodies seen), as in a normal male. Karyotyping is necessary when the Barr body screening test is ambiguous or inconclusive. In a young woman of short stature and average intelligence who has never menstruated, there is a strong indication that one of the forms of

Turner's syndrome exists, and the presence of one Barr body indicates that the patient has XX in some percentage of cells. About 10 percent of all Turner's syndrome patients show a mosaic pattern, with some cells having XO/XX or XO/XXX patterns. In this example, the patient is likely to be XO/XX by the formula $1 = 2 - 1$. In Turner's mosaics, the likelihood of developing a seminoma or gonadoblastoma is higher than expected, and gonadectomy may be indicated.

63. The answer is D. *(Robbins, 5/e, pp 160–162, 1156–1157.)* Sexual ambiguity arises when there is disagreement between the various ways of determining sex. Genetic sex is determined by the presence or absence of a Y chromosome. Gonadal sex is based upon the histologic appearance of the gonads. Ductal sex depends on the presence of derivatives of the müllerian or wolffian ducts. Phenotypic or genital sex is based on the appearance of the external genitalia. True hermaphroditism refers to the presence of both ovarian and testicular tissue. Pseudohermaphroditism is a disagreement between the phenotypic and gonadal sex. A female pseudohermaphrodite has ovaries but external male genitalia, while a male pseudohermaphrodite has testicular tissue, resulting from an XY genital sex karyotype, but female external genitalia. Female pseudohermaphroditism results from excessive exposure to androgens during early gestation; most often this is the result of congenital adrenal hyperplasia. Male pseudohermaphroditism results from defective virilization of the male embryo, most commonly caused by complete androgen insensitivity syndrome, also called *testicular feminization.* Turner's syndrome, which has a 45,X0 karyotype, is characterized by a female phenotype and bilateral streak ovaries. Mixed gonadal dysgenesis consists of one well-defined testis and a contralateral streak ovary. It is a cause of ambiguous genitalia in the newborn.

64. The answer is E. *(Robbins, 5/e, pp 443–444. Rubin, 2/e, pp 209–211.)* TORCH is an acronym referring to a group of microorganisms that produce similar changes during fetal or neonatal infection. The *T* stands for toxoplasma, the *O* for others, the *R* for rubella, the *C* for cytomegalovirus, and the *H* for herpes simplex virus. The "others" include syphilis, tuberculosis, and many other microorganisms. Manifestations of the TORCH complex include brain lesions, such as encephalitis and intracranial calcifications; ocular defects, including chorioretinitis; and cardiac abnormalities. Children born with congenital syphilis, caused by maternal infection with *Treponema pallidum,* initially show changes typical of the TORCH complex, but later they may develop characteristic lesions including flattening of the nose (saddle nose), notched incisors (Hutchinson's teeth), malformed molars (mulberry molars), outward bowing of the anterior tibia (saber shins), and progressive vascularization of the cornea (interstitial keratitis). The combination of deafness, interstitial keratitis, and notched incisors is referred to as *Hutchinson's triad.*

65. The answer is E. *(Rubin, 2/e, pp 1458, 1463, 1465, 1473.)* Retinopathy of prematurity, also called *retrolental fibroplasia,* is a cause of blindness in premature infants that is related to the therapeutic use of high concentrations of oxygen. The developing vessels in the retina become fibrosed, and the peripheral retina does not vascularize normally. The incidence of this complication has been markedly reduced due to close clinical monitoring of the concentration of administered oxygen. Presbyopia is an aging change resulting in loss of accommodation that affects most people at about the age of 40. Sun damage to the conjunctiva results in a yellow lesion at the limbus, a pinguecula. If the tissue encroaches on the cornea, it is called a *pterygium.* The macula has a large number of cones and is related to visual acuity. Degeneration of the macula occurs most often from age-related maculopathy, but it can also be caused by inherited disorders or drugs, such as chloroquine.

66. The answer is C. *(Robbins, 5/e, pp 446–449.)* Hemolytic disease of the newborn is characterized by anemia, jaundice, tissue edema, and hepatosplenomegaly. The transmission of maternal antibody (transplacental transmission) causes the disease because of incompatibility between maternal and fetal blood types. ABO incompatibilities occur often but are not severe; however, both ABO and Rh antigens may cause the disease. There are many Rh antigens that do not cause disease, but RhD is the usual antigen that causes mild to very severe disease, except in the first pregnancy. The frequency increases with repeat pregnancies as antibody level rises, and anti-RhD IgG must be given to a nonsensitized Rh-negative mother within 72 h of delivery or termination (abortion) of the first and of all subsequent pregnancies.

67. The answer is B. *(Robbins, 5/e, pp 171–174.)* Some features of leukocytes are specific for certain cells of the immune system. Some of these features involve substances on the surface of these cells. B lymphocytes are the type of leukocytes that have IgM on their surface. This surface immunoglobulin participates in the binding of B cells to many different antigens. The diversity of this binding and the subsequent production of many different immunoglobulins is obtained by rearrangement of the immunoglobulin genes from their germline configuration. This rearrangement occurs only in B lymphocytes, and thus, the presence of rearranged immunoglobulin genes in a lymphoid cell indicates that the cell is a B lymphocyte. Similarly, T lymphocytes have a surface antigen–binding receptor (TCR) that consists of CD3 proteins attached to a heterodimer composed of alpha, beta, gamma, or delta polypeptide chains. Demonstration of TCR gene rearrangement is a molecular marker of T lymphocytes. Macrophages, required to process antigen to T cells, have class II HLA antigens on their surface. They are also active phago-cytes and have receptors for the Fc portion of IgG and C3a. Dendritic cells, present in lymphoid tissue, and Langerhans cells, present in the epidermis, are antigen-presenting cells. They have large amounts of class II HLA antigens on their cell surfaces. Natural killer cells are identified by two cell surface molecules, CD16 and CD56.

68. The answer is A. *(Anderson, 9/e, p 492. Robbins, 5/e, pp 171–174, 635).* With the advent of monoclonal antibodies derived from hybridomas, it is now possible to identify cells of certain specificity. These antibodies recog-nize epitopes of antigens found on the cell surfaces that have been used to in-duce immunity within the mouse. Using an immunoperoxidase technique, the OKT (Leu series) identifies T cells. In addition specific markers will identify subsets of T cells. For example, all peripheral blood T cells react with OKT1, OKT3, and OKT11 cluster designations CD5, CD3, and CD2; OKT4 (Leu-3) reacts with mature T cells; OKT4 or CD4 identifies helper T cells; and OKT8 (CD8) reacts with suppressor cells. The normal T helper/suppressor ratio in humans is about 2. These antibodies do not label cells other than those in the T-lymphocyte system. T cells as a group function in immune regulation and act in concert with B lymphocytes and macrophages. T helper cells aid the cellular immune response in reaction to antigens, while T suppressor cells help in turning the immune response off. EAC rosette cells refer to B lympho-cytes that have surface receptors (C3b) that bind to sheep erythrocytes coated with IgM antibody and complement. B lymphocytes also express surface im-munoglobulin.

69. The answer is D. *(Robbins, 5/e, pp 172–173. Rubin, 2/e, p 101.)* B cells possess surface membrane IgM and IgD, with monomeric IgM the antigen re-ceptor of all B cells. B cells also express the pan-B-cell antigens CD19 and CD20, which is obviously of practical value in differentiating a chronic leukemia such as chronic lymphocytic leukemia (CLL) in which transformed B cells possess surface IgM and IgD and express CD19 and CD20 antigens, but not the early B cell antigen CD10. In contrast, CD8 and CD4 are on 30 percent and 60 percent of peripheral T cells, respectively. CD4 is a marker for T helper cells, and CD8 a marker for cytotoxic/suppressor T cells. B lympho-cytes have receptors for fixed complement components C3b and C3d and for the Fc portion of IgG. Immunologic diagnosis of B-cell lymphoid tumors by immunofluorescence or flow cytometry shows the cell surface immunoglobu-lins and cluster differentiation antigens through detection by monoclonal anti-bodies; molecular biology techniques reveal Ig gene rearrangements on the altered B cells.

70. The answer is B. *(Robbins, 5/e, pp 175–177. Rubin, 2/e, pp 103–104.)* The genes that code for antigens that evoke tissue rejection reactions if transplanted are called *histocompatibility genes*. The genes that code for the strongest transplantation antigens are clustered together on chromosome 6 and are called the *major histocompatibility complex (MHC)*, or the human leukocyte antigen (HLA) complex. The products of MHC are classified into three groups. Class I and class II genes encode for cell surface glycoproteins, while class III genes encode for components of the complement system. Class I molecules are associated with beta$_2$ microglobulin. The loci that encode for class I antigens are HLA-A, HLA-B, and HLA-C. Class I antigens are serologically defined by using antisera (antibodies) to specific HLA antigens. Some class II antigens, e.g., HLA-DQ and HLA-DR, may also be defined serologically using antibodies. Class II DQ and DR antigens can also be defined using the mixed lymphocyte reaction, which involves mixing the patient's lymphocytes with lymphocytes of known HLA type. The patient's lymphocytes will proliferate only in response to incompatible lymphocytes. The patient's cells are assigned the DQ or DR type of the compatible lymphocytes. Some class II antigens, e.g., HLA-DP, cannot be serologically determined, and instead the primed lymphocyte assay is used. In this test, cells that have been previously typed and are primed to react with specific DP antigens are mixed with the patient's cells. The primed cells will then proliferate only in response to the patient's cells that have that specific antigen.

71. The answer is A. *(Robbins, 5/e, pp 175–177.)* CD8+ cytotoxic T lymphocytes can recognize a foreign antigen only if that antigen is complexed to self-class I antigens. In general these class I molecules bind to proteins synthesized within the cell, one example of which is the cellular production of viral antigens. The CD8 molecule of the cytotoxic T cell binds to the nonpolymorphic portion of the class I molecule, while the T-cell receptor on the surface of the T lymphocyte binds to a complex formed by the peptide fragment of the antigen and the class I antigen. In contrast, CD4+ helper T lymphocytes can recognize a foreign antigen only if that antigen is complexed to self-class II antigens. In general, class II antigens present foreign antigens that have been processed within the cell in endosomes or lysosomes, one example of which is bacteria. Macrophages and neutrophils are active phagocytes and have receptors for the Fc portion of IgG and C3b; both of these substances are important opsonins. Macrophages also ingest and present antigens to T cells in conjunction with surface class II antigens.

72. The answer is A. *(Robbins, 5/e, pp 177, 1253–1254.)* A variety of different diseases have an association with certain HLA types. The exact mechanism of this association is unknown. These diseases can be grouped into three broad categories: inflammatory diseases, such as ankylosing spondylitis, and HLA-B27; inherited errors of metabolism, such as hemochromatosis, and HLA-A3; and autoimmune diseases, which are usually associated with the DR locus. Two examples of the last are the associations of rheumatoid arthritis with DR4 and insulin-dependent diabetes with DR3/DR4. Ankylosing spondylitis is one type of spondyloarthropathy that lacks the rheumatoid factor found in rheumatoid arthritis. Other seronegative spondyloarthropathies include Reiter's syndrome, psoriatic arthritis, and enteropathic arthritis. All of these are associated with an increased incidence of HLA-B27. Ankylosing spondylitis, also known as *rheumatoid spondylitis,* or *Marie-Strümpell disease,* is a chronic inflammatory disease that primarily affects the sacroiliac joints of adult males. Reiter's syndrome is the triad of arthritis, nongonococcal urethritis, and conjunctivitis. It may be related to previous gastrointestinal or genitourinary infections.

73. The answer is D. *(Robbins, 5/e, pp 178–190.)* The reaction in the question is a type 2 hypersensitivity reaction that is mediated by antibodies reacting against antigens present on the surface of cells, in this case blood group antigens or irregular antigens present on the donor's red blood cells. Type 2 hypersensitivity reactions result from attachment of antibodies to changed cell surface antigens or to normal cell surface antigens. Complement-mediated cytotoxicity occurs when IgM or IgG binds to a cell surface antigen with complement activation and consequent cell membrane damage or lysis. Blood transfusion reactions and autoimmune hemolytic anemia are examples of this form. Systemic anaphylaxis is a type 1 hypersensitivity reaction in which mast cells or basophils that are bound to IgE antibodies are reexposed to an allergen, which leads to a release of vasoactive amines that causes edema and broncho- and vasoconstriction. Sudden death can occur. Systemic immune complex reactions are found in type 3 reactions and are due to circulating antibodies that form complexes upon reexposure to an antigen, such as foreign serum, which then activates complement followed by chemotaxis and aggregation of neutrophils leading to release of lysosomal enzymes and eventual necrosis of tissue and cells. Serum sickness and Arthus' reactions are examples of this. Delayed-type hypersensitivity is type 4 and is due to previously sensitized T lymphocytes, which release lymphokines upon reexposure to the antigen. This takes time—perhaps up to several days following exposure. The tuberculin reaction is the best known example of this. T-cell–mediated cytotoxicity leads to lysis of cells by cytotoxic T cells in response to tumor cells, allogenic tissue, and virus-infected cells. These cells have CD8 antigens on their surfaces.

74. The answer is B. *(Robbins, 5/e, pp 187–189.)* Delayed-hypersensitivity reactions are mediated by T lymphocytes and other mononuclear cells. The reaction requires previous exposure to antigen, frequently a large protein, and takes from 1 to 3 days to develop fully. Only true palpable induration is considered a positive reaction.

75. The answer is C. *(Anderson, 9/e, pp 531–532.)* An allograft is also called a *homograft* and refers to a graft between members of the same species. An autograft is a tissue graft taken from one site and placed in a different site in the same individual. Isografts are grafts between individuals from an inbred strain of animals. A graft between individuals of two different species is a xenograft, or heterograft.

76. The answer is D. *(Henry, 18/e, pp 53–55. Robbins, 5/e, pp 200–201.)* Diagnostic specificity is defined as the probability of a negative diagnostic test result in the absence of the disease the test is designed to detect, or, simply, the ability of a screening test to correctly identify a person who is free of the specific disease. Two clinically useful tests specific for systemic lupus erythematosus (SLE) are the detection of antibodies to double-stranded DNA (anti-ds DNA) and to the nonhistone Smith (Sm) antigen, since these antibodies are rare in other autoimmune diseases. Positive testing for antinuclear antibody (ANA) occurs in virtually all patients with SLE (marked diagnostic sensitivity), but the test is *not specific* since positive results are frequent in other autoimmune diseases. In diffuse systemic sclerosis, positive antibodies to nucleolar RNA and Scl-70 antibody to nonhistone nuclear protein are specific. In the CREST syndrome of systemic sclerosis, an anticentromere antibody is specific. The best information from laboratory tests comes from their positive and negative predictive values (PVs) relating the results (+ or −) to prevalence of the disease in the population being studied.

77. The answer is E. *(Robbins, 5/e, pp 190–195.)* Histocompatible antigens (HLA) are responsible for rejection of transplanted organs in humans. Organ rejection requires both humoral and cell-mediated immunologic reactions involving T cells both from the donated organ and the patient's own CD4 T helper cells and CD8 cytotoxic T cells. Hyperacute rejection occurs within minutes after transplantation and consists of neutrophils within the glomerulus and peritubular capillaries. Acute rejection occurs within days after transplantation and is marked by vasculitis and interstitial lymphocytic infiltration. Subacute rejection vasculitis occurs during the first few months after transplantation and is characterized by the proliferation of fibroblasts and macrophages in the tunica intima of arteries. In chronic rejection tubular atrophy, mononuclear interstitial infiltration, and vascular changes are encountered, with the vascular changes being characteristic and probably reflecting an end stage of arteritis. The vascular obliteration leads to interstitial fibrosis and tubular atrophy with loss of renal function. However, the histologic picture is complicated by secondary ischemic damage, and it may be difficult to discern inflammation, fibrosis, and vascular changes as cause or effect.

78. The answer is B. *(Robbins, 5/e, pp 210–213.)* The constellation of Raynaud's phenomenon, acral sclerosis, and fibrotic tightening of the muscles of facial expression should raise the specter of progressive systemic sclerosis (scleroderma), a multisystem disease that involves the cardiovascular, gastrointestinal, cutaneous, musculoskeletal, pulmonary, and renal systems through progressive interstitial fibrosis. Small arterioles in the forenamed systems show obliteration caused by intimal hyperplasia accompanied by progressive interstitial fibrosis. Evidence implicates a lymphocyte overdrive of fibroblasts to produce an excess of rather normal collagen. Eventually, myocardial fibrosis, pulmonary fibrosis, and terminal renal failure ensue. Over half of all patients have dysphagia with solid food caused by the distal esophageal narrowing in the disease.

79. The answer is B. *(Robbins, 5/e, pp 217–219.)* Patients with isolated IgA deficiency, a very common immunodeficiency that affects about 1 in 600 persons in the United States, have very low levels of serum and secretory IgA. Patients commonly have recurrent sinopulmonary infections and diarrhea. These patients also have an increased incidence of respiratory tract allergy and autoimmune diseases. There is no increase in the incidence of lymphoma. Serum antibodies to IgA, however, are found in about 40 percent of these patients, who, if given blood containing normal IgA, may develop severe, possibly fatal anaphylaxis reactions. Tetany due to lack of parathyroid development is seen in patients with DiGeorge's syndrome. Angioedema, localized edema affecting the skin and mucous membranes, is seen with absence of C1 esterase inhibitor due to the excessive generation of vasoactive C2 kinin. Thrombocytopenia is part of the X-linked disorder Wiskott-Aldrich syndrome.

80. The answer is B. *(Robbins, 5/e, pp 199–208.)* Renal failure, not heart disease, is the most common cause of death in SLE. Most cases show some renal abnormality (mild or marked) by immunofluorescence and by light and electron microscopy. Diffuse proliferative glomerulonephritis (GN) occurs in about 50 percent of cases and is the most common and most serious renal lesion. Subendothelial location of immune complex deposits is particularly characteristic of SLE. Membranous GN occurs in only 10 percent of cases and has a better prognosis, but may progress. Polyclonal B-cell activation occurs with increased production of autoantibodies and hypergammaglobulinemia. This B-cell activation may follow genetic B-cell abnormalities or loss of

T-suppressor cell influence. Most of the tissue lesions are mediated by the immune complex (type III hypersensitivity). Nonerosive arthritis occurs in about 90 percent of cases and often involves small peripheral joints. Lack of deformity and of synovial proliferation distinguish arthritis of SLE from rheumatoid arthritis.

81. The answer is C. *(Robbins, 5/e, pp 208–210.)* Sjögren's syndrome is characterized by dryness of the mouth (xerostomia) and eyes (keratoconjunctivitis sicca). Secondary Sjögren's syndrome is associated with rheumatoid arthritis (RA), or SLE, or systemic sclerosis. The primary form shows increased frequency of HLA-DR3, while association with RA shows a positive correlation with HLA-DR4. Anti-SSB antibodies are fairly specific, anti-SSA less so, and both may occur in SLE; rheumatoid factor is often present. Glomerular lesions are very rare but a mild tubulointerstitial nephritis is quite common and may result in renal tubular acidosis. In addition to the usual dense, lymphoplasmacytic infiltrate of salivary glands, the lymph nodes may show a "pseudolymphomatous" appearance. True B-cell lymphomas have developed with increased frequency in Sjögren's syndrome (relative risk of 44).

82. The answer is C. *(Rubin, 2/e, p 140.)* Ten to twenty percent or more of cases of polymyositis are associated with underlying visceral malignancies of virtually any organ. Although the cause of this association remains unknown, it has been postulated that some cancers either produce substances that are toxic to skeletal muscle or contain antigens that are cross-reactive with skeletal muscle.

83. The answer is D. *(Robbins, 5/e, pp 216–218.)* Common variable immunodeficiency (CVI) represents a heterogeneous group of disorders characterized by hypogammaglobulinemia. In contrast to X-linked agammaglobulinemia of Bruton, patients with CVI may be of either sex. They also have normal numbers of B cells in the blood and lymphoid tissue, and their symptoms develop later in life. The B cells cannot differentiate into plasma cells, and this leads to hyperplasia of the lymphoid follicles and hypogammaglobulinemia. Patients are prone to recurrent bacterial and viral infections and have an increased incidence of lymphoma and autoimmune diseases. Thymic aplasia or hypoplasia due to lack of development of the third and fourth pharyngeal pouches is seen in patients with DiGeorge's syndrome. About 40 percent of the patients with the autosomal recessive form of severe combined immunodeficiency disease (SCID) have a deficiency of the enzyme adenosine deaminase (ADA). The lack of ADA leads to the accumulation of substances that are toxic to immature lymphocytes, particularly the T lymphocytes.

84. The answer is C. *(Henry, 18/e, pp 689–690.)* Cytopenias occur in over 50 percent of patients with HIV infection either individually or as part of a pancytopenia. Suppression of hemopoiesis in the bone marrow as a result of mycobacterial, fungal, or protozoal infection; infiltration by lymphoma, leukemia, or Kaposi's sarcoma; and the effects of drugs (particularly zidovudine) may result in cytopenia. Anemia is seen in 80 to 85 percent of cases, usually in the pattern of anemia of chronic disease. Thrombocytopenia occurs in about 30 percent of cases and is thought to be a result of peripheral destruction of platelets, possibly by an immune mechanism. Neutropenia occurs in 40 percent of patients. Lymphopenia and a reduced ratio of CD4 to CD8 lymphocytes are characteristic of HIV infection. Atypical plasmacytoid lymphocytes are usually present in the peripheral blood smear. Examination of the bone marrow in cytopenic patients shows a normocellular or hypercellular pattern in more than 90 percent of cases.

85. The answer is D. *(Robbins, 5/e, pp 219–231.)* AIDS is caused by infection with the retrovirus human immunodeficiency virus (HIV) (formerly called HTLV III/LAV). The virus infects T helper cells, preventing function, destroying cells, and increasing susceptibility to and incidence of infection. Cytotoxic/suppressor T cells may be normal, slightly increased, or decreased in number, although they show a proportional increase in comparison to helper T cells, which are markedly decreased. In AIDS, the ratio of helper to suppressor cells is inverted, being approximately 1:2, instead of the normal 2:1. Wide defects of immune function in AIDS include defects in natural killer cells, in monocytes, and in virus-specific cytotoxic T cells and B cells. B cells are polyclonally activated, resulting in hypergammaglobulinemia. Patients with AIDS have an increased incidence of certain malignancies, including Kaposi's sarcoma and B-cell non-Hodgkin's lymphoma.

86. The answer is C. *(Joklik, 20/e, pp 774–775. Robbins, 5/e, p 308.)* Togaviruses, a family of helical, predominantly single-stranded RNA viruses, include the genus *Alphavirus* (mosquito-borne), which causes eastern equine encephalitis (EEE) and western equine encephalitis (WEE). Yellow fever, dengue fever, and St. Louis encephalitis are caused by Flaviviridae; these were part of the old group B arboviruses, which used to be in the genus *Flavivirus* of the Togaviridae. The causative agent of epidemic hemorrhagic keratoconjunctivitis is usually the type B adenovirus, an icosahedral double-stranded DNA virus. Herpes simplex keratoconjunctivitis, although frequently recurrent, is not epidemic.

87. The answer is C. *(Robbins, 5/e, pp 322–323, 347–350, 352.)* Influenza is caused by small RNA viruses, classified as myxoviruses. All the other viral illnesses listed in the question are caused by herpesviruses, which are relatively large, double-stranded DNA viruses. Shingles and chickenpox are caused by herpes zoster, which is identical to varicella. Cytomegalovirus causes cytomegalic inclusion disease, and Epstein-Barr (EB) virus causes mononucleosis.

88. The answer is B. *(Duchin, N Engl J Med 330: 949–955, 1994.)* The *Hantavirus* genus belongs to the Bunyaviridae family and includes the causative agent of a group of diseases that occur throughout Europe and Asia and are referred to as *hemorrhagic fever with renal syndrome*. The characteristic features of this syndrome are hematologic abnormalities, renal involvement, and increased vascular permeability. Respiratory involvement is generally minimal in these diseases. Although several species of rodents in the United States were known to be infected with *Hantavirus,* no human cases had been reported until an outbreak of severe, often fatal, respiratory illness occurred in the United States in May 1993 in the Four Corners area of New Mexico, Arizona, Colorado, and Utah. This illness resulted from a new member of the genus *Hantavirus* that caused a severe disease characterized by a prodromal fever, myalgia, pulmonary edema, and hypotension. The main distinguishing feature of this illness, which is called *Hantavirus* pulmonary syndrome, is noncardiogenic pulmonary edema resulting from increased permeability of the pulmonary capillaries. Laboratory features common to both *Hantavirus* pulmonary syndrome and hemorrhagic fever with renal syndrome include leukocytosis, atypical lymphocytes, thrombocytopenia, coagulopathy, and decreased serum protein concentrations. Abdominal pain, which can mimic an acute abdomen, may be found in both *Hantavirus* pulmonary syndrome and hemorrhagic fever with renal syndrome.

89. The answer is B. *(Henry, 18/e, pp 514–515, 1041–1045. Robbins, 5/e, pp 337–338.)* The pneumococcus (*Streptococcus pneumoniae*) is a gram-positive, encapsulated coccus, differentiated from other alpha-hemolytic streptococci by bile solubility or serologic typing. But inhibition of pneumococci by Optochin is easier and has about 90 percent specificity. Capsular polysaccharides form the basis for division into serotypes; when exposed to type-specific antisera they show a positive precipitin reaction or capsular swelling, the quellung reaction. Detection of pneumococcal capsular polysaccharides in sputum or body fluids by immunologic methods (CIE or latex agglutination) are other methods for presumptive diagnosis of infection, but cross reactions between pneumococci and other bacteria occur. So, immunologic diagnosis is less specific than bacteriologic diagnosis by capsular typing by the quellung reaction. Capsular polysaccharides protect pneumococci from phagocytosis and are virulence factors. M protein occurs in the cell walls of pathogenic group A beta-hemolytic streptococci (*S. pyogenes*) and functions as the principal virulence factor by inhibiting phagocytosis.

90. The answer is D. *(Anderson, 9/e, pp 2154–2156. Henry, 18/e, pp 448–451.)* In a patient who is suspected of having meningitis, microscopic examination of cerebrospinal fluid is of immediate importance. In the photomicrograph shown, all the cells are polymorphonuclear leukocytes and bacteria are visible in the cytoplasm. Neutrophils may be present in viral or tuberculous meningitis, but lymphocytes are more common. Demonstration of bacteria by Gram stain of the cerebrospinal fluid is the most valuable aid in establishing a diagnosis of early bacterial meningitis and is possible in more than 90 percent of cases.

91. The answer is C. *(Joklik, 20/e, pp 1060–1063. Rubin, 2/e, pp 341–344.)* Human parvovirus may cause a serious aplastic crisis in patients with an underlying chronic hemolytic anemia. In children, infection with parvovirus produces a characteristic rash, called *erythema infectiosum* or *fifth disease,* which first appears on the face and is described as a "slapped cheek" appearance. Human parvovirus infection in adults produces a nonspecific syndrome of fever, malaise, headache, myalgia, vomiting, and a transient rash. Arthralgia is more common in adults than in children. There are many types of rhinoviruses, which are causative agents of the common cold (coryza). This infection is characterized by rhinorrhea, pharyngitis, cough, and a low-grade fever. Parainfluenza viruses, single-stranded RNA viruses that kill ciliated respiratory epithelial cells, are the most common cause of croup, which is a disease of children characterized by a barking sound on inspiration. Rubeola virus, an RNA virus, is the cause of measles. After an incubation of 10 to 21 days, measles is characterized by fever, rhinorrhea, cough, skin lesions, and mucosal lesions (Koplik spots). Rubella virus, another RNA virus, produces a mild, acute febrile illness, but if the infection occurs in the first trimester of pregnancy it can produce developmental abnormalities such as cardiac lesions, ocular abnormalities, deafness, and mental retardation.

92. The answer is D. *(Henry, 18/e, pp 514–515. Robbins, 5/e, pp 337, 696–697.)* Most cases of lobar pneumonia are caused by *Streptococcus pneumoniae* (reclassification of the pneumococcus). Streptococcal or pneumococcal pneumonia involves one or more lobes and is often seen in alcoholics or debilitated persons. Type 3 pneumococcus (*S. pneumoniae*) causes a virulent lobar pneumonia characterized by mucoid sputum, which is also seen in *Klebsiella* pneumonia. *K. pneumoniae* (Friedländer's bacillus) usually produces a bronchopneumonia, rather than lobar pneumonia, but is clinically indistinguishable from pneumococcal lobar pneumonia. *Legionella* species cause a fibrinopurulent lobular pneumonia that tends to be confluent, almost appearing lobar.

93. The answer is D. *(Robbins, 5/e, pp 331, 360, 793–794.)* *Yersinia* (formerly called *Pasteurella*) is an important genus of gram-negative bacilli that causes a wide variety of human and animal disease, ranging from plague (*Y. pestis*) to acute mesenteric lymphadenitis (*Y. enterocolitica*) in older children and young adults. *Y. enterocolitica* infections also occur in the terminal ileum in young adults, causing an ileitis that produces inflammation not unlike that seen in some stages of Crohn's disease (regional enteritis). Since the organisms grow slowly on enrichment media, they may be overgrown by other coliforms at 37°C. The organisms may be isolated by means of cold enhancement at 4°C.

94. The answer is C. *(Henry, 18/e, pp 1049–1050. Robbins, 5/e, p 309. Rubin, 2/e, p 283.)* Listeriosis is a food-borne illness (e.g., via milk products, coleslaw) usually occurring in the immunocompromised, in pregnant women and their fetuses, and in the debilitated elderly. *Listeria monocytogenes* is a gram-positive, motile bacillus, often found within circulating lymphocytes (similar to *Legionella*). Maternal infection is mild; fetal infection is severe. Meningitis is predominant in neonatal infections and in opportunistic adult disease, and *Listeria monocytogenes* is responsible for about 2 percent of bacterial meningitis cases in this country. True epithelioid granulomas are rare, although macrophages may appear late, following neutrophil infiltration or abscesses in organs or lymph nodes.

95. The answer is D. *(Henry, 18/e, pp 1058–1059. Rubin, 2/e, pp 371–372.)* The *Vibrio* genus, including *V. cholerae,* is associated with gastrointestinal disease in the Far East, especially India, but is capable of inducing disease in the United States, as in pandemics occurring here around 1832 and in 1849. Along the coasts, especially the northeast and Gulf coasts of the United States, the vibrios increase in numbers in seawater and in seafood and are more likely to cause infections during the late summer and early autumn months. Patients with underlying liver disease, such as alcoholics, and those with immunosuppressive disorders are advised not to ingest raw shellfish during these months because of an increased incidence of disease with the vibrio organisms in these patients. The mycobacteria are acid-fast bacilli associated with tuberculosis and tuberculosis-like diseases; *M. avium-intracellulare* is known to be a frequent organism in AIDS. These organisms are not curved as the vibrios are.

96. The answer is C. *(Robbins, 5/e, pp 361–362, 1253, 1260.)* A localized skin rash in the summertime followed within a period of weeks by arthritis, especially involving less than three joints, should arouse suspicion of Lyme disease. This disorder was first described in the mid-1970s in Connecticut when small clusters of cases of children suffering from an illness resembling juvenile rheumatoid arthritis were first noted. The disease has now been shown to be caused by a spirochete, *Borrelia burgdorferi,* through the bite of a tick belonging to the genus *Ixodes.* The spirochete-infested ticks reside in wooded areas where there are deer and small rodents. The deer act as a wintering-over reservoir for the ticks. In the spring the tick larval stage emerges and evolves into a nymph, which is infective for humans if they are bitten. Adult ticks are also capable of transmitting the spirochete as well during questing. The bite is followed by a rash called *erythema chronicum migrans,* which may resolve spontaneously. However, many patients have a transient phase of spirochetemia, which may allow the spread of the spirochete to the meninges, heart, and synovial tissue. Originally thought to be confined to New England, Lyme disease has now been shown to be present in Europe and Australia as well. The spirochetes are sensitive to penicillin, erythromycin, and tetracycline. Reiter's disease does not present with a spreading rash, and a Baker's cyst produces swelling in the popliteal fossa behind the knee rather than joint effusions anteriorly.

97. The answer is C. *(Henry, 18/e, pp 1094–1096. Robbins, 5/e, p 344.)* Although the rapid plasma reagin (RPR), Kolmer, and Venereal Disease Research Laboratory (VDRL) tests are rapid and easily performed tests that can help confirm a diagnosis of active syphilis, they are associated with false positive reactions because of their low specificity for antibodies against treponemal or cardiolipin antigens. Therefore, RPR, Kolmer, and VDRL tests usually are used for screening programs. The *Treponema pallidum* immobilization (TPI) and the fluorescent treponemal antibody-absorption (FTA-ABS) tests have greater specificity for treponemal antigen but are technically more difficult to perform. The FTA-ABS test is generally the most sensitive and most specific procedure for diagnosis of syphilis.

98. The answer is E. *(Rubin, 2/e, pp 386–387, 390–396.)* Lymphogranuloma venereum, usually transmitted by sexual contact, is caused by obligate intracellular parasites that contain both RNA and DNA and belong to the genus *Chlamydia* (*C. trachomatis*). Chlamydial agents, originally thought to be viruses because they form inclusion bodies in infected cells, also cause trachoma, inclusion conjunctivitis, and psittacosis-ornithosis. The other infections listed are caused by spirochetes and are nonvenereal.

99. The answer is E. *(Robbins, 5/e, pp 307, 698–699.)* Mycoplasma pneumoniae, the causative agent of primary atypical interstitial pneumonia, belongs to the mycoplasma group of tiny pleuropneumonia-like organisms (PPLOs, or Eaton agents), which lack cell walls and are beyond the resolution of light microscopy. *M. pneumoniae* can cause up to 50 percent of pneumonias in college students and mainly affects adolescents and young adults. The interstitial pneumonia with mononuclear response is similar to viral pneumonia; pharyngitis and tracheobronchitis with persistent cough are common. Serum immunoglobulins that agglutinate human type O red cells at 4°C (cold agglutinins) are often present; this test is nonspecific but suggestive of *M. pneumoniae.*

100. The answer is C. *(Robbins, 5/e, pp 328–329.)* In the approximate center of the photomicrograph is the classic, refractile, double-walled spherule of the deep fungus *Coccidioides immitis,* which is several times the diameter of the largest inflammatory cell nearby. Coccidioidomycosis is endemic in California, Arizona, New Mexico, and parts of Nevada, Utah, and Texas, where it resides in the arid soils and is contracted by direct inhalation of airborne dust. If inhaled, it produces a primary pulmonary infection that is usually benign and self-limiting in immunologically competent persons, often with several days of fever and upper respiratory flulike symptoms. However, certain ethnic groups, such as some blacks, Asians, and Filipinos, are at risk of developing a potentially lethal disseminated form of the disease that can involve the central nervous system. If the large, double-walled spherule containing numerous endospores can be demonstrated outside the lungs (e.g., in a skin biopsy), this is evidence of dissemination. Antibodies of high titers are detectable by means of complement fixation studies in patients undergoing spontaneous recovery. Amphotericin B is usually reserved for treating high-risk and disseminated infection. The cultured mycelia of the organism on Sabouraud's agar present a hazard for laboratory workers.

101. The answer is E. *(Robbins, 5/e, pp 365–367.)* Lepromatous and tuberculoid leprosy, the major forms, are caused by *Mycobacterium leprae* and nerve involvement is most typical of the lepromatous form. Numerous bacilli in packets occupy histiocytes or lepra cells in the lesions of lepromatous leprosy. Polyclonal hypergammaglobulinemia often occurs in lepromatous leprosy, in which patients do not have the adequate cellular immune response of the tuberculoid form. Large amounts of anti-lepra antibody occur in the lepromatous form with frequent formation of antigen-antibody complexes and resultant disorders such as erythema nodosum. A "clear" zone between infiltrate and overlying epidermis is characteristic of lepromatous leprosy, unlike the encroachment on basal epidermis of the tuberculoid infiltrate.

102. The answer is C. *(Henry, 18/e, pp 1077–1099. Robbins, 5/e, pp 324–325.)* Pathogenic mycobacteria, including *M. tuberculosis,* have a known propensity for resistance to drying in the environment, survival for extended periods of time on inanimate surfaces, resistance to alkali and acids, and impermeability to routine tissue and Gram stains. Many of these features are thought to be related to the very high lipid and wax content of the bacilli, which makes up some 60 percent of the total dry weight. Mycolic acid is only one of many fatty acids present. Virulence is thought to be related to the presence of the mycoside trehalose 6-6 dimycolate (cord factor).

103. The answer is D. *(Anderson, 9/e, pp 438–439).* *Giardia lamblia,* a flagellate protozoan, is the most common cause of outbreaks of waterborne diarrheal disease in the U.S. and is seen frequently in Rocky Mountain areas. Ingestion of cysts from contaminated water results in trophozoites in duodenum and jejunum. Identification of the trophozoite stage is done by duodenal aspiration or small-bowel biopsy and of the cyst stage (intermittent) by examination of stool. The trophozoite may appear as a pear-shaped, binucleate organism ("two eyes"). Giardiasis may cause malabsorption but is often asymptomatic. Duodenal aspiration, immunofluorescence, and ELISA testing for *Giardia* antigens are diagnostic and therapy with metronidazole or quinacrine is effective. Lymph nodes often contain numerous parasites in trypanosomiasis and leishmaniasis. *Triatoma* is the vector of Chagas' disease (American trypanosomiasis). *Trichomonas vaginalis* is identified in cervicovaginal smears.

104. The answer is B. *(Anderson, 9/e, pp 464–465.)* In the photomicrograph, a cross section of an *Enterobius* adult worm is shown. Apparent morphologic features of this nematode include the bilateral crests, the meromyarial type of musculature, and the noncellular cuticle with spines. *Enterobius vermicularis,* the agent responsible for the helminthic infection most common in the United States, usually produces pruritus ani as the outstanding and most disturbing symptom of enterobiasis (pinworm infection). *Enterobius* worms often attach themselves to the cecal mucosa and contiguous regions, but the usual host sites for schistosomiasis, clonorchiasis, and filariasis are the veins of the large intestine, the bile ducts, and the lymphatics, respectively. Elephantiasis is a characteristic feature in filariasis, and infection by *Strongyloides stercoralis* usually produces hyperemia and edema of the mucosa of the small intestine.

105. The answer is E. *(Robbins, 5/e, pp 324–327.)* *Mycobacterium tuberculosis* is an obligate aerobe—thus its predilection for pulmonary infection. The high content of lipids in its cell wall is in part responsible for its acid-fast response to Ziehl-Neelsen staining. The frequency of occurrence of drug-resistant mutants in this organism has necessitated simultaneous use of multiple chemotherapeutic agents against it. Persons with silicosis have a high incidence of infection with *M. tuberculosis,* which on culture requires several weeks to grow.

106. The answer is D. *(Robbins, 5/e, p 310. Rubin, 2/e, pp 408–419.)* The deep fungal infections produce characteristic morphologic features in tissue sections. The two basic morphologic types of fungi are yeasts, which are oval cells that reproduce by budding, and molds, which are filamentous colonies consisting of branched tubules called *hyphae.* Some yeasts produce buds that do not detach. Instead they form long structures that resemble hyphae and are called *pseudohyphae.* This is characteristic of *Candida* species. Blastomyces is a larger, double contoured yeast that is characterized by broad-based budding. Aspergillus is characterized by septate hyphae with acute-angle branching of the filamentous colonies and occasional fruiting bodies. Irregular, broad, nonseptate hyphae with wide-angle branching is seen with mucormycosis (zygomycosis). Large spheres with external budding, referred to as a "ship's wheel," are seen with paracoccidioides, while large spheres with endospores are seen with coccidiomyces infection.

107. The answer is D. *(Anderson, 9/e, pp 462, 467–468.)* Eggs of the roundworm *Ascaris* are found in contaminated soil in the southeastern United States. When swallowed, these eggs hatch, reach the small intestinal vessels, and travel to the lungs, where they may produce clinical bronchial asthma and pneumonitis. The New World hookworm, *Necator americanus,* penetrates exposed skin through exposure to larvae-containing soil; these infective filariform larvae reach the pulmonary circulation via the lymphatic and vascular systems and cause alveolar hemorrhages and temporary bronchopneumonia. Rhabditiform *Strongyloides* soil larvae also gain access to the vascular system and pulmonary circuit through penetration of exposed skin and also cause intraalveolar pneumonitis and hemorrhages. *Wuchereria bancrofti* filariae gain access to the human lymphatics (endolymphangitis, elephantiasis) via bites of the *Culex* mosquito; this organism is not noted for producing a pulmonary phase, but it does produce characteristic spermatic cord granulomas.

108. The answer is C. *(Henry, 18/e, pp 154–155. Robbins, 5/e, p 1143.)* Parathyroid hormone (PTH), by affecting the kidneys, bones, and intestinal mucósa, is the principal regulator of plasma levels of phosphate and calcium. PTH, by its action on renal tubular cells, not only causes decreased phosphate reabsorption, it causes increased calcium reabsorption; these reciprocal processes result in a decrease in serum phosphate and a corresponding increase in extracellular calcium levels. Extracellular levels of calcium are also maintained by the release of calcium during PTH-induced osteocytic and osteoclastic osteolysis, a process that is regarded as the mobilization of calcium from bone. PTH also may induce the intestinal mucosa to absorb calcium derived from dietary sources.

109. The answer is A. *(Henry, 18/e, pp 264–265, 276–278. Robbins, 5/e, p 537.)* The levels of serum aspartate aminotransferase (AST), which is also called serum glutamic-oxaloacetic transaminase (SGOT) (curve II), become elevated within 12 h after nearly all acute myocardial infarctions; they generally reach a peak level within 48 h and return to normal within 4 to 5 days. After myocardial infarctions, creatine phosphokinase levels (curve I) rise and fall more rapidly than do SGOT levels. Lactic dehydrogenase levels (curve III) also become elevated within 1 day after infarctions, but they remain elevated for about 10 days. Alkaline phosphatase and 5′-nucleotidase levels, normal during infarctions, usually show marked increases in patients who have obstructive jaundice.

110. The answer is E. *(Henry, 18/e, pp 251, 274–276, 530–531.)* An elevated serum amylase level is usually associated with acute pancreatitis; it is practically diagnostic if it is more than three times normal, and if salivary gland disease and intestinal perforation or infarction are excluded. There may be increased amylase with parotitis alone, but increased lipase (more sensitive and much more specific) only with pancreatitis. Elevated amylase may be associated with biliary tract disease, and also with renal disease because of decreased clearance. Low serum amylase has been noted with serum protein loss in congestive heart failure. Amylase can be produced by certain tumors (lung, breast, ovarian cancer). In these and in acidotic states, the amylase must be distinguished from that of pancreatitis by isoenzyme analysis. P isoamylases arise from the pancreas; S isoamylases arise from nonpancreatic sources, as in diabetic ketoacidosis.

111. The answer is D. *(Henry, 18/e, pp 241–243, 260–262, 697.)* In polycythemia vera the serum alkaline phosphatase level is not increased. However, the neutrophil alkaline phosphatase is markedly elevated in 80 percent of patients with polycythemia vera, while this leukocyte alkaline phosphatase level is depressed in chronic myelogenous leukemia. Serum alkaline phosphatase is usually quite markedly elevated in such hepatobiliary diseases as obstructive jaundice, intrahepatic cholestasis, biliary cirrhosis, and infectious mononucleosis. Milder elevations occur in alcoholic cirrhosis and viral hepatitis. The placental alkaline phosphatase isoenzyme peaks during the third trimester and returns to normal post partum.

112. The answer is C. *(Robbins, 5/e, pp 1255–1259. Rubin, 2/e, pp 1335–1339.)* Hyperuricemia, prominent in gout, occurs most often secondary to disorders that increase production or reduce excretion of uric acid. These include myeloproliferative disorders and some cancers, such as leukemias and lymphomas, in which there is increased turnover of nucleic acid with resultant hyperuricemia. Reduced excretion of uric acid may arise from renal causes, or from competition by certain organic acids, as in starvation ketosis. Lesch-Nyhan syndrome, a rare X-linked disease caused by an absence of hypoxanthine-guanine phosphoribosyltransferase (HGPRT), is characterized by mental retardation, self-mutilation, hyperuricemia, and gouty arthritis. Chondrocalcinosis, or calcium pyrophosphate dihydrate (CPPD) deposition disease, is not associated with hyperuricemia.

113. The answer is A. *(Henry, 18/e, pp 266–270.)* The patient described probably has hepatitis, according to the values given for the five isoenzymes of lactic dehydrogenase (LDH). Liver cells contain higher proportions of LDH_4 and LDH_5 than do myocardium or red blood cells, both of which contain greater relative amounts of LDH_1 and LDH_2. Lung tissue is high in LDH_3, and brain tissue contains only small amounts of LDH_5. During the LDH increase following a myocardial infarction, levels of LDH_1 are usually higher than those of LDH_2. This pattern is called a "flipped" LDH.

114–115. The answers are 114-B, 115-E. *(Lever, 7/e, pp 433–435. Robbins, 5/e, pp 139, 140–142, 162–163.)* Fabry's disease, seen mostly in males, is characterized by accumulation of glycosphingolipid (trihexosylceramide) in the cardiovascular-renal system, skin, and eyes due to a deficiency of α-galactosidase A. Angiokeratomas of the skin (small, red, raised lesions) usually appear in childhood and increase with age, often in a "swimsuit" distribution on buttocks, back, genitalia, and inner thighs. Burning pain in hands and feet, triggered by exercise or stress, and diminished ability to sweat are common. Ocular abnormalities—tortuous conjunctival vessels and corneal opacity—are suggestive. Inheritance is X-linked recessive and female carriers develop angiokeratomas, eye changes, and burning pains, without the renal and cardiac problems of males. Renal dialysis and transplantation have now improved prognosis. Prenatal diagnosis is done by amniocentesis or chorionic villus sampling and the disorder occurs in about one in 40,000 persons.

Tay-Sachs disease (TSD), or G_{M2} gangliosidosis type I, is a storage disease in which this ganglioside accumulates in neurons of the central and autonomic nervous systems and retina because of deficient hexosaminidase A. Inherited as an autosomal recessive trait, TSD is found primarily but not exclusively among Ashkenazi Jews and among a group of non-Jewish French Canadians. Thousands of carriers of the TSD gene have been identified, and prenatal diagnosis is possible by assay for hexosaminidase A activity in cultured fetal cells. Major clinical features include mental-motor deterioration, blindness, a cherry-red spot in the macula, and death by 3 years of age.

116–119. The answers are 116-A, 117-B, 118-D, 119-C. *(Robbins, 5/e, pp 411–414, 420–425, 603–610. Rubin, 2/e, pp 328–332.)* Pyridoxine deficiency should be rare but is fairly common because of drugs that act as pyridoxine antagonists. Pyridoxal phosphate is important for numerous enzyme reactions in amino acid metabolism, in heme synthesis, and for normal neuronal excitability. Peripheral neuritis, seizures, microcytic anemia, and often dermatitis and glossitis suggest the deficiency. Many drugs may act as antagonists of vitamin B_6: estrogens inhibit its role in tryptophan metabolism, isoniazid can inhibit enzymes that use pyridoxine as a cofactor (thus inducing seizures), and penicillamine acts in the same way. A common cause of B_6 deficiency is chronic alcoholism.

Ascorbic acid, a redox agent, is essential in collagen synthesis, so deficiency in vitamin C means defective collagen synthesis resulting in fragile capillaries and hemorrhagic areas around hair follicles, abnormal hair development, splinter hemorrhages in the nail beds, and hematomas. The syndrome is common in elderly people living on a diet deficient in milk, fruits, and vegetables.

Folate deficiency may be present with scurvy and causes a macrocytic anemia similar to the megaloblastic anemia of vitamin B_{12} deficiency, but without gastric atrophy or neurologic changes. Deficiency occurs in chronic alcoholics, the elderly, and malabsorption syndromes (sprue) or with folate antagonists (methotrexate) used in cancer chemotherapy.

Thiamine deficiency occurs in alcoholics and prisoners of war because of poor diet, deficient absorption and storage, and accelerated destruction of thiamine diphosphate. Major manifestations are both cardiovascular, with tachycardia an early sign of peripheral vasodilatation, and neurologic, with resultant beriberi. Nystagmus, ataxia, and confusion—often with bilateral lateral rectus, or sixth nerve, palsies (ophthalmoplegia)—indicate Wernicke's encephalopathy. The lack of B_1 has caused damage to areas of thalamus, hypothalamus, midbrain, and cerebellar vermis. The classic triad of confusion, ataxia, and ophthalmoplegia is not common and some patients remain undiagnosed. Others who recover after thiamine administration from the acute encephalopathy are left with major defects in retrograde memory and learning (Korsakoff syndrome).

Night blindness is the earliest symptom of vitamin A deficiency, followed by conjunctival changes—xerophthalmia (dry cornea and conjunctiva) and keratomalacia. Deficiency also leads to squamous metaplasia in the trachea and bronchi, and such metaplasia in sebaceous and sweat glands of dry skin causes follicular hyperkeratosis and predisposes to acne.

120–123. The answers are 120-B, 121-C, 122-A, 123-D. *(Robbins, 5/e, pp 308, 327–328, 346, 355, 359–360. Rubin, 2/e, pp 396–397.) Histoplasma capsulatum* causes one of the three major fungal infections in the United States that may result in systemic infection (*Blastomyces* and *Coccidioides* are the other two.) Although it commonly produces asymptomatic primary disease, it can result in striking granulomatous inflammation with granulomatous lung disease and possibly sclerosing mediastinitis. Seen most frequently in the Midwest and inhaled from contaminated soil, it forms a yeastlike pathogenic phase in the host and may cause acute, chronic progressive, or asymptomatic disease, the last being the most common outcome.

Cryptococcal infection is the most common fungal DNA infection in the immunocompromised, especially in persons with AIDS or leukemia, lymphoma, and Hodgkin's disease. The soil-dwelling yeast is inhaled, but lung involvement is mild, at least in the nonimmunodeficient. Diagnosis of the dangerous cryptococcal meningitis is achieved by finding encapsulated yeasts in CSF preparations treated with India ink to expose the wide capsules by negative staining (positive in only 50 percent of cases in which diagnosis is eventually made). The CSF and serum should be tested for cryptococcal antigen by the latex cryptococcal agglutination test (LCAT), which is positive in more than 90 percent of cases. Cryptococcal meningitis varies from a chronic inflammatory and granulomatous infection to a noninflammatory meningitis with numerous yeasts massed, sometimes forming cystic "soap-bubble" lesions in the brain.

Rocky Mountain spotted fever is transmitted to man by ticks, as is Lyme disease. Rocky Mountain spotted fever—an acute infectious disease caused by *Rickettsia rickettsii* and characterized by muscle pain, high fever, and skin eruptions—is endemic throughout North America. Rickettsiae typically invade the walls of blood vessels with resultant hemorrhage and thrombosis.

Yellow fever is an acute infectious disease of variable severity and short duration. It is an arthropod-borne (*Aedes* mosquito), hemorrhagic disease of subtropical and tropical New World areas, caused by a single-stranded RNA togavirus. It results in hepatocellular damage (forming Councilman bodies) with jaundice and hematemesis.

Gram-negative bacteria have cell walls containing endotoxins (lipopolysaccharide-protein complexes) that are released from disintegrating bacteria to cause such effects of gram-negative sepsis as fever, increased capillary permeability with shock, and disseminated intravascular coagulation.

124–127. The answers are 124-C, 125-D, 126-E, 127-B. *(Robbins, 5/e, pp 365, 411–414, 921. Rubin, 2/e, pp 395, 1473.)* Long-standing diabetes mellitus is a major cause of blindness in the United States and Europe (25 percent of cases of acquired blindness in the U.S.). Diabetic retinopathy is the most common form, but cataracts and glaucoma occur also. Two major types of diabetic retinopathy, nonproliferative and proliferative, exist with the former characterized by microaneurysms, hemorrhages, and thickened retinal capillaries (microangiopathy). In proliferative retinopathy, new capillary formation and fibrosis eventually lead to blindness or decreased visual acuity.

Keratomalacia, which is due to severe, protracted vitamin A deficiency, is a major problem in Southeast Asia, Africa, and Central and South America, where it causes blindness in about one quarter million children annually. Dryness, softening, and destruction of the cornea occur, while characteristic eye changes include Bitot's spots—a localized form of keratomalacia with small gray plaques representing thickened, keratinized epithelium.

Trachoma, a common cause of blindness in hot, arid regions of the Third World, is caused by *Chlamydia trachomatis,* serotypes A to C. Conjunctival infection is followed by lymphoid follicular hyperplasia and, subsequently, pannus invades the cornea and leads to blindness.

Retinitis pigmentosa is a rare degeneration of the retinal outer receptor layer and underlying pigment epithelium; it is inherited as an autosomal dominant, or recessive, or sex-linked recessive trait. Losses of night vision and, eventually, central vision are prominent.

Silver-wire arterioles are seen in severe arteriosclerotic retinopathy when sclerotic opacity obscures intravascular blood completely.

128–131. The answers are 128-C, 129-E, 130-A, 131-D. *Henry, 18/e, pp 818–820. Robbins, 5/e, pp 178–182, 665–666, 956–957.)* All five immunoglobulins are polypeptides with two light and two heavy chains linked by disulfide bonds. The Ig molecule consists of two fragments of Fab, which are capable of binding antigen, and one Fc fragment. Light chains are two types, kappa and lambda. Heavy chains are of five major types forming five distinct immunoglobulin classes on the basis of the heavy chains that account for the antigenic differences.

IgA is synthesized by mucosal plasma cells of the GI tract, lung, and urinary tract—thus making it the immunoglobulin of "secretory immunity"—and is found in saliva, sweat, nasal secretion, and tears. It is secreted as dimer bound to a secretory piece that stabilizes the molecule against proteolysis. In IgA nephropathy (Berger's disease), circulating IgA immune complex is present in 50 percent of patients and a diffuse renal mesangial proliferation with IgA deposition occurs.

Local anaphylactic reactions include hay fever, bronchial asthma, certain food allergies, and urticarial reactions to drugs or injected antigens. Systemic anaphylaxis may result from injection of antisera or penicillin and may cause severe shock or death. Type I hypersensitivity (anaphylaxis) occurs when exposure to antigen leads to production of cytotropic IgE antibodies that become fixed by their Fc portions to mast cells and basophils. On reexposure, antigen combines with the cell-bound antibody and this is followed by mast cell degranulation with discharge of primary mediators (histamine). Secondary mediators (leukotrienes, prostaglandin) are released via cell membrane phospholipids.

IgM is the first immunoglobulin to respond to an antigenic stimulus and is the largest Ig. Waldenström's macroglobulinemia is a plasma cell dyscrasia characterized by infiltration of bone marrow, lymph nodes, liver, and spleen by neoplastic B cells that secrete a monoclonal IgM immunoglobulin, leading to macroglobulinemia. Serum electrophoresis shows an M-protein spike and diagnosis rests on the typical bone marrow findings and the M-protein spike due to IgM in the serum.

Most of the circulating human gamma globulin (80 percent) is of the IgG class. It crosses the placenta and is the major protective immunoglobulin in the neonate. IgG has Fc receptors and activates complement.

132–135. The answers are 132-C, 133-A, 134-D, 135-B. *(Robbins, 5/e, pp 231–233.)* Amyloid is a pathologic proteinaceous substance deposited in various body sites in a variety of disease processes. Many chemically distinct classes of amyloid fibril exist, each derived from a chemically related precursor protein. Amyloid light chain (AL) is the most common amyloid protein and is derived from immunoglobulin light chains. It is deposited in various immunocyte dyscrasias, most commonly multiple myeloma and including nodular malignant lymphoma.

Amyloid-associated (AA) protein is a polypeptide derived from serum amyloid-associated protein, which is produced in the liver. Systemic deposits of AA protein occur in reactive systemic amyloidosis, which complicates various chronic infections and inflammatory processes, most commonly rheumatoid arthritis and including other connective tissue diseases, bronchiectasis, and inflammatory bowel disease.

Beta$_2$ amyloid protein is a polypeptide that forms the amyloid found in the cores of cerebral plaques and in the blood vessels in Alzheimer's disease. Do not confuse beta$_2$ amyloid protein with beta$_2$ microglobulin, a component of the MHC class I molecule, which composes the amyloid protein that complicates long-term hemodialysis.

Transthyretin is a normal serum protein that binds and transports thyroxine and retinol. A mutant form of this protein is deposited as amyloid in both familial amyloid polyneuropathies and senile cardiac amyloidosis.

Medullary carcinoma of the thyroid is associated with amyloid deposits derived from calcitonin.

Hematology

DIRECTIONS: Each question below contains five suggested responses. Select the **one best** response to each question.

136. Which of the following red cell abnormalities is most indicative of hemolysis?

(A) Target cells
(B) Acanthocytes
(C) Schistocytes
(D) Basophilic stippling
(E) Heinz bodies

137. Intravascular hemolysis results in all the following EXCEPT

(A) elevated plasma hemoglobin (hemoglobinemia)
(B) hemoglobinuria
(C) hemosiderinuria
(D) jaundice
(E) splenomegaly

138. Which of the following laboratory findings is LEAST likely to be present in a patient with sickle cell anemia?

(A) Normochromic anemia
(B) Increased number of target cells
(C) Elevated reticulocyte count
(D) Elevated erythrocyte sedimentation rate
(E) Increased hemoglobin F

139. Two days after receiving the antimalarial drug primaquine, a 27-year-old black man developed sudden intravascular hemolysis resulting in a decreased hematocrit, hemoglobinemia, and hemoglobinuria. Examination of the peripheral blood revealed erythrocytes with a membrane defect forming "bite" cells; when crystal violet stain was applied, many Heinz bodies were seen. The most likely diagnosis is

(A) hereditary spherocytosis
(B) glucose-6-phosphate dehydrogenase deficiency
(C) paroxysmal nocturnal hemoglobinuria
(D) autoimmune hemolytic anemia
(E) microangiopathic hemolytic anemia

140. Which of the following tests best detects the presence of hemoglobin S?

(A) Osmotic fragility test
(B) Metabisulfite test
(C) Coombs test
(D) Sucrose hemolysis test
(E) Schilling test

141. The graph below depicts the results of a red cell osmotic fragility test. The broken-line curve represents which of the following?

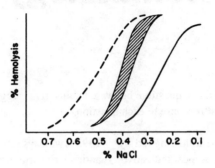

(A) Glucose-6-phosphate dehydrogenase deficiency
(B) Thalassemia
(C) Hereditary spherocytosis
(D) Drug-induced hemolytic anemia
(E) Normal response

---

142. An anemic patient has the following red cell indexes: mean corpuscular volume, 70 μm³(normal: 90 ±7); mean corpuscular hemoglobin, 22 g/dL (normal: 29 ±2); and mean corpuscular hemoglobin concentration, 34 percent (normal: 34 ±2). These values are most consistent with a diagnosis of

(A) folic acid deficiency anemia
(B) iron deficiency anemia
(C) pernicious anemia
(D) sideroblastic anemia
(E) thalassemia minor

143. Which one of the following gene abnormalities is associated with a relative excess production of β-globin chains?

(A) Promoter region mutation of β-globin chain gene
(B) Chain terminator mutation of β-globin chain gene
(C) Splicing mutation of α-globin chain gene
(D) Deletion of one β-globin chain gene
(E) Deletion of three α-globin chain genes

144. The neutrophil in the photomicrograph shown below was obtained from peripheral blood and is most likely to be found in association with

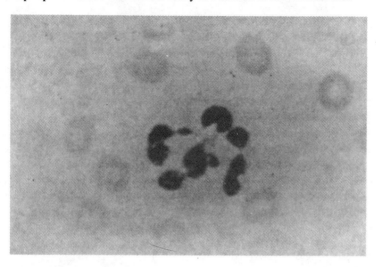

(A) folic acid deficiency
(B) infection
(C) iron deficiency
(D) malignancy
(E) ingestion of a marrow-toxic agent

---

145. An anemic patient is found to have hypochromic, microcytic red cells. Additional tests reveal the serum iron levels, the total iron-binding capacity, and the transferrin saturation to all be reduced. A bone marrow biopsy reveals the iron to be present mainly within macrophages. The most likely diagnosis is

(A) iron deficiency
(B) thalassemia trait
(C) anemia of chronic disease
(D) sideroblastic anemia
(E) pernicious anemia

146. A 25-year-old woman with known systemic lupus erythematosus presents with jaundice, splenomegaly, peripheral blood schistocytes, and a reticulocyte count of 24 percent. The antibody most likely to be responsible for this complex reacts in vitro at

(A) 5°C
(B) 20°C
(C) 25°C
(D) 37°C
(E) 56°C

147. The photomicrograph below is from the bone marrow of a patient with weakness. All the following may be associated with this abnormality EXCEPT

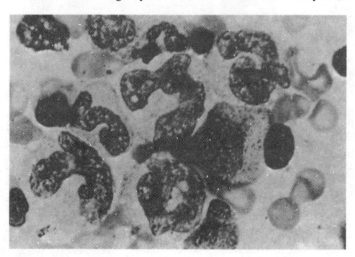

(A) pernicious anemia
(B) hyperthyroidism
(C) celiac disease
(D) HTLV
(E) alcoholism

---

148. True statements regarding hemochromatosis include all the following EXCEPT

(A) it characteristically causes a micronodular pigment cirrhosis
(B) it is complicated by carcinoma of the liver in 15 to 30 percent of cases with cirrhosis
(C) it causes diabetes with severity unrelated to the degree of pancreatic iron deposition
(D) it can be diagnosed by liver biopsy showing raised amounts of hemosiderin
(E) it is associated with skin pigmentation due entirely to deposition of hemosiderin

149. Transferrin shows all the following characteristics EXCEPT

(A) normally about 33 percent saturation with iron
(B) increased saturation in hemochromatosis
(C) increased saturation in severe liver disease
(D) decreased saturation in marrow hypoplasia
(E) decreased saturation in iron deficiency anemia

150. Megaloblasts are the result of impaired synthesis of

(A) DNA
(B) RNA
(C) glutathione
(D) β-globin chains
(E) decay accelerating factor

151. The causes of secondary aplastic anemia include all the following EXCEPT

(A) whole body irradiation
(B) alkylating agents
(C) chloramphenicol
(D) myelophthisic anemia
(E) viral hepatitis

152. The most common type of disordered porphyrin metabolism (porphyria) is

(A) intermittent acute porphyria
(B) variegate porphyria
(C) protoporphyria
(D) congenital erythropoietic porphyria
(E) porphyria cutanea tarda

153. True statements concerning the hemolytic-uremic syndrome (HUS) in young children include all the following EXCEPT

(A) endothelial injury is an initiating pathologic event
(B) prior infection with *E. coli* is common
(C) hypertension exists in about half the patients
(D) involvement of the CNS is a dominant feature
(E) acute, anuric renal failure occurs in over 50 percent of cases

154. A 37-year-old woman who has a clinical picture of fever, splenomegaly, varying neurologic manifestations, and purplish ecchymoses of the skin is found to have a hemoglobin level of 10.0 g/dL, a mean corpuscular hemoglobin concentration (MCHC) of 48, peripheral blood polychromasia with stippled macrocytes, and spherocytes, with a blood urea nitrogen level of 68 mg/dL. The findings of coagulation studies and the patient's fibrin-degraded products are not overtly abnormal. Which of the following is most closely identified with these findings?

(A) Idiopathic thrombocytopenic purpura
(B) Thrombotic thrombocytopenic purpura
(C) Disseminated intravascular coagulopathy
(D) Submassive hepatic necrosis
(E) Waterhouse-Friderichsen syndrome

155. Acute idiopathic thrombocytopenic purpura (ITP) is characterized by

(A) an insidious onset
(B) being more common in females of childbearing age
(C) a history of recent viral infection
(D) megakaryocytic hypoplasia in the bone marrow
(E) a high mortality

156. A woman who is 5 weeks post partum (normal delivery, healthy child) develops bleeding episodes with oliguria and hematuria. No fever or neurologic manifestations are present. The blood urea nitrogen level is 65 mg/dL; a peripheral blood smear is presented in the photomicrograph below. This patient most likely has

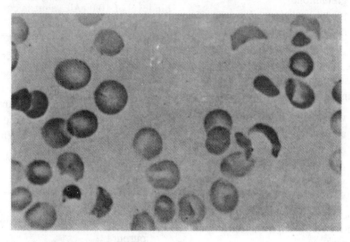

(A) thrombotic thrombocytopenic purpura
(B) autoimmune thrombocytopenic purpura
(C) hemolytic uremic syndrome
(D) disseminated intravascular coagulopathy
(E) sickle cell crisis

---

157. An adult patient suffers from recurrent bleeding from the gums, intermittent GI bleeding, and excessive bleeding from minor trauma to the skin. A prolonged bleeding time is discovered, but the platelet count is normal. Which of the following levels or activities would probably be abnormal in this patient?

(A) Prothrombin time
(B) Plasma fibrinogen
(C) Factor VIII:R
(D) Factor IX
(E) Factor XIII

158. A patient presents with fever, weakness, and pain and tenderness over the left deltoid muscle. A biopsy of this area reveals *Trichinella spiralis.* The peripheral blood of this patient most likely would show an increase in the number of

(A) neutrophils
(B) eosinophils
(C) basophils
(D) monocytes
(E) lymphocytes

159. The photomicrograph below was taken from a soft tissue swelling in the cheek and mandible of a 17-year-old girl. The cytoplasmic vacuoles would react with which one of the following?

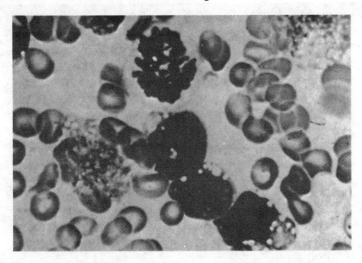

(A) Myeloperoxidase
(B) Oil red O
(C) Nonspecific esterase
(D) Chloracetate esterase
(E) Periodic acid–Schiff (PAS)

---

160. A 20-year-old man presents in the emergency room with a lymphoma involving the mediastinum that is producing respiratory distress. The lymphocytes are most likely to have cell surface markers characteristic of which of the following?

(A) B cells
(B) T cells
(C) Macrophages
(D) Dendritic reticulum cells
(E) Langerhans cells

161. A 19-year-old man presents with a sore throat, malaise, and cervical lymphadenopathy. Peripheral blood film shows lymphocytosis with many lymphocytes that show atypical nuclei and abundant basophilic cytoplasm. The most appropriate course of action is

(A) lymph node biopsy
(B) bone marrow biopsy
(C) prompt treatment with ampicillin
(D) monospot test
(E) blood cultures

162. The non-Hodgkin's lymphoma pictured in the photomicrograph below may be characterized by which of the following?

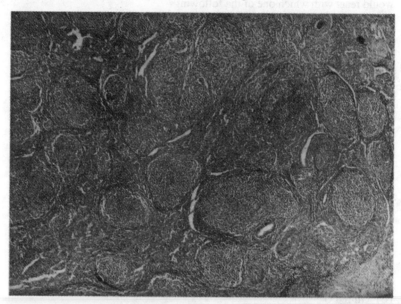

(A) Increased frequency in adolescents
(B) Lymphoblastic lymphoma
(C) B lymphocytes
(D) Tingible-body macrophages within nodules
(E) Well-differentiated lymphocytic lymphoma

163. Typical findings in a patient with von Willebrand's disease include all the following EXCEPT

(A) decreased levels of factor VIII
(B) normal platelet count
(C) prolonged bleeding time
(D) frequent hemarthrosis and spontaneous joint hemorrhage
(E) menorrhagia

164. True statements regarding nodular sclerosing Hodgkin's disease include that it

(A) is more common in males
(B) usually affects elderly people
(C) is characterized by the presence of lacunar cells
(D) is characterized by the presence of "popcorn" cells
(E) usually involves infradiaphragmatic lymph nodes

165. An elderly woman enters the hospital with an abdominal mass, anemia, and weakness. At surgery, an infiltrating retroperitoneal mass is found involving the mesenteric lymph nodes and right kidney. A biopsy specimen from one of the lymph nodes is shown and is compatible with large-cell immunoblastic lymphoma. This neoplasm is associated with all the following EXCEPT

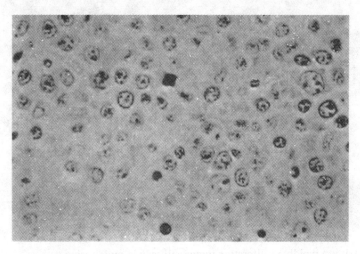

(A) predominant B-cell origin
(B) prior immunologic disorder
(C) typical "starry sky" pattern
(D) rapid death if untreated
(E) plasmacytoid or polymorphous features

166. Chronic myeloid leukemia is LEAST likely to be associated with

(A) splenomegaly
(B) basophilia
(C) translocation t (8;14)
(D) thrombocytosis
(E) low leukocyte alkaline phosphatase (LAP)

167. All the following diseases involve abnormal proliferations of Langerhans cells EXCEPT

(A) histiocytosis X
(B) alpha-chain disease
(C) Letterer-Siwe syndrome
(D) Hand-Schüller-Christian disease
(E) eosinophilic granuloma

168. The binucleate or bilobed giant cell with prominent acidophilic "owl-eye" nucleoli shown in the photomicrograph below is correctly characterized by which of the following statements?

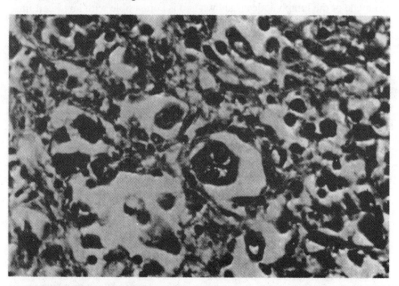

(A) It is a rapidly proliferating tumor cell seen in middivision
(B) It is sometimes referred to as the *lacunar cell*
(C) It is necessary but not sufficient for the diagnosis of Hodgkin's disease
(D) It is diagnostic of cytomegalic inclusion disease
(E) It is diagnostic of giardiasis

---

169. In polycythemia rubra vera (PRV),

(A) the bone marrow shows selective erythroid hyperplasia
(B) hemorrhagic phenomena are uncommon
(C) pruritus is common
(D) the platelet count is typically <150,000/mm³
(E) leukocyte alkaline phosphate levels are decreased

170. The presence in serum of a mu heavy-chain protein is associated with which of the following diseases?

(A) Chronic lymphocytic leukemia
(B) Lymphoblastic lymphoma
(C) Poorly-differentiated lymphocytic lymphoma
(D) Plasma cell myeloma
(E) Multiple myeloma

171. The photomicrograph below is of peripheral blood from a patient with splenomegaly, anemia, and pancytopenia. If hairy cell leukemia is suspected, which of the following would be useful in establishing the diagnosis?

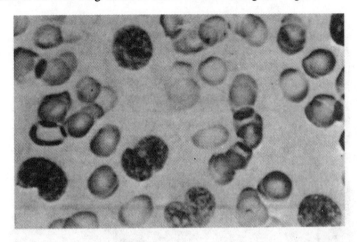

(A) Myeloperoxidase stain
(B) Sudan black B
(C) Acid phosphatase stain
(D) Leukocyte alkaline phosphatase
(E) Nonspecific esterase

172. An 11-year-old Jamaican boy develops a massive benign enlargement of the cervical lymph nodes associated with fever and leukocytosis. Which of the following lymph node disorders could account for these findings?

(A) Toxoplasmosis
(B) Histiocytic medullary reticulosis
(C) Burkitt's disease
(D) Sinus histiocytosis with massive lymphadenopathy (SHML)
(E) Angioimmunoblastic lymphadenopathy with dysproteinemia

173. A young child has recurrent bacterial infections, eczema, thrombocytopenia, lymphadenopathy, and the absence of delayed-type hypersensitivity. The most likely diagnosis is

(A) Pelger-Huët anomaly
(B) Wiskott-Aldrich syndrome
(C) Chédiak-Higashi syndrome
(D) chronic granulomatous disease of childhood
(E) Hodgkin's disease of nodular sclerosis subgroup

174. The cells seen in the photomicrograph below were removed from an anemic patient and stained with an iron stain. This patient is most likely to have

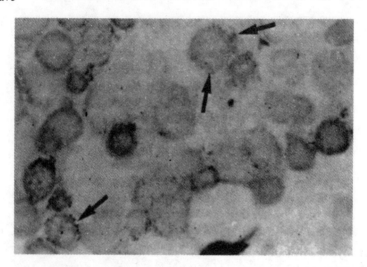

(A) iron deficiency anemia
(B) acute blood loss
(C) B_{12} deficiency
(D) B_2 deficiency
(E) pyridoxine deficiency

---

175. All the following are known to cause splenomegaly EXCEPT

(A) sickle cell disease
(B) Hodgkin's disease
(C) chronic lymphocytic leukemia (CLL)
(D) hairy cell leukemia
(E) polycythemia vera

176. During the induction of an immune response, which cell is thought to process the initiating antigen?

(A) Eosinophil
(B) Basophil
(C) Macrophage
(D) T cell
(E) B cell

177. The bone marrow biopsy shown below was performed because of splenomegaly and anemia in an adult. On the basis of the appearance of the bone marrow core, choose the most likely diagnosis.

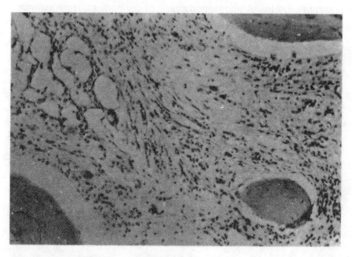

(A) Chronic myeloid leukemia (CML)
(B) Aplastic anemia
(C) Acute leukemia
(D) Myeloid metaplasia with myelofibrosis
(E) Microangiopathic hemolytic anemia

178. A bone marrow aspirate was obtained from a 70-year-old man whose symptoms included weakness, weight loss, and recurrent infections. Laboratory findings included proteinuria, anemia, and an abnormal component in serum proteins. A photomicrograph of the bone marrow aspirate is shown below. The most probable diagnosis is

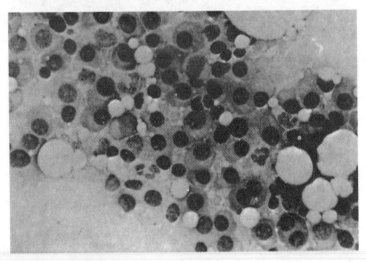

(A) monomyelocytic leukemia
(B) histiocytic leukemia
(C) multiple myeloma
(D) Gaucher's disease
(E) leukemic reticuloendotheliosis

179. In the disorder depicted below in which multiple, focal osteolytic skull lesions occur, all the following are common EXCEPT

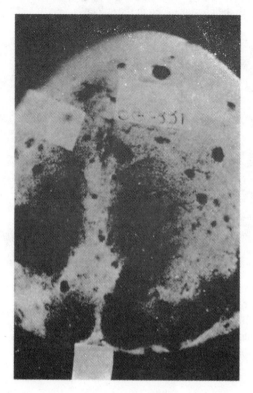

(A) a normal serum alkaline phosphatase level
(B) increased production of monoclonal immunoglobulin
(C) lymphadenopathy
(D) bone pain
(E) hypercalcemia

180. The photomicrograph below is of the spleen from an adult patient who had marked splenomegaly. Which of the following abnormalities is most compatible with the changes seen in the spleen?

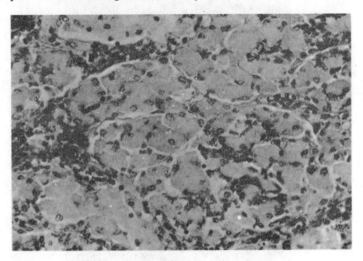

(A) Glucocerebrosidase deficiency
(B) Glucose-6-phosphate dehydrogenase deficiency
(C) Glucuronidase deficiency
(D) Lysosomal glucosidase deficiency
(E) α-Galactosidase deficiency

181. The cell in the photomicrograph below was found in a bone marrow aspirate from a 25-year-old man. Such a cell is generally considered pathognomonic for

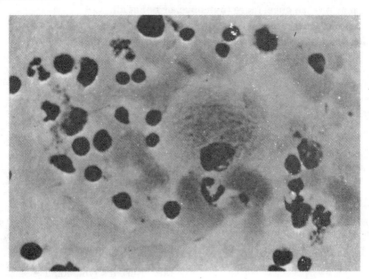

(A) Niemann-Pick disease
(B) histiocytic lymphoma
(C) megaloblastic anemia
(D) Gaucher's disease
(E) myelogenous leukemia

DIRECTIONS: The groups of questions below consist of lettered headings followed by a set of numbered items. For each numbered item select the **one** lettered heading with which it is **most** closely associated. Each lettered heading may be used **once, more than once, or not at all.**

Questions 182–185

For each description below, choose the type of leukemia with which it is most likely to be associated.

    (A) Acute lymphoblastic leukemia

    (B) Acute myeloblastic leukemia (M1)

    (C) Acute promyelocytic leukemia (M3)

    (D) Chronic lymphocytic leukemia

    (E) Hairy cell leukemia

182. Multiple Auer rods are frequently present in the leukemic cells

183. It is associated with diffuse intravascular coagulation

184. It occurs in older adults, produces relatively few symptoms, and is similar to small lymphocytic lymphoma

185. The enzyme TdT is often present in leukemic cells; lymphadenopathy is characteristic and striking

Questions 186–188

For each disease listed below, choose the appropriate chromosomal translocation and associated oncogene.

    (A) t8;14, c-*myc*

    (B) t8;21, c-*mos*

    (C) t9;22, c-*abl*

    (D) t15;17, c-*fes*

    (E) t15;18, *bcl*-2

186. Follicular lymphoma

187. Chronic myeloid leukemia

188. Burkitt's lymphoma

Hematology

Answers

136. The answer is C. *(Henry, 18/e, pp 585–590. Rubin, 2/e, pp 1012–1013.)* Abnormalities of red cells can help to identify a disease process. Schistocytes, which are red cell fragments, indicate the presence of hemolysis, and they can occur in hemolytic anemia, megaloblastic anemia, or severe burns. Red cell shapes characteristic of hemolysis include triangular cells and helmet cells. Target cells—red cells with a central dark area—are the result of excess cytoplasmic membrane material and are found in patients with liver disease, such as obstructive jaundice, or in any of the hypochromic anemias. Acanthocytes are irregularly spiculated red cells found in patients with abetalipoproteinemia or liver disease. Ecchinocytes, in contrast, have regular spicules (undulations) and may either be artifacts (crenated cells) or found in hyperosmolar diseases such as uremia. Basophilic stippling of red cells—irregular basophilic granules within erythrocytes—vary from fine granules, seen in young reticulocytes (polychromatophilic cells), to coarse granules, seen in diseases with impaired hemoglobin synthesis, such as lead poisoning and megaloblastic anemia. Heinz bodies are formed by denatured hemoglobin and are not seen with routine stains. They are found in patients with glucose-6-phosphatase dehydrogenase deficiency and the unstable hemoglobinopathies.

137. The answer is E. *(Robbins, 5/e, pp 587–589.)* Destruction of red cells, hemolysis, may occur within the vascular compartment (intravascular hemolysis) or within the mononuclear-phagocyte system (extravascular hemolysis). In both cases, the hemolysis will lead to anemia, and the breakdown of hemoglobin will lead to jaundice, which is increased indirect bilirubin. Intravascular hemolysis releases hemoglobin into the blood (hemoglobinemia), which then binds to haptoglobin. When haptoglobin levels are depleted, free hemoglobin is oxidized to methemoglobin, and then both hemoglobin and methemoglobin are secreted into the urine (hemoglobinuria and methemoglobinuria). Within the renal tubular epithelial cells, hemoglobin is reabsorbed, hemosiderin is formed, and when these cells are shed into the urine, hemosiderinuria results. Since extravascular hemolysis does not occur within the vascular compartment, hemoglobinemia, hemoglobinuria, methemoglobinuria, and hemosiderinuria do not occur. The breakdown of the red cells within the phagocytic cells causes anemia and jaundice, just as with intravascular hemolysis, and since hemoglobin escapes into the blood from the phagocytic cells, plasma haptoglobin levels are also reduced. Unlike intravascular hemolysis, the erythrophagocytosis causes hypertrophy and hyperplasia of the mononuclear phagocytic system, which in turn may lead to splenomegaly.

138. The answer is D. *(Lee, 9/e, pp 30–31, 1077–1078.)* Blood from patients who have sickle cell anemia exhibits a low erythrocyte sedimentation rate (ESR). The irregular shape of sickle cells prevents the rouleaux formation that is prerequisite for a normal ESR. Sickle cell anemia is classifed as a normocytic, normochromic, and hemolytic anemia in which target cells, found in increased numbers, can compose up to 30 percent of peripheral blood cells, and in which reticulocytosis—as a reflection of an increased rate of erythropoiesis in the hyperplastic bone marrow—is persistently 10 percent above normal. In addition, electrophoretic findings reveal an elevation of hemoglobin F up to 40 percent, the presence of hemoglobin S in a range of 60 to 99 percent, and the absence of hemoglobin A.

139. The answer is B. *(Robbins, 5/e, pp 589–592, 601–603.)* Glucose-6-phosphate dehydrogenase (G6PD) is an enzyme of the hexose monophosphate shunt pathway that maintains glutathione in a reduced (active) form. Glutathione normally protects hemoglobin from oxidative injury. If the erythrocytes are deficient in G6PD, as occurs in G6PD deficiency, exposure to oxidant drugs, such as the antimalarial drug primaquine, denatures hemoglobin, which then precipitates with erythrocytes as Heinz bodies. Macrophages within the spleen remove these bodies, producing characteristic "bite" cells. These red cells then become less deformable and are trapped and destroyed within the spleen (extravascular hemolysis). The gene for G6PD is located on the X chromosome and has considerable pleomorphism at this site. Two variants are the A type, which is found in 10 percent of American blacks and is characterized by milder hemolysis of younger red cells, and the Mediterranean type, which is characterized by a more severe hemolysis of red cells of all ages. Hereditary spherocytosis (HS), an autosomal dominant disorder, is characterized by an abnormality of the skeleton of the red cell membrane that makes the erythrocyte spherical, less deformable, and vulnerable to splenic sequestration and destruction (extravascular hemolysis). In HS, there is a defect in the spectrin molecule, which then has less binding to protein 4.1. This disorder can be diagnosed in the laboratory by the osmotic fragility test. Paroxysmal nocturnal hemoglobinuria (PNH), an acquired clonal stem cell disorder, is characterized by abnormal red cells, granulocytes, and platelets. The red cells are abnormally sensitive to the lytic activity of complement due to a deficiency of GPI (glycosyl phosphatidyl inositol) linked proteins, namely decay-accelerating factor (DAF, or CD55), membrane inhibitor of reactive lysis (CD59), or CD59 (a C8 binding protein). Complement is activated by acidosis, such as with exercise or sleep, which can produce a red morning urine. Complications of PNH include the development of frequent thromboses and possibly acute leukemia. Autoimmune hemolytic anemia is caused by anti-red cell antibodies and is diagnosed using the Coombs antiglobulin test. Microangiopathic hemolytic anemia refers to hemolysis of red cells caused by narrowing within the microvasculature and is seen in patients with prosthetic heart valves or those with disseminated intravascular coagulation, thrombotic thrombocytopenic purpura, or hemolytic-uremic syndrome.

140. The answer is B. *(Henry, 18/e, pp 634, 644–646, 652, 668.)* The metabisulfite test is used to detect the presence of hemoglobin S, but it does not differentiate the heterozygous sickle cell trait from the homozygous sickle cell disease. The test is based on the fact that erythrocytes with a large proportion of hemoglobin S sickle in solutions of low oxygen content. Metabisulfite is a reducing substance that enhances the process of deoxygenation. The osmotic fragility test is a diagnostic test for hereditary spherocytosis. Spherocytes will lyse at a higher concentration of salt than will normal cells, thus causing an increased osmotic fragility. The direct antiglobulin test (DAT), or Coombs test, is used to differentiate autoimmune hemolytic anemia (AIHA) due to the presence of anti-red cell antibodies from other forms of hemolytic anemia. In this test, antibodies to human immunoglobulin cause the agglutination (clotting) of red cells if these anti-red cell antibodies are present on the surface of the red cells. In patients with paroxysmal nocturnal hemoglobinuria, the erythrocytes are excessively sensitive to complement-mediated lysis in low ionic environments (the basis for the sucrose hemolysis test) or in acidotic conditions, such as sleep, exercise, or the Ham acid hemolysis test. The Schilling test, which measures intestinal absorption of vitamin B_{12} with and without intrinsic factor, is used to diagnose decreased vitamin B_{12} caused by pernicious anemia, which is characterized by a lack of intrinsic factor.

141. The answer is C. *(Henry, 18/e, pp 644–645. Robbins, 5/e, pp 589–591.)* Spherocytes in a peripheral blood smear show a smaller diameter than normal and an apparent increase in hemoglobin concentration because of a decrease in cell surface, with consequent deeper staining for hemoglobin. Spectrin lacks the ability to bind protein 4.1 in this autosomal dominant disorder, yielding a skeleton defect of the red cell membrane. Other proteins that help maintain the shape of the red cell include protein 3 and ankyrin, which bridges the spectrin and the cell membrane protein 3. The disorder can be diagnosed in the laboratory by the osmotic fragility test (the shaded area in the graph reflects a normal response to a hypotonic solution). Spherocytes will lyse at a higher concentration of sodium chloride than will normal red cells. Flat hypochromic cells, as those in thalassemia, have a greater capacity to expand in dilute salt solution and thus lyse at a lower concentration (which is seen in the unbroken curve to the far right). The longer the incubation of the red cells in these salt concentrations, the greater the response to osmotic change.

142. The answer is E. *(Henry, 18/e, pp 657, 670.)* Both thalassemia minor and iron deficiency anemia are microcytic disorders in which the mean corpuscular hemoglobin is usually found to be reduced. Red blood cell indexes may be useful in differentiating the two disorders, for while the mean corpuscular hemoglobin concentration (MCHC) is often normal or only slightly reduced in association with thalassemia minor, the MCHC is often definitely reduced in association with iron deficiency anemia. Both pernicious and folate deficiency anemias lead to megaloblastic changes in erythrocytes.

143. The answer is E. *(Robbins, 5/e, pp 596–601. Rubin, 2/e, pp 1020–1022.)* The thalassemia syndromes are characterized by a decreased or absent synthesis of either the α- or the β-globin chain of hemoglobin A $(\alpha_2\beta_2)$. β Thalassemias result from reduced production of β-globin chains, while α-thalassemias result from reduced synthesis of α-globin chains. β Thalassemias are associated with a relative excess production of α-globin chains, while α thalassemias are associated with a relative excess production of non-α-globin chains. In the fetus these are γ-globin chains, but in the adult they are β-globin chains. Most of the β thalassemias result from point mutations involving the β-globin gene, while α thalassemias result from deletions of one or more of the four α-globin genes. The amount of β-globin produced depends upon the location of the point mutation. Promoter region mutations result in decreased production of β-globin. This is called β+ thalassemia. Chain terminator mutations generally produce no functional β-globin. This is called β0 thalassemia. Splicing mutations may result in either β0 or β+ thalassemia. The severity of α thalassemia depends on the number of α genes deleted. Deletion of three α-globin genes results in excess production of β-globin chains, which then form β tetramers (Hb H); this disease is called *hemoglobin H disease.*

144. The answer is A. *(Robbins, 5/e, pp 603–605.)* In contrast to a normal, mature neutrophil, which has from two to five nuclear lobes, the neutrophil shown has at least six lobes and is an illustration of neutrophilic hypersegmentation. Granulocytic hypersegmentation is significant and among the first hematologic findings in the peripheral blood of patients who have megaloblastic anemia in its developmental stages. Neutrophilic hypersegmentation is generally considered a sensitive indicator of megaloblastic anemia, which can be caused by a deficiency either in vitamin B_{12}, in folate, or in both.

145. The answer is C. *(Henry, 18/e, pp 628–631, 636, 641, 669–671.)* The four main causes of microcytic/hypochromic anemias are iron deficiency, anemia of chronic disease (AOCD), thalassemia, and sideroblastic anemia. Additional laboratory tests can differentiate between these four diseases. The serum iron and percentage of saturation are decreased in both iron deficiency anemia and AOCD, increased in sideroblastic anemia, and may be normal or increased in thalassemia. The total iron-binding capacity (TIBC) is increased only in iron deficiency. It is normal or decreased in the other diseases. An additional differentiating test for these four diagnoses is evaluation of the bone marrow iron stores. In iron deficiency, iron stores are decreased or absent. In AOCD, iron is present, but is restricted to and increased within macrophages. It is decreased in amount within marrow erythroid precursors. Marrow iron is increased in patients with sideroblastic anemia. The iron levels in patients with thalassemia trait are generally within normal limits. Approximately one-third of the normoblasts in the normal bone marrow contain ferritin granules and are called *sideroblasts*. In sideroblastic anemia, because of the deficiency of pyridoxine and ferritin, the production of globin or heme is markedly reduced, and ferritin granules accumulate within the mitochondria that rim the nucleus. This produces the characteristic ring sideroblast.

146. The answer is D. *(Robbins, 5/e, pp 601–603.)* The autoimmune hemolytic anemias are important causes of acute anemia in a wide variety of clinical states and can be separated into two main types: those secondary to "warm" antibodies and those reactive at cold temperatures. Warm-antibody autoimmune hemolytic anemias react at 37°C in vitro, are composed of IgG, and do not fix complement. They are found in patients with malignant tumors, especially leukemia-lymphoma; with use of such drugs as alpha methyldopa; and in the autoimmune diseases, especially lupus erythematosus. Cold-antibody autoimmune hemolytic anemia reacts at 4 to 6°C, fixes complement, is of the IgM type, and is classically associated with mycoplasma pneumonitis (pleuropneumonia-like organisms). These antibodies are termed *cold agglutinins* and may reach extremely high titers and cause intravascular red cell agglutination.

147. The answer is D. *(Robbins, 5/e, pp 603–610.)* The photomicrograph in the question shows the presence of megaloblasts accompanied by unusually large neutrophils and precursors. These abnormalities may be caused by either a deficiency or lack of absorption of vitamin B_{12} or of folic acid. In addition to diets deficient in these two substances, any condition leading to poor absorption of them will also lead to megaloblastic anemia. Thus malabsorption (as in celiac disease), gastrectomy, infiltrative disorders of the bowel (including lymphoma and collagen vascular disease such as scleroderma), infections by the fish tapeworm, and metabolic disorders (such as hyperthyroidism and increased demand for folic acid as in advanced stages of malignancy) all will lead to reduced levels of vitamin B_{12} and folic acid. A deficiency of either vitamin B_{12} or folic acid will lead to maturational arrest of the red cell precursors, which yields large and apparently immature red cell precursors—hence the name *megaloblastic*. The nuclei of red cell precursors are in an immature stage for the maturation of the cytoplasm, which results in an unusually large nucleus.

148. The answer is E. *(Robbins, 5/e, pp 861–863.) Hemochromatosis* is a generic term for disorders of iron overload marked by increases in total body iron and deposition of ferritin and hemosiderin in various organs with morphologic and functional damage to those organs. The pathogenesis is not fully understood but involves altered intestinal handling of iron with decreased postabsorption excretion, and alterations in iron metabolism and storage in reticuloendothelial cells. It causes a micronodular pigment cirrhosis with hemosiderin deposition in parenchymal, Kupffer, and bile duct epithelial cells, which is highlighted on Prussian blue staining. Hepatocellular carcinoma is a frequent (15 to 30 percent) complication of pigment cirrhosis. The pancreas shows intense pigmentation with atrophy and loss of parenchymal cells and diffuse interstitial fibrosis. Diabetes is a major feature of the clinical syndrome but is poorly correlated to the degree of iron deposition in the islets. Other tissues and organs that suffer major deposition of iron include the myocardium, the endocrine glands, skin (melanin and hemosiderin), and testes. Various tests useful in diagnosis reveal increased serum ferritin and plasma iron and decreased iron-binding capacity, reflecting increased body iron load. Liver biopsy is definitive when it shows elevated hemosiderin content. Skin pigmentation is mainly due to increased amounts of melanin, seen with various types of cirrhosis.

149. The answer is D. *(Henry, 18/e, pp 669–671. Robbins, 5/e, pp 610–613.)* Intravascular iron is bound to transferrin, which is usually about 33 percent saturated with iron. Increased saturation occurs in states of iron overload (hemochromatosis), in severe liver disease, hemolytic conditions, and marrow hypoplasia (reduced iron utilization). Iron deficiency is associated with low serum iron levels, increased iron-binding capacity, and decreased saturation.

150. The answer is A. *(Robbins, 5/e, pp 591, 596, 601, 603–605.)* Deficiency of either vitamin B_{12} or folate will result in megaloblastic anemia. Their deficiency impairs DNA synthesis and delays mitotic division. This in turn causes the nuclei to be enlarged. The synthesis of RNA and cytoplasmic elements is not affected, however, so there is nuclear-cytoplasmic asynchrony. These cellular changes affect all rapidly proliferating cells in the body, but in the bone marrow, they result in enlarged erythroid precursors, which are referred to as *megaloblasts*. These abnormal cells produce abnormally enlarged red cells, which are called *macroovalocytes*. These megaloblasts also undergo autohemolysis within the bone marrow, resulting in ineffecctive erythropoiesis. Granulocyte precursors are also enlarged and are called *giant metamyelocytes*. These abnormal cells produce enlarged hypersegmented neutrophils. The megakaryocytes are large and have nuclear abnormalities, but although the platelet count is decreased, the platelets are not enlarged. Abnormalities of glutathione production are seen in patients with glucose-6-phosphate dehydrogenase deficiency, while decreased synthesis of β-globin chains is seen in patients with β thalassemia. Abnormalities of decay accelerating factor are seen in patients with paroxysmal nocturnal hemoglobinuria.

151. The answer is D. *(Robbins, 5/e, pp 613–615.)* Hematopoietic stem cell failure occurs in aplastic anemia, probably because of defective stem cells or their immunologic suppression. Pancytopenia results, although selective suppression with pure red cell aplasia, agranulocytosis, or thrombocytopenia may occur. In 50 percent of cases, aplastic anemia is idiopathic or primary, but there are many physical and chemical causes of secondary aplastic anemia. Whole body irradiation is the major physical cause. Chemical causes include many drugs, such as alkylating agents, antimetabolites, and the antibiotic chloramphenicol. Severe aplastic anemia may occur following viral hepatitis C (non-A, non-B) or following infectious mononucleosis. An inherited form of aplastic anemia is seen in patients with Fanconi's anemia. In myelophthisic anemia, marrow failure is due to marrow replacement by metastatic tumor or other lesions, but no association with stem cell defects exists.

152. The answer is E. *(Lee, 9/e, pp 1272–1290.)* The porphyrias are inherited or acquired disorders of heme biosynthesis with varied patterns of overproduction, accumulation, and excretion of heme synthesis intermediates. Major characteristics include intermittent neurologic dysfunction and skin sensitivity to sunlight, but intermittent acute porphyria shows no skin photosensitivity, unlike the other types. Porphyria cutanea tarda is the most common type and has chronic skin lesions (face, forehead, forearms) and frequent hepatic disease. Excess urinary porphobilinogen excretion occurs in variegate porphyria and inter n.ctent acute porphyria. Detection of porphobilinogen in the urine forms the basis for a positive Watson-Schwartz reaction in the diagnosis of variegate and intermittent acute porphyria.

153. The answer is D. *(Anderson, 9/e, pp 826, 827. Robbins, 5/e, pp 979–981.)* Endothelial injury is considered to be an initiating pathologic event, especially in HUS associated with gram-negative infections, predominantly infection with verocytotoxin-producing *E. coli*. The verocytotoxins of *E. coli*, which infects up to 75 percent of the patients, are cytotoxic to endothelium and are similar to the shigatoxins produced by *Shigella*. Hypertension exists in about 50 percent of the patients, but the relative lack of CNS involvement helps to distinguish HUS from thrombotic thrombocytopenic purpura in which there is usually more general involvement with thrombi formed in several organs.

154. The answer is B. *(Robbins, 5/e, pp 117–121, 619–620, 981.)* A fulminating septic state should always be considered whenever the constellation of fever, deteriorating mental status, skin hemorrhages, and shock develops. Such conditions can be seen in gram-negative rod septicemia caused by any of the coliforms (gram-negative endotoxic shock) or fulminant meningococcemia (Waterhouse-Friderichsen syndrome). However, a form of nonbacterial vasculitis termed *thrombotic thrombocytopenic purpura (TTP)* is notorious for producing a clinical syndrome very similar to fulminating infective states. It is characterized by arteriole and capillary occlusions by fibrin and platelet microthrombi and is usually unassociated with any of the predisposing states seen in disseminated intravascular coagulopathy (DIC), such as malignancy, infection, retained fetus, and amniotic fluid embolism. Macrocytic hemolytic anemia, variable jaundice, renal failure, skin hemorrhages, and central nervous system dysfunction are all seen in TTP and are related to the fibrin thrombi, which can be demonstrated with skin, bone marrow, and lymph node biopsies. There is less coagulopathy in TTP than is found in DIC, and hemolytic anemia is generally not found in idiopathic or autoimmune thrombocytopenic purpura. The condition of patients with TTP may be improved by plasmapheresis, with 80 percent survival.

155. The answer is C. *(Robbins, 5/e, pp 617–619.)* In acute idiopathic thrombocytopenic purpura (ITP), which occurs predominantly in children under 8 years of age, there is an acute onset about 2 weeks after a viral infection (rubella, viral hepatitis, infectious mononucleosis). There is no female predominance as seen in chronic ITP, which is most frequent in women 20 to 50 years old and is characterized by an insidious onset. Both acute and chronic forms are associated with increased platelet destruction and normal or increased megakaryocytes in bone marrow. Most patients with acute ITP make a spontaneous recovery in 4 to 6 weeks.

156. The answer is C. *(Anderson, 9/e, pp 826–827. Robbins, 5/e, pp 619–620, 980–981.)* A woman who manifests a hemorrhagic diathesis following childbirth should be considered to have intravascular coagulopathy until proof to the contrary is obtained—for instance, the condition may be due to retained products of conception. However, the peripheral blood smear depicted in the question shows, in addition to thrombocytopenia (three to four platelets are normally present in every high-power field), remarkably misshaped red blood cells (poikilocytosis) in the form of schistocytes (fragments of red cells), spherocytes, and, importantly, "helmet" red cells, so named because of their similarity in shape to military or football helmets. Helmet cells imply the presence of microangiopathic hemolytic anemia and are thought to form through hemolytic-mechanical red cell membrane disruption by passing through arteriole-capillary beds that have fibrin thrombin meshes. Disorders that cause microangiopathic hemolytic anemia are childhood and adult hemolytic uremic syndrome and thrombotic thrombocytopenic purpura (TTP). The lack of jaundice and neurologic symptoms in this case rules out TTP. The combination of microangiopathic hemolytic anemia and renal insufficiency strongly suggests hemolytic uremic syndrome.

157. The answer is C. *(Henry, 18/e, pp 745–747.)* Von Willebrand's disease is not as rare as once thought, and numerous subtypes, which are delineated by two-dimensional electrophoresis, have been described. The disease is characterized clinically by mucocutaneous bleeding, menorrhagia, and epistaxis. Milder forms of the disease may not be diagnosed until the patient is older. Factor VIII is a complex of several components that can be discerned electrophoretically. Of all the factor VIII components, factor VIII:R, or ristocetin cofactor, is most apt to be abnormal in von Willebrand's disease. The coagulant (C) and the related antigen (Ag) forms of factor VIII may sometimes be normal in various autosomal dominant types. Most patients even with the milder forms will have decreased factor VIII:R. Prothrombin time, fibrinogen levels, and factors IX and XIII are not affected in this disorder.

158. The answer is B. *(Robbins, 5/e, pp 631–632. Rubin, 2/e, pp 1030–1033.)* Leukocytosis, increased numbers of leukocytes in the peripheral blood, is a reaction seen in many different disease states. The type of leukocyte that is mainly increased may be an indicator of the type of disease process present. Eosinophilia is associated with cutaneous allergic reactions;

allergic disorders, such as bronchial asthma or hay fever; Hodgkin's disease; some skin diseases, such as pemphigus, eczema, and dermatitis herpetiformis; and parasitic infections, such as trichinosis, schistosomiasis, and strongyloidiasis. The most common cause of eosinophila is probably allergy to drugs such as iodides, aspirin, and sulfonamides, but eosinophilia is also seen in collagen vascular diseases. Marked eosinophilia occurs in hypereosinophilic syndromes (Loeffler's syndrome and idiopathic hypereosinophilic syndrome), which may be treated with corticosteroids. Neutrophilic leukocytosis (neutrophilia) may be the result of acute bacterial infections or tissue necrosis, such as is present with myocardial infarction, trauma, or burns. Basophilia is most commonly seen in immediate-type (type I) hypersensitivity reactions. Both eosinophils and basophils may be increased in patients with any of the chronic myeloproliferative syndromes. Monocytosis is seen in chronic infections, such as tuberculosis, some collagen vascular diseases, neutropenic states, and some types of lymphomas. Lymphocytosis may be seen along with monocytosis in chronic inflammatory states or in acute viral infections, such as viral hepatitis or infectious mononucleosis.

159. The answer is B. *(Henry, 18/e, pp 701, 710–711. Robbins, 5/e, p 641.)* Burkitt's lymphoma, or undifferentiated lymphoma, is characterized by a rapid proliferation of primitive lymphoid cells with thick nuclear membranes, multiple nucleoli, and intensely basophilic cytoplasm when stained with Wright's stain. The cells are often mixed with macrophages in biopsy, giving a starry-sky appearance. The vacuoles contain lipid and this would be reflected by a positive oil-red-O reaction. PAS stain is nonspecific but does mark neutrophils and acute lymphoblastic leukemia cells. Nonspecific esterase is found predominantly within monocytes but also in megakaryocytes. Chloracetate esterase and myeloperoxidase are primarily found within the lysosomes of granulocytes, including neutrophils, promyelocytes, and faintly in rare monocytes.

160. The answer is B. *(Robbins, 5/e, p 641.)* T-cell lymphomas occurring in the thoracic cavity in young patients usually arise in the mediastinum and have a particularly aggressive clinical course with rapid growth in the mediastinum impinging upon the trachea or mainstem bronchi and leading to marked respiratory deficiency, which can in turn lead to death in a relatively short period of time if not treated. These unique lymphomas are characterized by rapid cell growth and spread into the circulation, where they produce elevated total white counts reflected by circulating lymphoma cells. As T cells they have characteristics of rosette formation with sheep blood cells. T cells also have subtypes and subsets, which can be delineated by monoclonal antibodies as CD4 helper, CD8 suppressor (cellular differentiation) T-cell surface antigens. The tumor cells also express IL-2 receptor. FC receptors occur on B cells and macrophages. Class II HLA antigens can be found on macrophages, Langerhans cells, and dendritic reticulum cells.

161. The answer is D. *(Robbins, 5/e, pp 347–349.)* Infectious mononucleosis is a benign lymphoproliferative disorder caused by the Epstein-Barr virus (EBV). It typically occurs in young adults and presents with systemic symptoms, lymphadenopathy, and pharyngitis. Hepatosplenomegaly may be present. Peripheral blood shows an absolute lymphocytosis, and many lymphocytes are atypical with irregular nuclei and abundant basophilic vacuolated cytoplasm. These represent CD8+ T-killer cells induced by EBV-transformed B lymphocytes. These atypical lymphocytes are usually adequate for diagnosis, along with a positive heterophil or monospot test (increased sheep red cell agglutinin). Administration of ampicillin for a mistaken diagnosis of streptococcal pharyngitis results in a rash in many patients.

162. The answer is C. *(Robbins, 5/e, pp 634–636. Rubin, 2/e, pp 1074–1076. Silverberg, 2/e, pp 383–384.)* The Rappaport classification has separated NHL into nodular and diffuse categories; this is of major importance since the nodular pattern, independent of the cytologic subtype, is associated with a much better prognosis than is the diffuse type. The nodular lymphomas are composed of neoplastic B cells. Unlike the diffuse lymphomas, which often occur in children and adolescents, nodular lymphomas are rare in those under 20. They affect males and females equally, while diffuse lymphomas are much more common in males. Well-differentiated lymphocytic lymphoma and lymphoblastic lymphoma occur only in the diffuse form. Tingible-body macrophages are present within germinal centers of reactive, nonneoplastic lymph nodes.

163. The answer is D. *(Lee, 9/e, pp 1432–1437. Robbins, 5/e, p. 622.)* In contrast to factor VIII deficiency, hemarthroses are uncommon in patients who have von Willebrand's disease. Von Willebrand's disease is characterized by quantitative or qualitative abnormalities of von Willebrand's factor. A prolonged bleeding time affects most of the patients, and there is a moderate deficiency in coagulation factor VIII. Decreased retention of platelets in glass bead filters, normal numbers of platelets, and menorrhagia are usual findings, but petechiae rarely occur. The most common symptoms include epistaxis, increased susceptibility to bruises, and excessive bleeding from wounds.

164. The answer is C. *(Robbins, 5/e, pp 643–648.)* Hodgkin's disease is broadly divided into four histologic subtypes, the most common of which is the nodular sclerosis variant. This is characterized morphologically by the presence of the lacunar variant of Reed-Sternberg (RS) cells and by bands of fibrous tissue that divide the lymph node into nodules. Unlike the other subtypes of Hodgkin's disease, it is more common in females. Young adults are classically affected and the disease typically involves the cervical, supraclavicular, or mediastinal lymph nodes. Involvement of extranodal lymphoid tissue is unusual. Variant RS cells with a multilobed, puffy nucleus ("popcorn" cell) are seen in the lymphocyte-predominant subtype.

165. The answer is C. *(Robbins, 5/e, pp 640–642.)* The large-cell immunoblastic lymphoma is one of the three high-grade lymphomas, which also include lymphoblastic lymphoma and small, noncleaved lymphomas, such as Burkitt's lymphoma. Lymphoblastic lymphoma occurs predominantly in adolescents, is closely related to T-cell acute lymphoblastic leukemia, and, in addition to a mediastinal mass, disseminates early to bone marrow and blood. In contrast, large-cell immunoblastic lymphoma is predominantly of B-cell origin (5 to 10 percent are T cell) and occurs in much older people, many of whom had a prior immune or lymphoproliferative disorder (Sjögren's syndrome, AIDS, or renal transplant immunosuppression). Bone marrow involvement is uncommon except in late stages; extranodal tumor (retroperitoneum) is common. The tumor is aggressive and rapidly fatal if untreated. The cells appear plasmacytoid (B immunoblasts) or show multilobed, polymorphous nuclei (T immunoblasts), but molecular studies are essential to differentiate T-cell receptor gene rearrangement from the immunoglobulin gene rearrangements of B immunoblasts. A "starry sky" pattern is produced by the digestion of cellular debris by benign macrophages and is typically seen in both lymphoblastic lymphoma and Burkitt's lymphoma.

166. The answer is C. *(Robbins, 5/e, pp 264–265, 654–655.)* Chronic myeloid leukemia (CML) is one of the four chronic myeloproliferative disorders, but, unlike myeloid metaplasia or polycythemia vera, CML is associated with the Philadelphia chromosome translocation t (9;22) in over 90 percent of cases. Association with the translocation t (8;14) is characteristic of Burkitt's lymphoma. In differentiating CML from a leukemoid reaction, several other features are important: lack of alkaline phosphatase in granulocytes, increased basophils and eosinophils in the peripheral blood, and, often, increased platelets in early stages followed by thrombocytopenia in late or blast stages. Other well-known features of CML include marked splenomegaly, leukocyte counts greater than 50,000/mm^3, and mild anemia.

167. The answer is B. *(Robbins, 5/e, pp 666–667. Rubin, 2/e, pp 1034–1036.)* Langerhans cell histiocytosis is a complex of three syndromes affecting the reticuloendothelial system: Letterer-Siwe syndrome, Hand-Schüller-Christian disease, and eosinophilic granuloma. An unknown pathogenesis and an abnormal proliferation of a type of histiocyte called a Langerhans cell are characteristics common to all three syndromes and provide the basis for the designation of Langerhans cell histiocytosis. The Langerhans cells contain Birbeck granules ultrastructurally, which have a characteristic tennis-racket appearance. Alpha-chain disease, seen in the Mediterranean, involves abnormal proliferations of lymphocytes and plasma cells in the lamina propria of the small intestines.

168. The answer is C. *(Robbins, 5/e, pp 643–648.)* The diagnosis of Hodgkin's disease depends on the total histologic picture and the presence of binucleated or bilobed giant cells with prominent acidophilic "owl-eye" nucleoli known as Reed-Sternberg (RS) cells. However, cells similar in appearance to RS cells may also be seen in infectious mononucleosis, mycosis fungoides, and other conditions. Thus, while RS cells are necessary for histologic confirmation of the diagnosis of Hodgkin's disease, they must be present in the appropriate histologic setting of lymphocyte predominance, nodular sclerosis, mixed cellularity, or lymphocyte depletion.

169. The answer is C. *(Robbins, 5/e, pp 658–660.)* Polycythemia rubra vera (PRV) is one of the myeloproliferative diseases characterized by excessive proliferation of erythroid, granulocytic, and megakaryocytic precursors derived from a single stem cell. In PRV the erythroid series dominates, but there is hyperplasia of all elements. There is plethoric congestion of all organs. The liver and spleen are typically moderately enlarged and may show extramedullary hemopoiesis. Thrombotic complications are an important cause of morbidity and mortality, and major and minor hemorrhagic complications are also frequent. The red cell count is elevated with hematocrit >60 percent. The white cell count and platelet count are also elevated. Leukocyte alkaline phosphatase (LAP) activity is elevated in contrast to chronic myeloid leukemia, where it is reduced. Pruritus and peptic ulceration are common, possibly in relation to increased histamine release from basophils.

170. The answer is A. *(Robbins, 5/e, p 666. Silverberg, 2/e, pp 452–453.)* The finding of mu heavy-chain proteins in the serum is diagnostic generally of macroglobulinemia and specifically of mu heavy-chain disease. This form of macroglobulinemia has been detected in patients with chronic lymphocytic leukemia without findings of lymphadenopathy or bone marrow infiltrates of lymphocytes and plasma cells, which are typical of Waldenström's macroglobulinemia. Hepatomegaly and splenomegaly are usually present.

171. The answer is C. *(Robbins, 5/e, pp 656–658.)* Hairy cell leukemia, a type of chronic B-cell leukemia, should be suspected in patients with splenomegaly; pancytopenia, including thrombocytopenia; bleeding; fatigue;

and leukemic lymphocyte-like cells in the peripheral blood demonstrating cytoplasmic projections at the cell periphery ("hairy" cells). These cells stain for acid phosphatase, and the reaction is refractory to treatment with tartaric acid (tartrate-resistant acid phosphatase, or TRAP).

172. The answer is D. *(Anderson, 9/e, pp 1436, 1440–1442. Rubin, 2/e, p 1033.)* Clinicians and pathologists alike should be familiar with the benign syndrome of lymph node enlargement called *sinus histiocytosis with massive lymphadenopathy.* This is a self-limiting, invariably benign disorder found classically in young, black, African and Caribbean patients, but it has been found in others as well. It is characterized clinically by profound enlargement of regional cervical lymph nodes, fever, and leukocytosis. Histologically, the lymph nodes show marked histiocytic proliferation within the sinuses, with engulfment of lymphocytes within the histiocytes. There may be skin involvement, and histiocytes containing phagocytosed lymphocytes may be present in the skin biopsy specimen. The patients predictably revert to normal within a period of months. Histiocytic medullary reticulosis is a disease in which a form of malignant histiocytes is found in lymph node sinuses, with engulfed red cells found within the neoplastic histiocytes (erythrophagocytosis). Primitive, round lymphoblastic tumor cells are found in tissue taken from patients with Burkitt's lymphoma.

173. The answer is B. *(Robbins, 5/e, pp 64, 218–219.)* The findings given are consistent with Wiskott-Aldrich syndrome. The Pelger-Huët anomaly involves leukocytes that have dumbbell-shaped nuclei but function normally. Some of the listed clinical features occur in the Chédiak-Higashi syndrome, but delayed hypersensitivity reactions are normal. In chronic granulomatous disease, leukocytes are unable to kill phagocytized bacteria, but delayed hypersensitivity reactions and platelet counts are normal. In patients who have Hodgkin's disease, a different constellation of symptoms occurs.

174. The answer is E. *(Henry, 18/e, pp 630, 641–642.)* Seen in the photomicrograph are sideroblasts that are demonstrating distinctive rings of Prussian blue–positive granules that indicate iron. Approximately 35 percent of normoblasts in normal bone marrow contain ferritin granules under normal conditions of iron metabolism. Heme synthetase mediates the attachments of iron onto protoporphyrin for the synthesis of hemoglobin. In sideroblastic anemia the production of globin or of heme is markedly reduced because of the deficiency of pyridoxine and ferritin, which contains iron accumulations with sideroblasts without progression into hemoglobin. The accumulation of these ferritin granules takes place in the mitochondria, where heme synthetase is located, and then can be seen rimming the nucleus of the normoblast—

hence the name *ring sideroblasts.* This is the opposite abnormality from iron deficiency anemia. This type of anemia may be seen in patients suffering from alcoholism, selective deficiencies of pyridoxine, and myelodysplastic syndromes (MDS).

175. The answer is A. *(Robbins, 5/e, pp 592–596.)* Homozygous expression of hemoglobin S results in nearly all the hemoglobin in the red blood cell's being of the S type. Thus, most of the circulating red cells have the abnormal sickling forms that are sequestered by the spleen and produce sludging within the splenic capillaries and consequent multiple and continuing infarctions. Eventually the spleen becomes small as it is replaced by fibrous tissue. This is sometimes referred to as 'autosplenectomy." Multiple crises contribute to this event. Massive enlargements of the spleen may be found in neoplastic blood disorders. Chronic lymphocytic leukemia (CLL) produces some very large spleens late in the disease, but massive splenomegaly has been seen in many examples of leukemias and lymphomas, including hairy cell leukemia. Even conversion from cutaneous T-cell lymphoma (mycosis fungoides) may result in a transformed immunoblastic-like sarcoma state.

176. The answer is C. *(Anderson, 9/e, pp 494–495. Robbins, 5/e, p 173.)* While the exact interactions between different cells are not totally understood, there is current evidence that an initiating antigen is first processed by a macrophage. The macrophage interacts with helper T cells and B cells in a conceptual triangular fashion with helper T cells functioning in the recognition of the carrier component of the antigen on the macrophage as well as recognizing the major histocompatibility complex (MHC) marker (Ia) on the macrophage surface. The macrophage appears to concentrate the antigen, thereby orchestrating interactions between itself and the T and B lymphocytes. After stimulation, the B cell may differentiate into antibody-producing plasma cells. Eosinophils and basophils function in type I reactions (anaphylaxis) by degranulation and binding of IgE.

177. The answer is D. *(Robbins, 5/e, pp 660–662.)* Myeloid metaplasia with myelofibrosis is a myeloproliferative disorder in which the bone marrow is hypocellular and fibrotic and extramedullary hematopoiesis occurs, mainly in the spleen (myeloid metaplasia). Marked splenomegaly with trilinear proliferation of normoblasts, immature myeloid cells, and large megakaryocytes occurs. Giant platelets and poikilocytic (teardrop) red cells are seen in the peripheral smear. Clinically, myeloid metaplasia may be preceded by polycythemia vera or chronic myeloid leukemia. Biopsy of the marrow is essential for diagnosis. In contradistinction to chronic myeloid leukemia, levels of leukocyte alkaline phosphatase are elevated or normal in myeloid metaplasia;

in CML, levels are low or absent. In 5 to 10 percent of cases of myeloid meta-plasia, acute leukemia occurs. In aplastic anemia the marrow is very hypocel-lular, but consists largely of fat cells, not fibrosis. There is no splenomegaly. Microangiopathic and other hemolytic anemias that result from trauma to red cells show many erythrocytic abnormalities (helmet and burr cells, triangle cells, and schistocytes) in the peripheral smear.

178. The answer is C. *(Robbins, 5/e, pp 663–665.)* The bone marrow aspi-rate exhibits a proliferation of plasma cells that are characterized by well-defined perinuclear clear zones and by dense cytoplasmic basophilia due to increased RNA accumulations. Weakness, weight loss, recurrent infections, proteinuria, anemia, and abnormal proliferation of plasma cells in the bone marrow are findings that highly suggest the presence of multiple myeloma, a plasma cell dyscrasia. The more definitive diagnostic criteria are findings of M-component in the results of serum electrophoresis and plasma cell levels above 20 percent in the bone marrow. Multiple myeloma, which occurs more commonly in males than in females, shows an increasing incidence with in-creasing age, and most patients are in their seventies.

179. The answer is C. *(Robbins, 5/e, pp 662–666.)* Multiple myeloma has a peak incidence at 50 to 60 years of age and presents a classic triad of mar-row plasmacytosis; a serum or urine M (monoclonal) protein or both, which represent the immunoglobulin molecule (or heavy or light chain) produced by the tumor cells; and lytic bone lesions. Myeloma is a monoclonal malignancy of the B-lymphocyte system with bone pain the most common symptom; oste-olytic, punched-out bone lesions are characteristic, especially in the skull. Since the process is lytic, alkaline phosphatase is usually not raised. Lymphadenopathy occurs in Waldenström's macroglobulinemia, another ma-lignancy of lymphoplasmacytoid cells, but myeloma is not associated with lymphadenopathy. Hypercalcemia from bone resorption is frequent, as are re-current infections because of severe suppression of normal immunoglobulins. In about 55 percent of patients, the abnormal M component is IgG and in 25 percent it is IgA.

180. The answer is A. *(Robbins, 5/e, pp 143–144.)* The photomicrograph in the question shows the presence of lipid-laden macrophages that have replaced much of the splenic parenchyma. The macrophages have a some-what vacuolated cytoplasm, which is characteristic of Gaucher's disease. This is an autosomal recessive disease characterized by a reduction or a deficiency of glucocerebrosidase. Thus glucocerebroside accumulates mainly in the mononuclear phagocytic system. Three clinical types occur. The classic is type I, which occurs in adults and generally spares the central nervous system with the glucocerebrosides limited to the mononuclear phagocyte system of the spleen, liver, and bone marrow. This is mainly found in European Jewish patients and is the most common form of Gaucher's disease. Type II is the infantile form, which involves the brain and presents no detectable glucocerebrosidase activity. Death occurs at an early age. Type III may be thought of as being an intermediate between types I and II; it is found in adolescent patients and mainly involves the mononuclear phagocyte system early but will involve the brain by the third decade of life. α-Galactosidase deficiency (Fabry's disease), which is characterized by angiokeratomas of the skin, involves marked ceramide trihexoside accumulations within the endothelial and smooth muscle cells of blood vessels, ganglion cells, heart, renal tubules, and glomeruli. Glucosidase deficiency is type II glycogen storage disease, which is one of the variants of liver phosphorylase deficiency. Glucose-6-phosphate dehydrogenase deficiency results in hemolytic disease in both sexes, with the male more severely affected.

181. The answer is D. *(Robbins, 5/e, pp 140–143.)* The cell in the photomicrograph is known as Gaucher's cell, the pathognomonic histopathologic finding in Gaucher's disease, and is a histiocyte typically found in the spleen, liver, and bone marrow. The cytoplasm contains glucocerebroside in an increased concentration that is demonstrable by periodic acid–Schiff reagent staining and appears wrinkled or striated in ordinary light microscopy. Histochemical ultrastructure studies have revealed that the unique cytoplasmic wrinkles are due to the presence of many spindle-shaped bodies (Gaucher's bodies) that contain 90 percent glucocerebroside and that show increased acid phosphatase activity. A characteristic histopathologic (but not pathognomonic) finding in Niemann-Pick disease is the foam cell; this cell is found mainly in lymphoid tissues.

182–185. The answers are 182-C, 183-C, 184-D, 185-A. *(Robbins, 5/e, pp 649–658.)* Multiple Auer rods are often prominent in the hypergranular promyelocytes of acute promyelocytic leukemia since they are formed from the abnormal azurophilic granules. Myeloblasts predominate in acute myeloblastic leukemia (AML) and, therefore, only a few granules, or occasional Auer rods, are present. Acute promyelocytic leukemia is associated with widespread petechiae and ecchymoses, cutaneous or mucosal, from disseminated intravascular coagulation. The vitamin A derivative all-*trans*-retinoic acid has been used to treat patients with M3 AML. The M1 and M3 classes refer to the French-American-British (FAB) classification of AML: M1 is AML in which myeloblasts predominate and M3 is acute promyelocytic leukemia with promyelocytes numerous. Myeloperoxidase is present in both, especially in M3. AML occasionally follows chemotherapy and radiotherapy for Hodgkin's disease.

Chronic lymphocytic leukemia occurs most frequently after the age of 50 (90 percent of cases) and is similar in many aspects to small lymphocytic lymphoma. It is associated with long survival in many cases and the few symptoms are related to anemia and the absolute lymphocytosis of small, mature cells. Splenomegaly may be noted. Some patients are asymptomatic.

Acute lymphoblastic leukemia (ALL) primarily affects children and young adults with marked lymphadenopathy, some splenomegaly, and hepatomegaly. Since chemotherapy at present results in complete remission in 90 percent of children, with more than 50 percent alive 5 years later, it is essential to differentiate ALL from acute myeloblastic leukemia in which prognosis is poor. Cytochemical differentiation includes PAS-positive blasts in most cases of ALL and the presence of terminal deoxynucleotidyl transferase (TdT) in 95 percent of cases of ALL, but in less than 5 percent of acute myeloblastic leukemias.

Hairy cell leukemia and chronic lymphocytic leukemia (CLL) are considered to be chronic lymphoproliferative disorders. CLL is a neoplasm of B cells, like most other lymphoid malignancies. Through molecular analysis, hairy cells are now known to rearrange and express immunoglobulin genes, assigning them also to B-cell lineage.

186–188. The answers are 186-E, 187-C, 188-A. (*Robbins, 5/e, pp 264–265.*) Chromsomal translocations are present in some malignancies, which suggests they have a possible role in malignant transformation. In some cases the translocation has been shown to involve proto-oncogenes, which raises the possibility of proto-oncogene activation. Eighty to ninety percent of cases of follicular non-Hodgkin's lymphoma contain the t14;18 transloaction. In these cases the immunoglobulin heavy chain locus is the site of a translocation involving the *bcl*-2 proto-oncogene on chromosome 18 with consequent overexpression of the *bcl*-2 protein.

More than 90 percent of cases of chronic myeloid leukemia exhibit the Philadelphia chromosome, a reciprocal translocation from the long arm of chromosome 22 to chromosome 9. The segment of chromosome 9 involved in translocation contains the proto-oncogene c-*abl*, which is rearranged in proximity to a break point cluster region (*bcr*) on chromosome 22. The resultant chimeric c-*abl/bcr* gene encodes a protein with tyrosine kinase activity.

More than 90 percent of cases of Burkitt's lymphoma have a translocation involving the c-*myc* proto-oncogene on chromosome 8 and the immunoglobulin heavy chain locus on chromosome 14. This change results in activation of the c-*myc* oncogene and overexpression of its gene product.

Cardiovascular System

DIRECTIONS: Each question below contains five suggested responses. Select the **one best** response to each question.

189. Atherosclerosis, the most prevalent form of arterial disease in humans, is first manifested by an innocuous fatty streaking of the intima and is characterized by all the following EXCEPT

(A) onset in mid-life
(B) formation of essential lesions in the intima
(C) disintegration of the internal elastic lamina in advanced lesions
(D) relatively numerous lesions in larger arteries and fewer in smaller arteries
(E) plaque formations that cause little reduction in the luminal size of large arteries

190. Major risk factors associated with development of coronary and generalized atherosclerosis (AS) include all the following EXCEPT

(A) cigarette smoking
(B) elevated high-density lipoprotein (HDL) levels
(C) diabetes mellitus
(D) hypertension
(E) hypercholesterolemia

191. Type II hyperlipidemia (familial hypercholesterolemia) results from a defect in

(A) lipoprotein lipase
(B) low-density lipoprotein (LDL) receptor
(C) apolipoprotein E
(D) apolipoprotein CII
(E) lipoprotein(a)

192. The form of vascular disease responsible for malignant hypertension is

(A) medial calcific sclerosis
(B) arteriosclerosis obliterans
(C) hyperplastic arteriolosclerosis
(D) hyaline arteriolosclerosis
(E) thromboangiitis obliterans

193. A factor that causes decreased peripheral resistance and decreased blood volume is

(A) angiotensin I
(B) angiotensin II
(C) aldosterone
(D) atriopeptin
(E) renin

194. If the coronary arteries on dissection at autopsy show severe atherosclerosis in a patient who had clinically acute (60-h) myocardial infarction, you would expect to find

(A) gross evidence of myocardial scarring
(B) coronary thrombosis in 90 percent of cases
(C) coronary thrombosis in 65 percent of cases
(D) a plaque with ulceration, fissure, or hemorrhage
(E) rupture of a papillary muscle

195. A factor that stimulates the proliferation of smooth muscle cells and also relates to the pathogenesis of atherosclerosis is

(A) platelet-derived growth factor (PDGF)
(B) transforming growth factor β (TGF-β)
(C) interleukin 1 (IL-1)
(D) interferon α
(E) tumor necrosis factor (TNF)

---

196. An 82-year-old woman complaining of headaches, visual disturbances, and muscle pain has a biopsy of the temporal artery. The changes revealed by the biopsy specimen are shown in the photomicrograph below. The next course of action is to

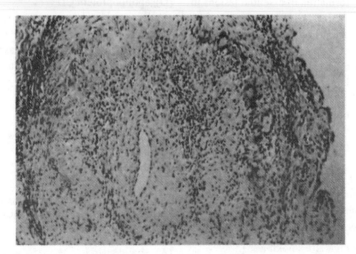

(A) administer corticosteroids
(B) verify with a repeat biopsy
(C) administer anticoagulants
(D) perform angiography
(E) order a test of the erythrocyte sedimentation rate (ESR)

197. The necrotizing inflammation of the small gastrointestinal artery shown in the photomicrograph below is most likely due to

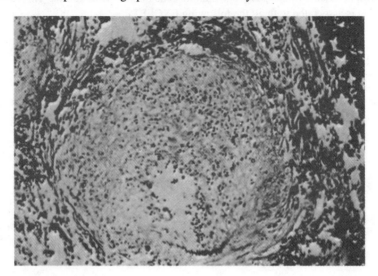

(A) myasthenia gravis
(B) polyarteritis nodosa
(C) atherosclerosis
(D) dissecting aneurysm
(E) syphilis

---

198. In a patient with vasculitis, the finding of serum antineutrophil cytoplasmic autoantibodies that react by immunofluorescence staining in a perinuclear pattern is most suggestive of

(A) giant cell arteritis
(B) classic polyarteritis nodosa
(C) Wegener's granulomatosis
(D) Churg-Strauss syndrome
(E) microscopic polyangiitis

199. A very painful lesion found under the nail of the second finger of the hand is most likely which one of the following lesions of blood vessels or lymphatics?

(A) Kaposi's sarcoma
(B) Capillary hemangioma
(C) Glomus tumor
(D) Angiosarcoma
(E) Cystic hygroma

200. The biopsy specimen shown below reveals a dermal vascular tumor with angular, slitlike spaces and spindle cells in the dermal stroma. This lesion is associated with all the following EXCEPT

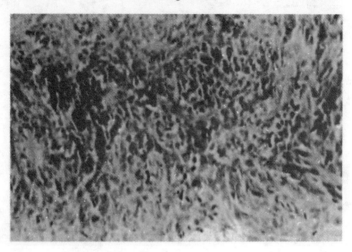

(A) several clinically distinct forms
(B) immunosuppression
(C) depletion of T-suppressor cells
(D) early histologic resemblance to granulation tissue
(E) tumor origin from vascular endothelium

---

201. Which of the following conditions is most likely to predispose to thrombosis and embolism?

(A) Atrial fibrillation
(B) Pulmonary stenosis
(C) Ventricular septal defect
(D) Aortic stenosis
(E) Atrial septal defect

202. A posterior myocardial infarction that involves the posterior portion of the left ventricle and the posterior one-third of the interventricular septum is caused by occlusion of the

(A) left coronary artery
(B) right coronary artery
(C) circumflex artery
(D) left anterior descending (LAD) artery
(E) posterior descending artery

203. A 56-year-old woman died in a hospital where she was being evaluated for shortness of breath, ankle edema, and mild hepatomegaly. Because of the gross appearance of the liver at necropsy in the photograph below, one would also expect to find

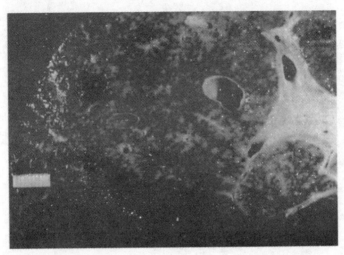

(A) a pulmonary saddle embolus
(B) right heart dilatation
(C) portal vein thrombosis
(D) biliary cirrhosis
(E) splenic amyloidosis

---

204. The mortality from myocardial infarction is most closely related to the occurrence of

(A) a pericardial effusion
(B) pulmonary edema
(C) coronary artery thrombosis
(D) an arrhythmia
(E) systemic hypotension

205. Unexpected sudden cardiac death is a very rare complication of

(A) severe coronary artery disease
(B) myocarditis
(C) cardiac tamponade
(D) mitral valve prolapse
(E) dilated or hypertrophic cardiomyopathy

206. The pathology evident in the photomicrograph below usually first appears after which of the following lengths of time following a myocardial infarction?

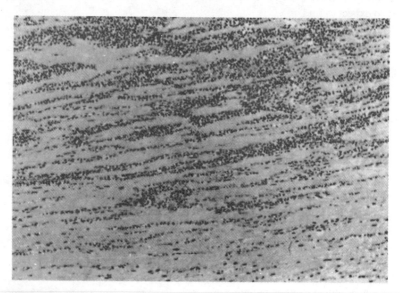

(A) 12 h
(B) 3 days
(C) 7 days
(D) 14 days
(E) 28 days

207. Following development of an acute myocardial infarction (MI), the LEAST likely complication is

(A) cardiac arrhythmia
(B) cardiogenic shock
(C) sudden cardiac death
(D) cardiac rupture
(E) thromboembolism

208. The most frequent cause of aortic valve incompetence and regurgitation is

(A) latent syphilis
(B) infective endocarditis
(C) rheumatic fever
(D) aortic dissection
(E) congenital

209. Severe mitral stenosis, as shown in the photograph below, is frequently accompanied by all the following EXCEPT

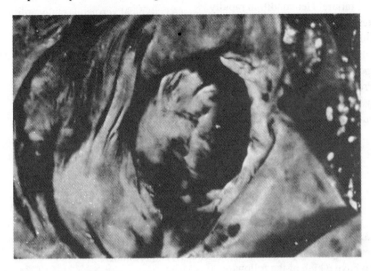

(A) aortic valve disease
(B) antecedent rheumatic fever
(C) left atrial enlargement with atrial fibrillation
(D) pulmonary valvular stenosis
(E) chronic passive pulmonary congestion

---

210. Manifestations of rheumatic fever that are of major diagnostic value include all the following EXCEPT

(A) subcutaneous nodules
(B) migratory arthritis of large joints
(C) fever
(D) erythema marginatum
(E) chorea minor

211. The most characteristic feature of chronic rheumatic heart disease is

(A) endocarditis
(B) myocarditis
(C) pericarditis
(D) mitral valvulitis
(E) pulmonic valvulitis

212. A 23-year-old woman develops the sudden onset of congestive heart failure. Her condition rapidly deteriorates and she dies in heart failure. At autopsy, patchy interstitial infiltrates composed mainly of lymphocytes are found, some of which surround individual myocytes. The most likely cause of this patient's heart failure is

(A) viral myocarditis
(B) bacterial myocarditis
(C) giant cell myocarditis
(D) hypersensitivity myocarditis
(E) beriberi

213. Bacterial endocarditis constitutes the greatest threat to patients who have which of the following forms of congenital heart disease?

(A) Atrial septal defect
(B) Ventricular septal defect
(C) Pulmonic stenosis
(D) Tetralogy of Fallot
(E) Patent ductus arteriosus

214. Acute infective endocarditis differs from subacute endocarditis in all the following respects EXCEPT

(A) the time required for the lesion to develop
(B) the nature of the preponderant organism
(C) embolization and dissemination
(D) the nature of valvular vegetations
(E) the causative organism

215. A synonym for *nonbacterial thrombotic endocarditis* is

(A) atypical verrucous endocarditis
(B) marantic endocarditis
(C) Libman-Sacks endocarditis
(D) viridans endocarditis
(E) rheumatic endocarditis

216. A 37-year-old woman complained of prolonged cramps, nausea, vomiting, diarrhea, and episodic flushing of the skin. At autopsy, pearly-white, plaquelike deposits were found on the tricuspid valve leaflets. These cardiac lesions most likely were due to

(A) rheumatic heart disease
(B) amyloidosis
(C) iron overload
(D) hypothyroidism
(E) carcinoid heart disease

217. An elderly man treated for congestive heart failure for years with digitalis and furosemide dies of pulmonary edema. A postmortem examination of the heart would most likely show

(A) severe left ventricular hypertrophy
(B) right and left ventricular hypertrophy
(C) right ventricular infarction
(D) aortic and mitral valve stenosis
(E) a dilated, globular heart with thin walls

218. The heart in the gross photograph below came from a patient who

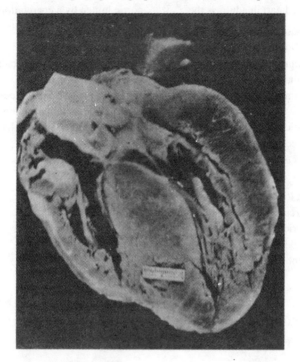

(A) suffered from alcohol toxicity
(B) had Libman-Sacks endocarditis
(C) may have had a family history of similar cardiac involvement
(D) frequently had obstructive symptoms
(E) had a hypocontractile heart

---

219. Features of tetralogy of Fallot include all the following EXCEPT

(A) obstruction to the pulmonary outflow
(B) hypertrophy of the right ventricle
(C) aortic dextroposition in 50 percent of cases
(D) development of cyanosis before 1 year of age
(E) ventricular septal defect

220. Which of the following is an atrial septal defect (ASD) that is located in the upper portion of the atrial septum above the fossa ovalis near the superior vena cava?

(A) Ostium primum defect
(B) Ostium secundum defect
(C) Patent foramen ovale
(D) Sinus venosus defect
(E) Persistent AV canal

221. The most common primary tumor of the heart in adults is the

(A) rhabdomyoma
(B) rhabdomyosarcoma
(C) papillary fibroelastoma
(D) lipoma
(E) myxoma

222. Which one of the following is the most common congenital heart defect to cause an initial left-to-right shunt?

(A) Tetralogy of Fallot
(B) Coarctation of the aorta
(C) Ventricular septal defect
(D) Atrial septal defect
(E) Patent ductus arteriosus

223. Complete obliteration of the aortic lumen by a coarctation proximal to the ductus arteriosus is fatal unless

(A) the foramen ovale is closed
(B) the ductus is ligated
(C) pulmonary stenosis coexists
(D) the ductus remains patent
(E) the tricuspid valve is incompetent

DIRECTIONS: Each group of questions below consists of lettered headings followed by a set of numbered items. For each numbered item select the **one** lettered heading with which it is **most** closely associated. Each lettered heading may be used **once, more than once, or not at all.**

Questions 224–227

Match the following descriptive phrases with the appropriate lettered type of cardiomyopathy.

(A) Hypertrophic cardiomyopathy
(B) Dilated (congestive) cardiomyopathy
(C) Immune myocarditis
(D) Endocardial fibroelastosis
(E) Endomyocardial fibrosis

224. Associated with sudden cardiac death in up to 30 percent of patients

225. Associated with heavy alcohol intake

226. Associated with obstruction of left ventricular outflow of blood

227. Usually identified in Southeast Asia and Africa

Questions 228–230

For each cardiac condition, choose the infectious agent with which it is most likely to be associated.

(A) Coxsackievirus
(B) *Mycobacterium tuberculosis*
(C) *Streptococcus*
(D) *Treponemea*
(E) *Escherichia coli*

228. Rheumatic fever

229. Aortic aneurysms

230. Suppurative pericarditis

Questions 231–234

For each aneurysm, choose the disease or syndrome with which it is most likely to be associated.

(A) Ehlers-Danlos syndrome
(B) Kawasaki's disease
(C) Rheumatic disease
(D) Polycystic renal disease
(E) Takayasu's arteritis

231. Berry aneurysm

232. Dissecting aortic aneurysm

233. Coronary aneurysm

234. Abdominal and distal thoracic aortic aneurysms

Cardiovascular System
Answers

189. The answer is A. *(Anderson, 9/e, pp 757–766. Robbins, 5/e, pp 476–479.)* In atherosclerosis, primarily a disease of the arterial intima, disintegration of the internal elastic lamina is typical in advanced lesions, and necrosis commonly occurs at the base of the thickened intima. Essential lesions, occurring in the intima, are more numerous in larger than in smaller arteries. Although plaque formations cause little reduction in the size of the lumen of large arteries, atherosclerosis can lead to arterial dilatation and aneurysms. It is a progressive disease that begins early in life. Fatty streaks can be found in some children younger than 1 year of age and all children older than 10 years.

190. The answer is B. *(Anderson, 9/e, pp 618–621. Robbins, 5/e, pp 474–476.)* Hypercholesterolemia (serum cholesterol greater than 200 to 230 mg/dL) is one of the major risk factors for development of atherosclerosis. Hypercholesterolemia is associated with elevated low-density lipoprotein (LDL), which contains a high proportion of cholesterol. Men with cholesterol levels above 240 mg/dL have a threefold risk of death from myocardial infarct compared with men with cholesterol below 200. However, in contrast to the LDL fraction, the HDL fraction is inversely related to the incidence of coronary heart disease (CHD). The Framingham heart study found that low plasma levels of HDL are a potent risk factor for coronary artery disease. HDL levels are increased by exercise, small amounts of alcohol, and administration of estrogens, but cigarette smoking depresses plasma HDL levels. Other major risk factors for atherosclerosis include hypertension, cigarette smoking, and diabetes.

191. The answer is B. *(Robbins, 5/e, pp 135–137, 481–483.)* Lipids are transported in the blood complexed to proteins called *apolipoproteins.* Abnormalities of this lipid transport or metabolism result in hyperlipoproteinemias, which are responsible for most syndromes of premature atherosclerosis. The hyperlipidemias are divided into five distinct electrophoretic patterns. Type I hyperlipoproteinemia, caused by a mutation in the lipoprotein lipase gene, results in increased chylomicrons and triglycerides. Type II hyperlipoproteinemia, perhaps the most frequent mendelian disorder, is caused by a mutation in the low-density lipoprotein (LDL) receptor gene. This results in increased LDL and cholesterol. Homozygotes for this gene defect have markedly increased plasma cholesterol levels and develop severe atherosclerosis at an early age. Mutations in the apolipoprotein E gene result in type III hyperlipoproteinemia, which is characterized by increased intermediate-density lipoproteins (IDL), triglycerides, and cholesterol. Type IV hyperlipoproteinemia causes increased very low-density lipoproteins (VLDL) and triglycerides. The genetic defect causing this is presently unknown. Type V hyperlipoproteinemia, caused by a mutation in apolipoprotein CII, results in increased VLDL, chylomicrons, triglycerides, and cholesterol. Lipoprotein(a) is an altered form of LDL that contains the apolipoprotein B100 linked to apolipoprotein(a). Increased levels of lipoprotein(a) are associated with an increased incidence of coronary and cerebral vascular disease, independent of the total LDL level.

192. The answer is C. *(Robbins, 5/e, pp 484, 488–489, 498, 976–978.)* *Malignant hypertension* refers to dramatic elevations in systolic and diastolic blood pressure often resulting in early death from cerebral and brainstem hemorrhages. Pathologically the renal vessels demonstrate a concentric obliteration of arterioles by an increase in smooth muscle cells, and protein deposition in a laminar configuration that includes fibrin material, which leads to total and subtotal occlusion of the vessels. Hyaline arteriolosclerosis as seen in diabetes is presumably caused by leakage of plasma components across the endothelium with or without hypertension. Medial calcific sclerosis (Mönckeberg's arteriosclerosis) is characterized by dystrophic calcification in the tunica media of muscular arteries. There is no narrowing of the lumen of the affected vessels. Thromboangiitis obliterans (Buerger's disease) is occlusion by a proliferative inflammatory process in arteries of heavy cigarette smokers and is often associated with HLA-A9, B5 genotypes.

193. The answer is D. *(Robbins, 5/e, pp 485–487. Rubin, 2/e, pp 483–484.)* Blood pressure is dependent on the product of cardiac output times peripheral resistance of the blood vessels. Factors that cause increased peripheral resistance will result in increased blood pressure. One of the major mechanisms involved in this regulation of blood pressure is the renin-angiotensin system. Renin splits angiotensinogen into angiotensin I, which is converted into angiotensin II by angiotensin-converting enzyme (ACE). Angiotensin II causes increased aldosterone secretion by the adrenal, which leads to sodium and fluid retention, increased cardiac output, and increased blood pressure. This renin-angiotensin-aldosterone system is countered by the actions of atrial natriuretic factor (ANF), or atriopeptin, a hormone secreted by specialized cells in the atria of the heart. ANF, secreted in response to volume expansion, causes vasodilation and increased renal excretion of sodium, leading to decreased blood and extracellular volume.

194. The answer is D. *(Robbins, 5/e, pp 529–530, 533, 536.)* At autopsy, coronary artery thrombosis has been found in less than 50 percent of cases of myocardial infarction (MI). However, when coronary angiography is done within 4 h of MI onset, a thrombosed artery is found in almost 90 percent of cases; occlusion is found in only about 60 percent when angiography is delayed for 12 to 24 h. Therefore, lysis occurs or there is relaxation of spasm, or both. Also, intravenous or intracoronary fibrinolysis restore flow to thrombosed arteries in more than 75 percent of recent MIs. These findings are proof of coronary thrombosis, whether it is found at autopsy or not. Ulcerated, fissured, or hemorrhagic atheromas are usually found beneath the thrombus, whether still attached or lysed. Following an infarction, granulation tissue forms at 10 days to 2 weeks, and this is followed by fibrous scarring.

195. The answer is A. *(Robbins, 5/e, pp 479–481. Rubin, 2/e, pp 466–470.)* The pathogenesis of atherosclerosis depends in part on the inflammatory function of macrophages, which involves the release of numerous cytokines. Platelet-derived growth factor (PDGF) is mitogenic and chemotactic for smooth muscle cells. This may explain the recruitment and proliferation of smooth muscle cells in atherosclerosis. Other macrophage products participate in the pathophysiology of atherosclerosis by other means. Interleukin 1 (IL-1) and tumor necrosis factor (TNF) transform the normally anticoagulant endothelial surface into a procoagulant surface by stimulating endothelial cells to produce platelet activating factor (PAF), tissue factor (TF), and plasminogen activator inhibitor (PAI). Interferon α and transforming growth factor β inhibit cell proliferation. This could explain the failure of endothelial cells to repair endothelial defects. These defects could then either provide entry areas for lipoproteins and plasma-derived factors or serve as an area where thrombi are formed.

196. The answer is A. *(Robbins, 5/e, pp 492–493. Rubin, 2/e, pp 488–489.)* Giant cell arteritis (temporal arteritis), although not a major public-health problem, is an important disease to consider in the differential diagnosis of patients of middle to advanced age who present with a constellation of symptoms that may include migratory muscular and back pains (polymyalgia rheumatica), dizziness, visual disturbances, headaches, weight loss, anorexia, and tenderness over one or both of the temporal arteries. The cause of the arteritis (which may include giant cells, neutrophils, and chronic inflammatory cells) is unknown, but the dramatic response to corticosteroids suggests an immunogenic origin. The disease may involve any artery within the body, but involvement of the ophthalmic artery or arteries may lead to blindness unless steroid therapy is begun. Therefore, if temporal arteritis is suspected, the workup to document it should be expedited and should include a biopsy of the temporal artery. Frequently, the erythrocyte sedimentation rate (ESR) is markedly elevated to values of 90 or greater. Whereas tenderness, nodularity, or skin reddening over the course of one of the scalp arteries, particularly the temporal, may show the ideal portion for a biopsy, it is important to recognize that the temporal artery may be segmentally involved or not involved at all even when the disease is present.

197. The answer is B. *(Robbins, 5/e, p 494.)* Classic polyarteritis nodosa—a necrotizing inflammation that occurs in episodes at random locations within or on the walls of medium-sized and small arteries—has been reported in about 0.1 percent of autopsies and affects, in order of increasing frequency, the arteries associated with peripheral and central nerves, skeletal muscles, pancreas, gastrointestinal tract, liver, heart, and kidneys. Proceeding in stages, the inflammatory reaction features acute necrosis, with fibrinoid deposition and neutrophilic infiltration, and leads to thrombosis of the lumen and destruction of the internal elastic membrane. Polyarteritis nodosa probably could be more accurately called "panarteritis nodosa," because *all* vascular coats are subject to inflammation. A remnant of the internal elastic membrane is visible in the photomicrograph.

198. The answer is B. *(Robbins, 5/e, pp 490–491. Rubin, 2/e, pp 489, 853–854.)* Antineutrophil cytoplasmic antibodies (ANCA) may be found in patients with certain inflammatory vascular diseases or glomerular diseases, and their presence is of clinical importance for diagnosing these diseases. Immunofluorescence reveals ANCA to have two different patterns. One is directed toward myeloperoxidase of neutrophils and is found in a perinuclear location (P-ANCA). This pattern is seen in patients with classic polyarteritis nodosa (PAN) or idiopathic crescentic glomerulonephritis without systemic disease. The other pattern reveals the antibodies to be directed against neutral leukocyte protease (proteinase 3) and results in a cytoplasmic staining pattern (C-ANCA). This pattern is seen in patients with Wegener's granulomatosis, microscopic polyangiitis, and Churg-Strauss syndrome.

199. The answer is C. *(Robbins, 5/e, pp 506–512.)* Tumors of vessels may originate from either blood vessels or lymphatics and may be either benign or malignant. Glomus tumors (glomangiomas) are exquisitely painful tumors derived from the glomus body and are found in the distal regions of the fingers and toes, possibly in a subungual location. Hemangiomas, benign tumors of blood vessels, may be subclassified into capillary hemangiomas and cavernous hemangiomas. "Birthmarks" are caused by capillary hemangiomas, while port wine stains are caused by cavernous hemangiomas of the skin. The juvenile (strawberry) hemangioma is a fast-growing lesion first appearing in the first few months of life, but it regresses completely by the age of 5. Cystic hygromas are cystic lymphangiomas, typically occurring in the neck or axilla. They may be found in patients with Turner's syndrome. Angiosarcomas are rare malignant tumors of blood vessels. In the liver they have been related to exposure to thorium dioxide (Thorotrast), arsenic, and vinyl chloride.

200. The answer is C. *(Robbins, 5/e, pp 511–512.)* Kaposi's sarcoma (KS) comprises four distinct forms. The classic, or European, form has been known since 1862. It occurs in older men of Eastern European or Mediterranean origin (predominantly Italian or Jewish) and is characterized by purple maculopapular skin lesions of the lower extremities and visceral involvement in only 10 percent of cases. The African form occurs in younger people and is more aggressive; it often involves lymph nodes in children. The rare form in immunosuppressed recipients of renal transplants often regresses when immunosuppression stops. In the epidemic form associated with AIDS, skin lesions may occur anywhere and include dissemination to mucous membranes, GI tract, lymph nodes, and viscera. Histologic determination is difficult, but all four clinical types appear similar. Early, irregular, dilated epidermal vascular spaces, extravasated red cells, and hemosiderin (like granulation tissue or stasis dermatitis) are characteristic. Later, more characteristic lesions show spindle cells around slit-spaces that are angular and contain red cells—a picture like that of angiosarcoma. The tumor cells are almost certainly of vascular endothelial origin (blood vessel or lymphatic or both). This often multifocal disease is rarely fatal, but death may be caused by frequent opportunistic infections or, less often, lymphoma, leukemia, or myeloma. There is depletion of T-helper cells, but T-suppressor cells are normal or increased.

201. The answer is A. *(Robbins, 5/e, pp 105–108.)* Stasis of blood in fibrillating atria predisposes to thrombosis and embolism. Systemic embolization from left atrial thrombi may cause infarction in the brain, lower extremities, spleen, and kidneys. Endocardial mural thrombi occur as a consequence of myocardial infarction, bacterial endocarditis, or nonbacterial (marantic) endocarditis.

202. The answer is B. *(Robbins, 5/e, pp 518–519. Rubin, 2/e, p 506.)* The right and left main coronary arteries originate around the sinuses of Valsalva of the aortic valve. The left coronary artery divides into the left anterior descending artery (LAD) and the left circumflex artery. The LAD supplies the anterior left ventricle, the anterior right ventricle, and the anterior two-thirds of the interventricular septum. The left circumflex artery supplies the lateral wall of the left ventricle. The right coronary artery supplies the remainder of the right ventricle, the posteroseptal portion of the left ventricle, and the posterior one-third of the interventricular septum. The posterior descending artery is usually a branch of the right coronary artery. This anatomic relationship is called a *right coronary dominant distribution.* Posterior (inferior or diaphragmatic) infarcts result from occlusion of the right coronary artery; anterior infarcts from occlusion of the LAD; and posterolateral infarcts from occlusion of the left circumflex artery.

203. The answer is B. *(Robbins, 5/e, pp 97–98, 520–523.)* The photograph shows the classic pattern of hepatic congestion around central veins, which leads to necrosis and degeneration of the hepatocytes surrounded by pale peripheral residual parenchyma. This is the pattern arising in the liver from chronic passive congestion as a result of right heart failure ("nutmeg liver"). Mitral stenosis with consequent pulmonary hypertension leads to right heart failure, as does any cause of pulmonary hypertension, such as emphysema (cor pulmonale). Right heart failure also leads to congestion of the spleen and transudation of fluid into the abdomen (ascites) and lower extremity soft tissues (pitting ankle edema) as a result of venous congestion. Portal vein thrombosis is most often seen in association with hepatic cirrhosis.

204. The answer is D. *(Robbins, 5/e, pp 537–540.)* In myocardial infarction, life-threatening arrhythmias occur in approximately 45 percent of patients without shock and in more than 90 percent of patients with shock. The most common arrhythmias are expressed as ventricular extrasystoles, but atrial extrasystoles, sinus tachycardia, and sinus bradycardia also occur. Even without arrhythmias, nearly two-thirds of patients with acute myocardial infarcts develop heart failure and pulmonary edema. Sudden death (death within 24 h of onset of symptoms and signs) occurs in about 20 to 25 percent of acute attacks.

205. The answer is D. *(Robbins, 5/e, pp 541, 545–547. Rubin, 2/e, p 542.)* The most common cause of sudden death in the adult is cardiac arrhythmia (usually ventricular fibrillation) due to severe coronary artery disease, with or without acute myocardial infarction. Ventricular fibrillation is also often due to primary cardiomyopathy, myocarditis, or congestive heart failure. However, sudden death is a rare complication of mitral valve prolapse (MVP), floppy valve syndrome, or the systolic click-murmur syndrome. In MVP the major complication is mitral insufficiency with left ventricular failure; however, MVP is asymptomatic in the majority of patients. Echocardiography has shown MVP to be common (5 to 10 percent of the general population). It is usually of unknown cause, but 10 to 15 percent of cases are familial with autosomal dominant inheritance. It is fairly frequent in Marfan's syndrome or cystic medial necrosis. There is excess mitral valve tissue and elongated chordae and the echocardiogram shows posterior displacement of the posterior (rarely anterior) mitral leaflet late in systole. Another interesting, but rare, noncardiac cause of sudden unexpected death is unrecognized anaphylaxis from insect stings. Postmortem sera should be examined for elevated venom-specific IgE antibodies, and laryngeal and pulmonary edema noted at autopsy.

206. The answer is B. *(Robbins, 5/e, pp 533–537.)* Usually by 3 days after a myocardial infarction, the predominant microscopic features that develop and that can be seen in a stained section of the affected myocardium include coagulation necrosis of fibers and evidence of extensive neutrophilic exudation. Interstitial edema may also be observed in microscopy, and the cross-striations of fibers may appear less recognizable. In gross examination 3 days after the infarction, the infarct has a hyperemic border surrounding a central portion that is yellow-brown and soft as the result of fatty change.

207. The answer is D. *(Robbins, 5/e, pp 537–538.)* Cardiac rupture, whether of free wall, septum, or papillary muscle, occurs in only 1 to 5 percent of cases following acute myocardial infarction. It occurs usually within the first week of infarction when there is maximal necrosis and softening (4 to 5 days) and is very rare after the second week. Rupture of the free wall results in pericardial hemorrhage and cardiac tamponade. Rupture of the interventricular septum causes a left-to-right shunt. Serious mitral valve incompetence results from rupture of anterior or posterior papillary muscles. Other common complications include arrhythmias such as heart block, sinus arrhythmias, or ventricular tachycardia or fibrillation. These occur in 90 percent of complicated cases. Next in importance, but not in frequency (only 10 percent), is cardiogenic shock from severe left ventricular contractile incompetence. Milder left ventricular failure with lung edema occurs in 60 percent, while mural thrombosis with peripheral emboli may occur in up to 40 percent. Ventricular aneurysm forms a "bulge" of the left ventricular chamber; it consists of scar tissue, does not rupture, but may contain thrombus. Sudden cardiac death occurs within 2 h in 20 percent of patients with acute myocardial infarction.

208. The answer is C. *(Anderson, 9/e, pp 650–652, 675–676.)* Aortic regurgitation (AR) is rheumatic in origin in approximately 70 percent of cases. Much less frequently it is due to syphilis, ankylosing spondylitis (rarely), infective endocarditis, aortic dissection, or aortic dilatation from cystic medial necrosis. Congenital forms of aortic stenosis occur fairly frequently but AR is rarely congenital in origin. In chronic AR, patients remain asymptomatic for many years, but clinical manifestations will include exertional dyspnea, angina, and left ventricular failure. Owing to the rapidly falling arterial pressure during late systole and diastole, there is often wide pulse pressure, Corrigan's "water-hammer" pulse, capillary pulsations at the nail beds, and a pistol-shot sound over the femoral arteries. A blowing diastolic murmur is heard along the left sternal border. Volume overload of the heart is the basic defect and results in left ventricular dilatation and hypertrophy.

209. The answer is D. *(Anderson, 9/e, pp 672–673.)* Mitral stenosis is most often associated with aortic valve disease and occasionally with tricuspid valve disease, especially in people with antecedent rheumatic fever. Occasionally, both aortic and mitral disease result from atherosclerosis. Pulmonary valvular stenosis is rarely caused by either aortic or mitral disease. Since severe mitral stenosis prevents significant regurgitation, left ventricular enlargement would not be expected. Left atrial enlargement and chronic pulmonary congestion are common in mitral disease.

210. The answer is C. *(Robbins, 5/e, pp 547–550.)* Rheumatic fever (RF) is a systemic disease with the major findings of migratory polyarthritis of large joints, carditis, erythema marginatum of skin (although skin involvement is not very common), subcutaneous nodules, and Sydenham's chorea, a neurologic disorder with involuntary, purposeless, rapid movements, most likely to occur in adolescent females and during pregnancy. There is no relation to Huntington's chorea. Fever is a minor characterization, although quite frequent. Rheumatic nodules may develop over pressure points during the later stages and seldom occur in cases without cardiac involvement. RF usually follows a pharyngeal infection with group A β-hemolytic streptococci because of an autoimmune mechanism based on cross-reactions between cardiac antigens and antibodies evoked by one of the many streptococcal antigens, e.g., streptococcal M protein. Immunofluorescence shows immunoglobulins and complement along sarcolemmal sheaths of cardiac myofibers, but Aschoff bodies seldom contain immunoglobulins or complement.

211. The answer is D. *(Robbins, 5/e, pp 547–550.)* Rheumatic fever (RF) produces both acute and chronic manifestations. Acute RF produces a pancarditis of all three layers of the heart. It is manifested by myocarditis, which is characterized by the Aschoff body; pericarditis, which is referred to as "bread and butter" pericarditis; and verrucous endocarditis. In contrast, chronic RF produces damage to cardiac valves. The mitral valve is most commonly involved, followed by the aortic valve. The stenotic valve has the appearance of a "fish mouth" or "buttonhole." An additional finding in chronic RF is a rough portion of the endocardium of the left atrium, called a *MacCallum's patch.*

212. The answer is A. *(Robbins, 5/e, pp 562–566. Rubin, 2/e, pp 543–545.)* Inflammation of the myocardium, myocarditis, has numerous causes, but most of the well-documented cases of myocarditis are of viral origin. The most common viral causes are coxsackieviruses A and B, ECHO virus, and influenza virus. Patients usually develop symptoms a few weeks after a viral infection. Most patients recover from the acute myocarditis, but a few may die from congestive heart failure or arrhythmias. Sections of the heart will show patchy or diffuse interstitial infiltrates composed of T lymphocytes and macrophages. There may be focal or patchy acute myocardial necrosis. Bacterial infections of the myocardium produce multiple foci of inflammation composed mainly of neutrophils. Giant cell myocarditis, which was previously called *Fiedler's myocarditis,* is characterized by granulomatous inflammation with giant cells and is usually rapidly fatal. In hypersensitivity myocarditis, which is caused by hypersensitivity reactions to several drugs, the inflammatory infiltrate includes many eosinophils, and the infiltrate is both interstitial and perivascular. Beriberi, one of the metabolic diseases of the heart, is a cause of high-output failure and is characterized by decreased peripheral vascular resistance and increased cardiac output. Patients have dilated hearts, but the microscopic changes are nonspecific. Hyperthyroid disease and Paget's disease are other causes of high-output failure.

213. The answer is B. *(Robbins, 5/e, pp 573–579.)* Even though children and infants who have small, isolated ventricular septal defects are usually asymptomatic, and even though two-thirds of infants who have uncomplicated lesions will have spontaneous closure of their ventricular septal defects by the age of 5, the main risk for these patients is bacterial endocarditis. Protection against bacteremia with antibiotics during routine but potentially infectious procedures is therefore required.

214. The answer is D. *(Robbins, 5/e, pp 550–554.)* Infective endocarditis, unlike rheumatic endocarditis, continues to be a clinical problem even in the antibiotic era, with such new factors as intravenous drug abuse and immunosuppression contributing to its persistence. The successful outcome of treatment is directly dependent on early recognition and diagnosis, since with time the infective organisms (such as yeast, bacteria, rickettsiae) tend to be covered with fibrin and platelets, thereby preventing access of antibiotics to the organisms. In addition, delayed treatment allows time for local valvular destruction. Acute endocarditis (AC) tends to develop within days on previously normal valves (60 percent of cases), whereas subacute endocarditis (SEC) takes more time to develop, may be clinically silent, and may be manifested only by the patient's complaint of not being "up to par." The organism causing AC tends to be pathogenic (e.g., *Staphylococcus aureus* or gonococcus); the organism causing SEC tends to be relatively innocuous (e.g., microaerophilic streptococci, *Streptococcus viridans,* and even diphtheroids). Bacterial embolization from the valves to other organs occurs mainly in AC and is much less common in SEC. Despite small differences, such as the smaller vegetations in SEC than in AC, it is not usually possible to distinguish SEC vegetations from AC vegetations through only structural criteria.

215. The answer is B. *(Anderson, 9/e, pp 652–655. Robbins, 5/e, pp 554–555.)* Nonbacterial thrombotic endocarditis is a form of endocarditis involving the mitral and aortic valves especially, characterized by resemblance to the verrucous-like protuberances of rheumatic valvulitis, which are usually large and friable; smooth and polypoid and shaggy forms are also encountered. These also may resemble the vegetations of bacterial endocarditis, but the lesions are sterile and contain no microorganisms. Both surfaces of the valves are not involved, as they may be in Libman-Sacks endocarditis seen in systemic lupus erythematosus. *Viridans endocarditis* is a synonym for *subacute bacterial endocarditis.* Nonbacterial thrombotic endocarditis is also referred to as *terminal* or *marantic endocarditis* and is associated in this country with advanced stages of cachexia, such as found in advanced malignancy or starvation. It occurs in many other terminal wasting diseases but has recently been described in well-nourished persons who have died acutely; thus, the older terms *marantic* and *terminal* are probably not appropriate. The pathogenesis is not clear, although there is evidence for increased coagulability in some patients, and the disorder may be associated with disseminated intravascular coagulation.

216. The answer is E. *(Robbins, 5/e, pp 549, 555–556, 565–566.)* Plaques or vegetations are found in characteristic locations within the heart in several diseases. The carcinoid syndrome is characterized by episodic flushing, diarrhea, bronchospasm, and cyanosis. These symptoms are caused by the release of vasoactive amines, such as serotonin, from carcinoid tumors. These substances are inactivated by enzymes such as monoamine oxidase, which are found in the liver, lung, and brain. Therefore cardiac symptoms are found only in patients with liver metastases, which bypass the inactivation of the liver itself. The cardiac lesions are found on the right side of the heart since the active metabolites secreted by the tumor are inactivated in the lung and do not reach the left side of the heart. The cardiac lesions consist of fibrous plaques found on the tricuspid and pulmonic valves. In contrast, plaques in the left atrium are seen in chronic rheumatic heart disease and are called *MacCallum's* *patches.* Vegetations also occur in rheumatic heart disease; these are small and are found in a row along the lines of closure of the valve. Amyloid deposits may be found in the heart secondary to multiple myeloma, or as an isolated event, such as in senile cardiac amyloidosis. Grossly the walls of the heart may be thickened, and there may be multiple, small nodules on the left atrial endocardial surface. Iron overload can affect the heart as a result of hereditary hemochromatosis or hemosiderosis. Grossly the heart is a rust-brown color and resembles the heart in idiopathic dilated cardiomyopathy. In hypothyroidism the heart is characteristically flabby, enlarged, and dilated, which results in decreased cardiac output. This reduced circulation results in a characteristic symptom of hypothyroidism, cold sensitivity. Histologically there is an interstitial mucopolysaccharide edema fluid within the heart.

217. The answer is E. *(Robbins, 5/e, pp 520–523.)* The morphological changes of clinical congestive heart failure cannot always be correlated with necropsy findings of the heart because there may be hypertrophy, dilatation, a combination of both, or even an absence of both. Many patients with long-standing congestive heart failure after decompensation will have hearts that are maximally dilated, with thinned and unusually soft myocardium rather than hypertrophic ventricular myocardium. This thinning of the myocardium occurs after a long period of compensatory hypertrophy and reflects a state in which the capacity of the myocardium to compensate has been exceeded. The first response of the myocardium to a demand for increased work (load) is to undergo hypertrophy according to Starling's law, leading to an increase in stroke volume. Eventually, this mechanism is exceeded under states of increased oxygen demand or demand for more cardiac output, and cardiac decompensation results, with the worst complication being acute pulmonary edema as a consequence of left ventricular failure.

218. The answer is C. *(Robbins, 5/e, pp 560–561.)* The cardiomyopathy shown in the photograph is designated *hypertrophic cardiomyopathy* with the synonyms of *idiopathic hypertrophic subaortic stenosis (IHSS), hypertrophic obstructive cardiomyopathy,* and *asymmetric septal hypertrophy (ASH).* It is characterized by a prominent and hypertrophic interventricular septum that is out of proportion to the thickness of the left ventricle. Histologically the myocardial fibers have disarray, caused by wide fibers with unusual orientation, and prominent hyperchromatic nuclei. There is increased incidence within families and there is evidence that it may be an autosomal dominant disorder. Patients may have dyspnea, light-headedness, and chest pain, especially upon physical exertion; however, many patients appear to be asymptomatic although a sudden, unexpected death occurs not infrequently, especially following or during physical exertion. There may be abnormalities of the coronary arteries. The mitral valve may be thickened and patients may experience endocarditis on it. Cardiac output can be markedly reduced in some patients because of reduced volume of the left ventricle. As the patient ages, however, cardiac dilatation often improves the reduced left ventricular volume. Chronic alcoholism and a flabby, hypocontractile heart occur with dilated (congestive) cardiomyopathy.

219. The answer is C. *(Robbins, 5/e, pp 575–576. Rubin, 2/e, p 517.)* Tetralogy of Fallot consists of subaortic ventricular septal defect, obstruction to right ventricular outflow, aortic override of the ventricular septal defect (aortic dextroposition), and moderate right ventricular hypertrophy. The obstruction to right ventricular outflow may be caused by infundibular stenosis of the right ventricle or stenosis of the pulmonic valve. A right-sided aorta occurs in about 25 percent of cases with tetralogy. Most patients are cyanotic from birth or develop cyanosis by the end of the first year of life, since even mild obstruction to right ventricular outflow is progressive. Tetralogy of Fallot is the most common cause of cyanosis after 1 year of age and causes 10 percent of all forms of congenital heart disease. Hypoxic attacks and syncope are serious complications, forming the commonest mode of death from this disease during infancy and childhood. Other complications include infectious endocarditis, paradoxical embolism, polycythemia, and cerebral infarction or abscess.

220. The answer is D. *(Robbins, 5/e, pp 573–574. Rubin, 2/e, pp 514–515.)* Atrial septal defects (ASDs) are located in the atrial wall at different locations based on the development of the interatrial septum. The initial connection between the left and right atria (ostium primum) is closed starting at the fifth week of gestation by the septum primum, which extends down from the roof of the atrium to join with the inferior endocardial cushions. Before these form a complete septum, a second connection between the atria (ostium secundum) develops in the septum primum. A second septum (septum secundum) develops to the right of the septum primum and grows downward toward the endocardial cushions to close this ostium secundum. A patent foramen is left, however, at the midportion of the septum and is called the *foramen ovale.* This foramen is sealed off after birth and is then called the *fossa ovalis.* The most common ASD is the ostium secundum type, which is located in the middle portion of the septum at the level of the fossa ovalis. A combination of a septum secundum ASD with mitral stenosis is called Lutembacher's syndrome. Other types of ASDs may be located high in the atrial septum near the superior vena cava (sinus venosus defect) or low in the atrial septum (ostium primum type). A persistent AV canal combines atrial and ventricular septal defects.

221. The answer is E. *(Robbins, 5/e, pp 569–570. Rubin, 2/e, pp 551–552.)* Most tumors involving the heart are secondary to metastases, most commonly from bronchogenic carcinoma or breast carcinoma, and usually involve the pericardium. Primary tumors of the heart are quite rare; the most common in the adult is the myxoma. These tumors occur most often in the left atrium, and if pedunculated, they may interfere with the mitral valve by a "ball-valve" effect. Histologically they are composed of stellate cells in a loose myxoid background. Rhabdomyomas are the most common primary cardiac tumor in infants and children and often occur in association with tuberous sclerosis. Histologically, so-called spider cells may be seen. Papillary fibroelastomas usually are incidental lesions found at the time of autopsy and are probably hamartomas rather than true neoplasms.

222. The answer is C. *(Robbins, 5/e, pp 571–575. Rubin, 2/e, pp 511–515, 520.)* Congenital heart defects may or may not have shunting of blood between systemic and pulmonary circulations. Examples of defects with no shunts include coarctation of the aorta, Ebstein malformation (a downward displacement of an abnormal tricuspid valve into an underdeveloped right ventricle), and transposition of the great vessels. Examples of defects that initially involve a left-to-right shunt, from the higher pressure left side to the lower pressure right side, include ventricular septal defects (the most common of all heart defects), atrial septal defects, patent ductus arteriosus, and persistent truncus arteriosus. These defects initially are not cyanotic, but cyanosis may develop later (tardive cyanosis) if the shunt shifts to right to left because of increased pulmonary vascular resistsance (Eisenmenger complex). A defect that initially involves a right-to-left shunt is the tetralogy of Fallot. This is the most common cyanotic congenital heart disease of older children and adults.

223. The answer is D. *(Robbins, 5/e, pp 577–578.)* Coarctation of the aorta occurs in 6 to 14 percent of cases of congenital heart disease. In its infantile form, coarctation takes place in the root of the aorta proximal to the ductus arteriosus, which, if patent, serves as a bypass to allow blood flow to the arterial system. Usually, surgical intervention is necessary for infants who have this anomaly, which may cause death soon after birth or within the first year of life.

224–227. The answers are 224-A, 225-B, 226-A, 227-E. *(Robbins, 5/e, pp 557–562.)* The cardiomyopathies (CMP) may be classified into primary and secondary forms. The primary forms are mainly idiopathic (unknown cause). The causes of secondary CMP are many and range from alcoholism (probably the most common cause in the United States) to metabolic disorders to toxins and poisons. Whereas there are not many gross organ and microscopic anatomic features of CMP, a few rather characteristic hallmarks are well recognized in separating the types. However, extensive clinical, historical, and laboratory data contribute as much if not more to classification of the type of CMP present than does biopsy or even the postmortem heart examination.

Hypertrophic CMP encompasses those cases in which the major gross abnormality is to be found within the interventricular septum, which is usually thicker than the left ventricle. If there is obstruction of the ventricular outflow tract, there will be moderate hypertrophy in the left ventricles as well, but the septum usually remains thicker, yielding an appearance of asymmetric hypertrophy. This form of CMP occurs in families (rarely sporadically) and is thought to be autosomal dominant. Up to one-third of these patients have been known to die sudden cardiac deaths, often under conditions of physical exertion. Histologically, the myofibers interconnect at angles and are hypertrophied.

In dilated (which is also called *congestive*) CMP, the ventricular chambers are markedly dilated, with the walls either of normal thickness or thinner than normal. Whereas many idiopathic cases exist, some patients have a history of heavy alcohol intake. The microscopic appearance is not distinctive. The ventricles may have mural thrombi.

Constrictive (restrictive) CMP is associated in the United States with amyloidosis and endocardial fibroelastosis and is so named because the infiltration and deposition of amyloid in the endomyocardium and the layering of collagen and elastin over the endocardium affect the ability of the ventricles to accommodate blood volume during asystole. The heart is more likely to be involved secondarily if the systemic amyloidosis is associated with primary systemic or plasma cell tumors (myeloma). Endocardial fibroelastosis occurs mainly in infants and in the first 1 to 2 years of life and causes a prominent fibroelastic covering to form over the endocardium of the left ventricle. There may be associated aortic coarctation, ventricular septal defects, mitral valve defects, and other abnormalities.

Endomyocardial fibrosis is a form of restrictive CMP found mainly in young adults and children in Southeast Asia and Africa, where it accounts for a not insignificant number of deaths in these age groups. It differs from endocardial fibroelastosis in the United States in that elastic fibers are not present. Its cause is unknown.

228–230. The answers are 228-C, 229-D, 230-B. (*Anderson, 9/e, pp 650–652, 659–661, 778–780. Robbins, 5/e, pp 501, 547–550.*) Primary myocarditis, an isolated lesion that is not secondary to a generalized disease, is most commonly caused by such agents as type B coxsackievirus, echoviruses, and *Toxoplasma gondii*.

Streptococci are generally considered the causative agents of rheumatic fever; and although group A β-hemolytic streptococci are most strongly implicated, viruses continue to be suspected as among the causes of this systemic nonsuppurative inflammatory disease. Abundant evidence supports the view that antibodies generated in the immunologic reaction to infection with group A β-hemolytic streptococcus cross-react with myocardial fibers, smooth muscle cells, and connective tissue glycoproteins. Aschoff bodies, produced in response to this cross-reaction, are regarded as pathognomonic for rheumatic fever.

Aortic aneurysms of luetic carditis constitute the tertiary manifestation of syphilis and become evident 15 to 20 years after persons have contracted infection with *Treponema pallidum*. Elastic tissue and smooth muscle cells of the media undergo ischemic destruction as a result of the treponemal infection. As a consequence of ischemia in the media, musculoelastic support is lost, leading to aortic aneurysms, widening of the aortic valve ring, and narrowing of the coronary ostia. Syphilitic aneurysms are almost always located in the thoracic aorta.

Suppurative pericarditis is a form of acute pericarditis that can be caused by *Mycobacterium tuberculosis* and is considered to invariably denote entry into the pericardium of bacterial, mycotic, or parasitic agents. In the suppurative pericarditis caused by *M. tuberculosis* (tuberculous pericarditis), tuberculosis of the mediastinal nodes has been a finding in the majority of affected adults. Up to 500 mL of thick fluid (typical of caseation necrosis) that contains granulocytes, erythrocytes, and, in 50 percent of patients, tubercle bacilli may be found in the pericardium.

231–234. The answers are 231-D, 232-A, 233-B, 234-E. *(Anderson, 9/e, pp 774–775. Robbins, 5/e, pp 132–135, 493–495, 499, 936, 1312–1313. Rubin, 2/e, p 490.)* Berry aneurysms in the circle of Willis have been noted in about one-sixth of patients with adult polycystic renal disease. Subarachnoid hemorrhage from these, because of hypertension, accounts for death in about 10 percent of patients with adult polycystic renal disease.

Ehlers-Danlos syndromes (EDSs) are a group of eight syndromes characterized by defects in collagen synthesis. In EDS IV there is deficient synthesis of type III collagen and a tendency to rupture of muscular arteries, including dissecting aneurysms of the aorta. A high incidence of dissecting aneurysm also occurs in Marfan's syndrome and it may occur in coarctation of the aorta.

Both Takayasu's and Kawasaki's diseases (mucocutaneous lymph node syndrome) are examples of arteritis. Kawasaki's disease was first recognized in Japan, but there have been several outbreaks in the continental U.S. and in Hawaii. A skin rash, lymphadenopathy, arthritis, and arteritis are predominant. Coronary arteritis results in aneurysms and is associated with myocarditis and sometimes infarction. The disease characteristically affects boys under 4 years old.

Takayasu's arteritis, or "pulseless disease," is most common in young women and affects large and medium arteries, especially the aorta and its larger branches. Aneurysms are common in the abdominal and distal thoracic aorta, especially in older patients. There may be thrombosis of vessels that arise from the aortic arch and many cases demonstrate the aortic arch syndrome. Marked weakening of the pulses in the upper extremities is noted. This arteritis has been known as *aortic arch syndrome, primary aortitis,* and *giant cell arteritis of the aorta,* in addition to other synonyms. Arterioscler-otic aneurysms are also common in the abdominal aorta; syphilitic aneurysm is practically limited to the thoracic segment.

Respiratory System

DIRECTIONS: Each question below contains five suggested responses. Select the **one best** response to each question.

235. Shown in the photomicrograph below is a section of alveolar tissue that was taken at autopsy of a 4-day-old premature infant. The pathologic process that is evident is consistent with

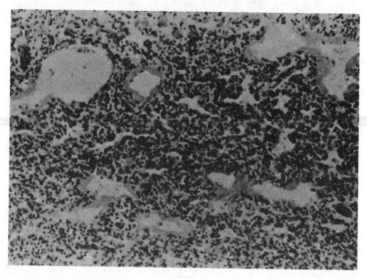

(A) pneumococcal pneumonia
(B) congenital pulmonary cystic malformation
(C) extralobar pulmonary sequestration
(D) primary fungal pneumonitis
(E) respiratory distress syndrome (hyaline membrane disease)

236. All the following conditions can produce a histopathologic condition in the lungs of adults that is similar to the histopathology of respiratory distress syndrome of the newborn (hyaline membrane disease) EXCEPT

(A) viral pneumonia
(B) uremia
(C) pulmonary irradiation
(D) severe bacterial infection
(E) tuberculosis

237. A young woman succumbed after an 8-month course of severe dyspnea, fatigue, and cyanosis that followed an uneventful delivery of a healthy infant. At necropsy, small atheromas were present in the large and small branches of the pulmonary arteries. Which of the following findings can be predicted in the histologic slides of the lungs?

(A) Diffuse hemorrhage and infarctions
(B) Diffuse alveolar hyaline membranes
(C) Severe atelectasis and edema
(D) Marked medial hypertrophy of pulmonary arterioles
(E) Multiple pulmonary emboli

238. Alpha$_1$-antitrypsin deficiency is associated with

(A) thalassemia
(B) nephrotic syndrome
(C) panlobular emphysema
(D) centrilobular emphysema
(E) anthracosis

239. A 24-year-old man who is being evaluated for infertility complains of recurrent sinusitis and a productive cough. He is found to be sterile, and situs inversus of his organs is noted. The most likely diagnosis for his pulmonary disease is

(A) asthma
(B) bronchiolitis
(C) bronchiectasis
(D) chronic bronchitis
(E) emphysema

240. All the following are presently used clinically for the diagnosis of sarcoidosis EXCEPT

(A) chest x-ray
(B) Kveim skin test
(C) conjunctival biopsy
(D) cultures of affected tissue
(E) blood levels of angiotensin-converting enzyme

241. The major pathologic injury in interstitial lung disease is generally accepted to be

(A) diffuse pneumonia
(B) bronchopneumonia
(C) bronchiolitis
(D) bronchitis
(E) alveolitis

242. Horner's syndrome is associated with

(A) lymphangitis carcinomatosa
(B) bronchial carcinoid
(C) exophthalmos
(D) tumor of the superior sulcus
(E) thoracocervical venous dilatation

243. The organism that is most likely to cause the necrotizing pulmonary lesion shown in the photomicrograph below is

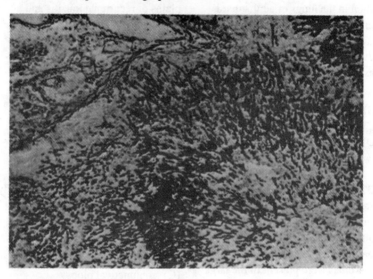

(A) *Pseudomonas aeruginosa*
(B) *Mycobacterium tuberculosis*
(C) *Pneumocystis carinii*
(D) *Trichinella spiralis*
(E) *Candida albicans*

---

244. Common tumors or cysts in the superior mediastinum include

(A) schwannoma
(B) bronchogenic cyst
(C) thymoma
(D) neurofibroma
(E) pericardial cyst

245. The most common benign tumor of the lung is the

(A) fibroma
(B) hemangioma
(C) hamartoma
(D) leiomyoma
(E) carcinoid

246. Which of the following bronchogenic carcinomas is most frequently associated with production of parathormone-like substances?

(A) Acinar adenocarcinoma
(B) Papillary adenocarcinoma
(C) Bronchioloalveolar carcinoma
(D) Squamous cell carcinoma
(E) Oat cell carcinoma

247. Acute lymphoblastic leukemia was diagnosed in a 10-year-old child. When this child later developed a patchy pulmonary infiltrate and respiratory insufficiency, a lung biopsy was performed. The material obtained by biopsy was then stained with Gomori's methenamine-silver stain and is shown in the photomicrograph below. In consideration of the patient's signs and microscopic evaluations, the prognosis is now complicated by

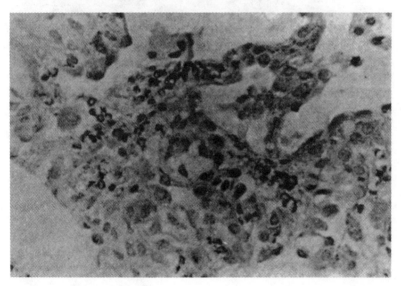

(A) *Pseudomonas* pneumonia
(B) *Aspergillus* pneumonia
(C) *Pneumocystis carinii* pneumonia
(D) pneumococcal pneumonia
(E) influenza pneumonia

248. The photomicrograph of the bronchial washing specimen shown below depicts

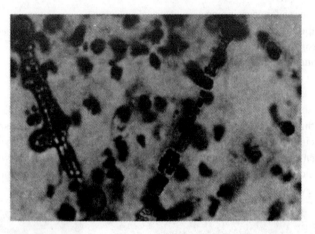

(A) Schaumann bodies
(B) ferruginous bodies
(C) cholesterol crystals
(D) *Candida* species
(E) silica particles

249. A 45-year-old man presents with shortness of breath, cough with mucoid sputum, and some weight loss and has diffuse, bilateral alveolar infiltrates on chest roentgenogram. Pulmonary function tests reveal decreased diffusing capacity and hypoxemia. The patient had worked for several years at grinding aluminum. The photomicrograph below is from a lung biopsy. Your diagnosis is

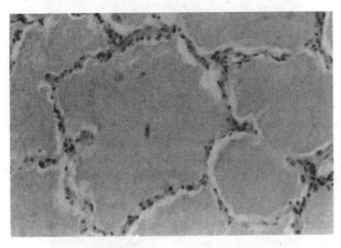

(A) *Pneumocystis carinii* pneumonia
(B) diffuse alveolar damage (DAD)
(C) pulmonary edema
(D) pulmonary alveolar proteinosis (PAP)
(E) lipid pneumonia

250. The condition seen below in the gross photograph of a sagittal section of the lung may occur in which of the following?

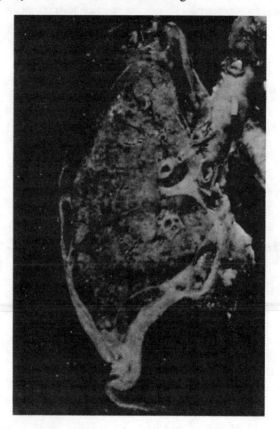

(A) Squamous cell carcinoma
(B) Oat cell carcinoma
(C) Metastatic carcinoma
(D) Benign spindle cell mesothelioma
(E) Malignant mesothelioma

DIRECTIONS: Each group of questions below consists of lettered headings followed by a set of numbered items. For each numbered item select the **one** lettered heading with which it is **most** closely associated. Each lettered heading may be used **once, more than once, or not at all.**

Questions 251–254

Match the most characteristic finding with each respiratory disorder.

(A) Neurosecretory granules
(B) Fungal infection
(C) Hemorrhagic interstitial pneumonitis
(D) Nasal mucosal ulcerations
(E) Asthmatic bronchitis

251. Wegener's granulomatosis

252. Oat cell carcinoma

253. Byssinosis

254. Goodpasture's syndrome

Questions 255–256

For each tumor, choose its most common site of origin.

(A) Nasal cavity
(B) Neuroendocrine cells of bronchi
(C) Submucosal bronchial glands
(D) Terminal bronchioles
(E) Bronchial blood vessels

255. Bronchial carcinoid

256. Bronchioloalveolar carcinoma

Questions 257–259

Match the pathologic or clinical findings with the appropriate organism.

(A) *Coccidioides immitis*
(B) Pathogenic staphylococci
(C) Group B streptococcus
(D) *Nocardia asteroides*
(E) *Legionella pneumophila*

257. Intracytoplasmic bacilli seen with silver stains

258. Acid-fast and aerobic presentation

259. Scalded skin syndrome

Respiratory System
Answers

235.   The answer is E.   *(Anderson, 9/e, pp 838–839, 925–926. Robbins, 5/e, pp 444–446.)* The photomicrograph shows classic hyaline membranes that are coating alveolar sacs and ducts and is diagnostic of the respiratory distress syndrome of the newborn. The eosinophilic, fibrinlike material is related to the alveolar surfactants. Atelectasis is usually also present, especially in premature infants. The deposited material appears not to form in utero, as it is found in infants who have breathed and is not found in stillborns. There is a direct correlation, however, between severity and the degree of prematurity.

236.   The answer is E.   *(Anderson, 9/e, pp 925–926, 960–962. Robbins, 5/e, pp 676–679.)* The presence of hyaline membranes indicates a diagnosis of acute alveolar injury, which can occur in all the conditions mentioned except tuberculosis. Indeed, the alveoli-lining, fibrinlike material may be found in multiple conditions of circulatory compromise and in poor perfusion states, such as hypovolemia; it may also be seen where 100% oxygen has been used for longer than 32 h (e.g., "shock lung" of Vietnam casualties). At autopsy, the lungs are relatively airless and heavy, and this finding is frequently accompanied by pulmonary edema and hemorrhage.

237.   The answer is D.   *(Robbins, 5/e, pp 680–682.)* Many pathologic pulmonary changes can be found in the lungs of patients who expire under conditions of progressive, unexplained dyspnea, fatigue, and cyanosis. These changes range from pulmonary fibrosis to hypersensitivity pneumonitis and to recurrent, multiple pulmonary emboli. Furthermore, traditional hospital treatment modalities for progressive pulmonary deterioration (including high oxygen delivery, overhydration, lack of pulmonary ventilation, irregular ventilation by mechanical respiratory assistance [PEEP], and superimposed nosocomially acquired pneumonitis) can complicate pulmonary pathologic findings. However, unremitting, progressive dyspnea, cyanosis, and fatigue in a young woman should suggest the diagnosis of primary pulmonary hypertension. Pulmonary vascular sclerosis is always associated with pulmonary hypertension primary or secondary to other states, such as emphysema and mitral stenosis.

238. The answer is C. *(Robbins, 5/e, pp 683–688.)* Patients who are homozygous for alpha$_1$-antitrypsin deficiency develop severe panlobular emphysema, often before the age of 40. This genetic disorder accounts for about 10 percent of cases of emphysema. Other factors in the pathogenesis of emphysema include air pollution and smoking. This disorder may result from variant alleles involving the Pi (proteinase inhibitor) locus on chromosome 14. Cigarette smoking greatly accelerates the emphysema in the homozygous (Pi ZZ) state.

239. The answer is C. *(Robbins, 5/e, pp 682–694.)* Chronic obstructive pulmonary disease (COPD) is a term that refers to a group of disorders characterized by dyspnea and airway obstruction. The spectrum of COPD includes all the diseases listed in the question. Patients with bronchiectasis have a persistent, productive cough due to abnormally dilated bronchi, which are the result of a chronic necrotizing infection. Patients with Kartagener's syndrome have the triad of bronchiectasis, recurrent sinusitis, and situs inversus. This syndrome is caused by abnormal motility of the cilia, which is due to abnormalities of the dynein arms. Males with this condition tend to be sterile because of the ineffective motility of the tail of the sperm. Patients with asthma suffer from episodic wheezing due to bronchial smooth muscle hyperplasia and excess production of mucus. Extrinsic (allergic) asthma may be related to IgE (type I) immune reactions; intrinsic (nonallergic) asthma may be triggered by infections or drugs. Clinically there is an elevated eosinophil count in the peripheral blood, and Curschmann's spirals and Charcot-Leyden crystals may be found in the sputum. Chronic bronchitis is characterized by a productive cough that is present for at least 3 months in at least 2 consecutive years. There is hyperplasia of mucous glands with hypersecretion due in large part to tobacco smoke. Emphysema is abnormal dilation of the alveoli due to destruction of the alveolar walls. Bronchiolitis is inflammation and scarring of bronchioles due mainly to tobacco smoke and air pollutants.

240. The answer is B. *(Henry, 18/e, p 274. Lever, 7/e, pp 252–256. Robbins, 5/e, pp 712–714.)* Sarcoidosis is a systemic disease characterized by noncaseating granulomas in multiple organs. The diagnosis of sarcoidosis depends upon finding these noncaseating granulomas in commonly affected sites. In 90 percent of cases, bilateral hilar lymphadenopathy or lung involvement is present and can be seen by chest x-ray or transbronchial biopsy. The eye and skin are next most commonly affected, so that both conjunctival and skin biopsies are clinical possibilities. Noncaseating granulomas may be found in multiple infectious diseases, such as fungal infections, but sarcoidosis is not caused by any known organism. Therefore, before the diagnosis of sarcoidosis can be made, cultures must be taken from affected tissues, and there must be no growth of any organism that may produce granulomas. Also in patients with sarcoid, blood levels of angiotensin-converting enzyme are increased, and this may be used as a clinical test. In the past, the Kveim skin test was used to assist in the diagnosis of sarcoid, but since it involves injecting into patients extracts of material from humans, it is no longer used.

241. The answer is E. *(Robbins, 5/e, pp 703–706.)* In diffuse interstitial lung disease (ILD) the early and major event is damage to the alveolar walls. First, an interstitial inflammation affects mainly the septae (interstitial alveolitis) with edema of the alveolar walls and an infiltrate of lymphocytes and monocyte-macrophages. The alveolar lining cells (mostly type I) are injured or become necrotic and are replaced by proliferating type II cells creating a cuboidal epithelial lining; alveolar endothelial cells are also injured, allowing exudation of fluid into the interstitium. If reversal does not occur, the changes become chronic with eventual fibrous scarring of alveolar walls, impaired respiratory function, and pulmonary hypertension. Causes of ILD include occupational exposure to inorganic dust (asbestos, silica), gases, aerosols, and organic dust, in addition to drugs (bleomycin, busulfan, nitrofurantoin) and infections (cytomegalovirus and tuberculosis). The major interstitial lung diseases of unknown cause include sarcoidosis and idiopathic pulmonary fibrosis (Hamman-Rich syndrome).

242. The answer is D. *(Robbins, 5/e, pp 571, 725.)* Horner's syndrome occurs with apical (superior sulcus) tumors of any type (Pancoast tumor). The syndrome is characterized by enophthalmos, ptosis, miosis, and anhidrosis on the same side as the lesion due to invasion of the cervical sympathetic nerves. Involvement of the brachial plexus causes pain and paralysis in the ulnar nerve distribution. Venous dilatation of the upper thorax and neck is seen in the superior vena cava syndrome because of compression or invasion by lung cancer or lymphoma. Lymphangitic carcinomatosis usually results from spread of metastatic tumors within subpleural lymphatics.

243. The answer is E. *(Anderson, 9/e, pp 411–413.)* Gomori's methenamine-silver staining technique emphasizes the pseudohyphae and yeast forms of *Candida* species. The pattern of vessel invasion is characteristic of many pathogenic fungi, including *Candida.* Such infections tend to occur in immunologically suppressed patients with other severe, usually neoplastic, diseases.

244. The answer is C. *(Robbins, 5/e, pp 727–728.)* The superior mediastinum consists of structures cephalad to the pericardial reflection of the heart. Metastatic carcinoma is fairly frequent in the superior mediastinum, arising often from lung or breast primaries, and less frequently from testis or kidney. Bronchogenic and pericardial cysts occur in the middle mediastinum, whereas neurogenic tumors such as neurofibroma and schwannoma are in the posterior mediastinum. Thymoma is found in the anterosuperior mediastinum. Lymphoma, especially Hodgkin's disease, is common in all mediastinal compartments and involves paratracheal lymph nodes in the superior mediastinum. Seminoma and metastatic choriocarcinoma from the testis are not uncommon. Parathyroid tumors and thyroid lesions occupy both the superior and anterior mediastinum. Retrosternal extension of a goiter, presenting as a superior mediastinal mass, is not unusual.

245. The answer is C. *(Anderson, 9/e, pp 573, 1015–1017, 1020–1021. Robbins, 5/e, pp 726–727.)* Pulmonary hamartomas, although infrequent, are still the most common of all benign lung tumors. Hamartomas consist of various tissues normally found in the organ where they develop, but in abnormal amounts and arrangement. In the lung, they consist of lobules of connective tissue often containing mature cartilage, fat, or fibrous tissue and separated by clefts lined by entrapped respiratory epithelium. The peak incidence is at age 60, and the tumor is usually found as a well-circumscribed, peripheral, "coin" lesion on routine chest x-ray. Unless the radiographic findings are . pathognomonic of hamartoma with "popcorn ball" calcifications, the lesion should be excised or at least carefully followed. Conservative excision is curative.

Bronchial carcinoids are tumors of low-grade malignancy with neuroendocrine differentiation confirmed by immunostaining for neuron-specific enolase, serotonin, calcitonin, or bombesin. They form intrabronchial polypoid growths but most of the tumor mass lies outside the bronchus. Most arise in central bronchi but 20 percent arise in small bronchi and appear as peripheral lung nodules. Surgical excision is curative in at least 90 percent, but 10 percent of carcinoids are aggressive with local invasion or metastases.

246. The answer is D. *(Robbins, 5/e, pp 295–296, 724–725.)* Squamous cell carcinoma, the most frequent type of bronchogenic carcinoma (25 to 30 percent), is the type most often associated with hypercalcemia. The hypercalcemia may be related to osteolytic bone metastases, but hypercalcemia as a paraneoplastic syndrome may occur in the absence of skeletal metastases. This form of hypercalcemia is caused by tumor production of parathormone-like substances, or prostaglandin E, or other calcium-mobilizing tumor products such as growth factors involved in the histogenesis of the tumor. These probably bind to the parathyroid hormone receptors in bone to mimic the calcium-mobilizing action of parathormone. Hypercalcemia is rare with oat cell tumors, which are much more likely to produce ACTH-like (Cushing's syndrome) or ADH-like substances.

247. The answer is C. *(Anderson, 9/e, p 948. Robbins, 5/e, p 357.)* Infection by the protozoan *Pneumocystis carinii* is characterized by the presence of oval and helmet-shaped organisms whose capsules are made more visible by use of Gomori's methenamine-silver staining technique. This organism, although it has low virulence, is opportunistic; it is often seen to attack severely ill, immunologically depressed patients. It is frequently the first opportunistic infection to be diagnosed in HIV-1 positive patients, and it is the leading cause of death in patients with AIDS.

248. The answer is B. *(Anderson, 9/e, pp 235, 587, 1003. Robbins, 5/e, pp 709–714.)* The segmented or beaded, often dumbbell-shaped bodies are ferruginous bodies that are probably asbestos fibers coated with iron and protein. The term *ferruginous body* is applied to other inhaled fibers that become iron-coated; however, in a patient with interstitial lung fibrosis or pleural plaques, ferruginous bodies are probably asbestos bodies. The type of asbestos mainly used in America is chrysotile, mined in Canada, and it is much less likely to cause mesothelioma or lung cancer than is crocidolite (blue asbestos), which has limited use and is mined in South Africa. Cigarette smoking potentiates the relatively mild carcinogenic effect of asbestos. Laminated spherical (Schaumann) bodies are found in granulomas of sarcoid and chronic berylliosis.

249. The answer is D. *(Robbins, 5/e, pp 718–719. Rubin, 2/e, pp 580–581.)* The alveolar spaces contain an intensely eosinophilic, proteinaceous, granular substance. Alveolar walls are relatively normal without inflammatory exudate or fibrosis, although type II pneumocytes may be hyperplastic. The process is often patchy, with groups of normal alveoli alternating with groups of affected alveoli. Acicular (cholesterol) clefts and densely eosinophilic bodies (necrotic cells) are found within the granular material. Distinction from edema fluid may be difficult, but PAP alveolar material stains with periodic acid–Schiff (PAS). At low power, alveolar material seen in *P. carinii* pneumonia may also mimic PAP, but with high power the foamy material seen with *Pneumocystis* is not present in PAP. In PAP the material is surfactant accumulation, either because of overproduction or failure of macrophage clearance. Causes of PAP include occupational exposure to silica or aluminum dusts. It also occurs in immunosuppressed patients and toxic drug reactions and is often associated with infections like nocardia, fungi, and TB (possible impaired macrophage killing). The treatment of choice is bronchoalveolar lavage to remove the proteinaceous debris.

250. The answer is E. *(Robbins, 5/e, pp 730–732.)* Malignant mesothelioma and adenocarcinoma are two neoplasms that may involve the pleural surfaces as seen in the gross photograph. Malignant mesothelioma arises from the pleural surfaces and develops with significant and chronic exposure to asbestos, usually occupationally incurred. As the malignant mesothelioma spreads, it lines the pleural surfaces including the fissures through the lobes of the lungs and results in a tight and constricting encasement. This restricts the excursions of the lungs during ventilation. Adenocarcinoma of the lung also may invade the pleural surfaces and spread in an advancing manner throughout the pleural lining. The differential diagnosis histologically between an epithelial type of malignant mesothelioma and an adenocarcinoma may be difficult and sometimes impossible without special techniques. A characteristic feature seen by electron microscopy is numerous, long microvilli on the surface of cells from mesotheliomas. Oat cell carcinoma usually arises in the central portions of the lungs near the hilum and does not invade the pleura in a spreading fashion. Benign spindle (fibrous) mesothelioma of the lung arises as a discrete mass that is spherical to ovoid in shape in a subpleural configuration and expands as this localized mass without spread over the surfaces.

251–254. The answers are 251-D, 252-A, 253-E, 254-C. *(Anderson, 9/e, p 1013. Robbins, 5/e, pp 496–497, 716–718, 723.)* Oat cell carcinomas, which are of neuroendocrine origin and display neurosecretory granules on electron microscopy, may cause a variety of syndromes, some from direct synthesis of hormones such as ACTH and serotonin. Other effects, not well understood, on the neuromuscular system include central encephalopathy and Eaton-Lambert syndrome, a myasthenic syndrome resulting from impaired release of acetylcholine and usually associated with pulmonary oat cell carcinoma. Oat cell carcincomas form 20 to 25 percent of primary lung tumors, occur most frequently in middle-aged or older men, have a strong association with cigarette smoking, and carry a poor prognosis.

Both Wegener's granulomatosis, a syndrome of necrotizing vasculitis with necrotizing granulomas of nasopharynx and lung, and Goodpasture's syndrome, a disease produced by autoantibodies directed against basement membranes, typically involve both the lung and kidney. Goodpasture's syndrome is characterized by development of a necrotizing hemorrhagic interstitial pneumonitis and rapidly progressing glomerulonephritis because of antibodies directed against the capillary basement membrane in alveolar septae and glomeruli. Prognosis for Goodpasture's syndrome has been markedly improved by intensive plasma exchange to remove circulating antibasement membrane antibodies and by immunosuppressive therapy to inhibit further antibody production. In Wegener's granulomatosis, the nose, sinus, antrum, and trachea often exhibit ulcerations. Originally lethal, prognosis is now much improved by immunosuppressive drugs.

Byssinosis, which is caused by inhalation of cotton, flax, or hemp dust, takes the form of an asthmatic bronchitis, rather than involving distal lung structures, as with other organic dusts that cause extrinsic allergic alveolitis. Prolonged exposure causes chronic lung disease with chronic bronchitis, emphysema, and interstitial granulomas.

255–256. The answers are 255-B, 256-D. *(Anderson, 9/e, p 1017. Robbins, 5/e, pp 725–727.)* Bronchial carcinoids form about 5 percent of lung tumors. Sex incidence is equal and many patients are under 40 years of age. No relation to cigarette smoking or environmental factors is known. The origin is the neuroendocrine argentaffin cells of bronchial mucosa (Kultschitzsky cells). The carcinoid syndrome (diarrhea, facial flushing, and cyanosis) rarely occurs in disease confined to the lung. Carcinoid belongs to the group of amine precursor uptake and decarboxylation (APUD) tumors.

Bronchioloalveolar carcinoma, a form of adenocarcinoma, arises from terminal bronchioles and extends to line alveolar spaces throughout peripheral lung tissue, often causing a pneumonia-like picture grossly and radiologically. Ultrastructurally it consists of mucin-secreting bronchiolar cells, Clara cells, and, rarely, type II pneumocytes.

Adenoid cystic carcinoma may arise at any level of the respiratory tract where there are mucous glands and is the most common tumor in the upper third of the trachea. Histopathologic appearance is similar to that of adenoid cystic carcinoma of minor salivary glands with a cribriform, lacelike pattern of either duct-lining secretory cells or myoepithelial cells. Pools of mucoid material are actually extracellular matrix.

Nasopharyngeal angiofibroma is a highly vascular tumor that can cause heavy bleeding and occurs in young males. Other rare, but distinctive nasal tumors include isolated plasmacytoma, lymphoepithelioma, olfactory neuroblastoma (esthesioneuroblastoma), inverted papilloma, and carcinomas of epidermoid and transitional cell types.

257–259. The answers are 257-E, 258-D, 259-B. *(Isselbacher, 13/e, pp 611–617, 621–622, 654–658, 696–698, 857–858.)* Legionnaire's disease is caused by the soil organism *Legionella pneumophila*, a weakly gram-negative aerobic bacillus (Legionellaceae, of over 25 species). The disease results from inhalation of infectious aerosols from hot water or air-conditioning systems of buildings (including hospitals); these aerosols contain legionellae, which are deposited in the lung alveoli. Legionellosis ranges from the fulminant pneumonia of Legionnaire's disease (first recognized in Philadelphia, 1976) to the mild, flulike Pontiac fever. Diarrhea, nausea, and vomiting are early symptoms as well as headache, fever, and often delirium. Chest x-ray shows dense infiltrates with pulmonary gross findings of a confluent bronchopneumonia with alveoli containing neutrophils and mononuclear phagocytes with many intracytoplasmic bacilli that may be seen by silver staining. Organisms are also detected by immunofluorescent staining and culture of lung tissue, pleural fluid, or transtracheal aspirate, but not sputum culture since other organisms overgrow legionellae. Erythromycin is the favored therapy.

Nocardia (Nocardia asteroides) and *Actinomyces* are classified as filamentous soil bacteria, although they are often described among the fungi. Nocardiae are aerobic and acid-fast in contrast to *Actinomyces,* which are strict anaerobes and not acid-fast. Inhaled nocardial bacteria produce lung or skin infections; progressive pneumonia with purulent sputum and abscesses is suggestive of nocardiosis, especially if dissemination to brain or subcutaneous tissue occurs. Patients developing nocardiosis are often immunosuppressed, and transplant rejection, steroid therapy, AIDS, and alveolar proteinosis are often antecedent. Organisms in sputum, pus, or bronchial lavage specimens are gram-positive. A modified acid-fast stain should be used for diagnosis. Actinomycosis has cervicofacial, abdominal, thoracic, and pelvic (some IUD use) forms and occurs in normal hosts, though trauma and devitalized tissues play a part. Both *Nocardia* and *Actinomyces* cause abscesses and the actinomycotic abscess contains yellow bacterial colonies ("sulfur granules"). *Nocardia* and *Actinomyces* both belong to the order Actinomycetales.

Coccidioidomycosis, caused by inhalation of *C. immitis* arthrospores from airborne dust, is prevalent in California (San Joaquin Valley), Arizona, West Texas, and New Mexico. Pulmonary infection with infiltrate, hilar adenopathy, or pleural effusion is prominent and may become chronic and progressive with dissemination to bone, skin, and meninges. This occurs in less than 1 percent of cases.

Factors that contribute to staphylococcal pathogenicity include production of coagulase, catalase, enterotoxin, and exotoxin. Some strains of coagulase-positive staphylococci (*S. aureus*) produce exotoxins that cause skin lesions (scalded skin syndrome) or multisystem dysfunction, as in toxic shock syndrome in which rash, fever, and hypotension are present. Coagulase and catalase help to protect staphylococci from destruction by phagocytosis. Some strains produce an enterotoxin that causes gastrointestinal disease.

Streptococcus agalactiae (group B) is associated with urinary tract infections, as well as neonatal pneumonia, meningitis, and sepsis.

Gastrointestinal System

DIRECTIONS: Each question below contains five suggested responses. Select the **one best** response to each question.

260. The lesion seen in the photomicrograph below is referred to as

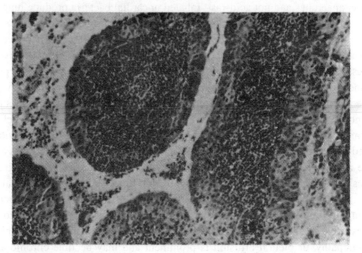

(A) adenoid cystic carcinoma
(B) lymphoepithelioma
(C) thyroglossal duct neoplasm
(D) Warthin's tumor
(E) sebaceous lymphadenoma

261. Carcinoma of the oral cavity

(A) is predominantly adenocarcinoma in type
(B) is more common in females
(C) is predisposed to by hairy leukoplasia
(D) is predisposed to by erythroplasia
(E) occurs most frequently on the hard palate

262. The photomicrograph below shows an esophageal biopsy taken 10 cm above the lower esophageal sphincter. The condition illustrated

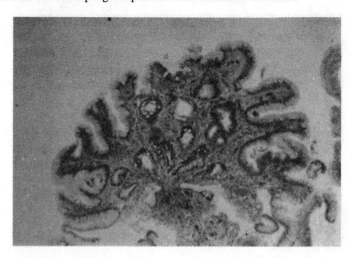

(A) is usually congenital in origin
(B) results from loss of esophageal myenteric ganglion cells
(C) is seen as a white patch at endoscopy
(D) increases the risk of carcinoma by a factor of 30 to 40
(E) is a common precursor of squamous cell carcinoma

---

263. Tumors of the salivary glands are correctly characterized by which of the following statements?

(A) They are principally mesenchymal in origin
(B) They metastasize early and pursue a rapid course when malignant
(C) They tend to have a similar clinical presentation regardless of histologic pattern
(D) They are less often malignant in the minor salivary glands than in the parotid
(E) They are more common in children than adults

264. A 45-year-old male alcoholic vomits blood and is hypotensive. The most likely cause of his bleeding episode is related to

(A) achalasia
(B) Plummer-Vinson syndrome
(C) sliding hiatal hernia
(D) Zenker's diverticula
(E) esophageal varices

265. All the following statements regarding *Helicobacter pylori* gastritis as illustrated in the photomicrograph below are true EXCEPT

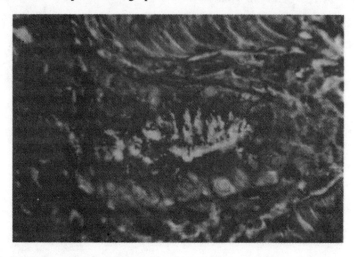

(A) it is present in the majority of patients with duodenal ulceration
(B) the inflammatory infiltrate is characteristically rich in eosinophils
(C) tissue invasion by microorganisms is inconspicuous
(D) organisms are absent from areas of intestinal metaplasia
(E) urease is an important virulence factor of *H. pylori*

---

266. All the following statements regarding carcinoma of the esophagus are true EXCEPT

(A) most carcinomas arising in the body of the esophagus are squamous
(B) squamous carcinomas begin as lesions in situ
(C) patients with Barrett's esophagus have approximately a 10 percent risk of carcinoma
(D) the most common morphological form is a polypoid fungating mass
(E) distant metastases are frequently present at the time of diagnosis

267. A 2-week-old infant presents with regurgitation and persistent, severe vomiting. An abdominal mass is felt during physical examination. The most likely diagnosis is

(A) congenital aganglionic megacolon
(B) congenital pyloric stenosis
(C) esophageal atresia
(D) hypertrophic gastropathy
(E) diaphragmatic hernia

268. All the following statements regarding the condition illustrated below are true EXCEPT

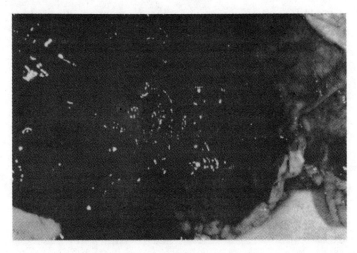

(A) over 95 percent of cases occur in the stomach or duodenum
(B) cases associated with Zollinger-Ellison syndrome are frequently atypical in location
(C) duodenal ulceration is associated with *H. pylori* infection
(D) gastric ulceration is associated with hypersecretion of acid
(E) size of gastric ulcer is not an accurate predictor of malignant potential

---

269. A 10-month old, previously healthy, male infant develops a severe, watery diarrhea 2 days after visiting the pediatrician for a routine checkup. The most likely diagnosis is

(A) rotavirus infection
(B) enterotoxogenic *E. coli* infection
(C) *Entamoeba histolytica* infection
(D) lactase deficiency
(E) ulcerative colitis

270. True statements regarding celiac disease (nontropical sprue) include that

(A) there is a strong association with HLA-B8 and HLA-DQw2 antigens
(B) severity of disease often correlates strongly with serum level of antibody to gliadin
(C) malignancy is unassociated
(D) many of the mucosal inflammatory cells express surface IgG antigliadin
(E) the distal small bowel shows the most severe involvement

271. Gastric tumors with the histologic appearance illustrated in the photomicrograph below

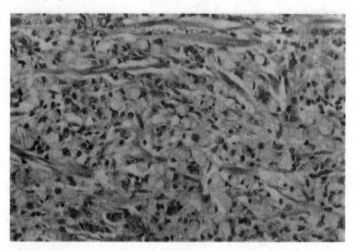

(A) usually fall into the category of early gastric carcinoma
(B) are most commonly located in the cardia
(C) often show a marked desmoplastic response
(D) carry a favorable prognosis
(E) belong to the category of neuroendocrine tumors

272. All the following statements concerning carcinoma of the stomach are true EXCEPT

(A) diffusely infiltrative carcinoma is associated with a striking desmoplastic reaction
(B) *early gastric carcinoma (EGC)* is synonymous with *carcinoma in situ*
(C) over 50 percent of gastric carcinomas are found in the pylorus and antrum
(D) there is a striking geographic variation in death rate from gastric carcinoma
(E) the death rate from gastric carcinoma has been decreasing for decades

273. The appearance of the small intestinal mucosa illustrated in the photomicrograph below indicates

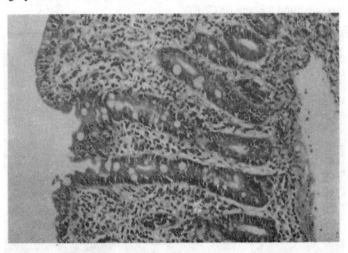

(A) small intestinal lymphoma
(B) Whipple's disease
(C) celiac disease
(D) Crohn's disease
(E) *Giardia lamblia* infestation

274. A 25-year-old schoolteacher was well until she attended a church bazaar where she heartily ate barbecued turkey. The following day she developed bloody diarrhea, crampy pain, and tenesmus. A gastroenterologist who did not take a history took a colon biopsy specimen that showed mucosal edema, congestion, and numerous lymphoid cells in the lamina propria. Which of the following differential diagnoses would apply?

(A) Staphylococcal gastroenteritis vs. Crohn's disease
(B) Viral gastroenteritis vs. acute diverticulitis
(C) Colonic endometriosis vs. amebic dysentery
(D) Early ulcerative colitis vs. salmonella colitis
(E) Bleeding hemorrhoids vs. Meckel's diverticulitis

275. The photomicrograph below shows the colonic wall 30 cm from the anal margin in a man with severe bloody diarrhea. All the statements regarding this condition are true EXCEPT

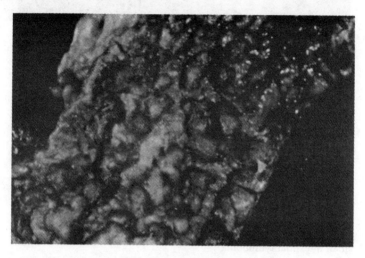

(A) inflammation is usually limited to the lamina propria
(B) multiple crypt abscesses are commonly seen
(C) atypical cytologic changes occur in the mucosa
(D) granulomas occur in the mucosa
(E) "skip" lesions are not present

276. Two subtotal colectomy specimens are sent to the laboratory with both showing a hemorrhagic cobblestone appearance of the mucosa. One, however, shows longitudinal grooving of the surface, which suggests

(A) ischemic bowel disease
(B) multiple polyposis syndrome
(C) ulcerative colitis
(D) Crohn's disease
(E) intestinal tuberculosis

277. A distinguishing feature when comparing ulcerative colitis with Crohn's disease is

(A) colonic involvement
(B) possible malignant transformation
(C) arthritis
(D) fistula formation
(E) absence of granulomas

278. The abnormality of the ileum illustrated below

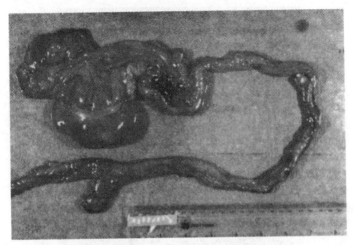

(A) is present in approximately 20 percent of normal persons
(B) is lined by heterotopic gastric mucosa in less than 2 percent of cases
(C) often shows mucosal ulceration
(D) is related to a persistence of the vitello-intestinal duct
(E) usually arises from the mesenteric border of the ileum

---

279. All the following statements concerning carcinoma of the colorectum are true EXCEPT

(A) 95 percent of all carcinomas of the colorectum are adenocarcinoma
(B) mucin secretion aids extension of the primary malignancy
(C) left-sided lesions tend to grow as polypoid fungating masses
(D) serum levels of carcinoembryonic antigen (CEA) are directly related to tumor size
(E) almost all carcinomas of the colorectum begin within adenomatous polyps

280. A 65-year-old man presents with episodes of facial flushing exacerbated by alcohol and associated with severe diarrhea. All the following findings may be expected on further investigation EXCEPT

(A) increased urinary levels of 5-hydroxyindoleacetic acid (5-HIAA)
(B) increased blood levels of 5-hydroxytryptamine (5-HT)
(C) areas of decreased uptake on liver scintillation scan
(D) right-sided cardiac valvular disease
(E) a small yellow nodule in the tip of the appendix

281. The lesion shown in the colon in the photograph below

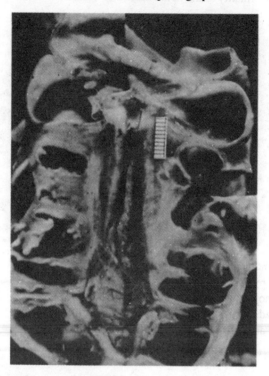

(A) is most prevalent under 50 years of age
(B) occurs most often in the ascending and transverse segments when it occurs in the colon
(C) occurs more often in the small intestine than the colon
(D) is more common in males
(E) is premalignant

282. Familial polyposis coli is characterized by

(A) autosomal recessive pattern of inheritance
(B) multiple hamartomatous polyps throughout the colon
(C) 100 percent risk of carcinoma
(D) an association with fibromatosis and multiple osteomas
(E) an association with tumors of the central nervous system

283. In the photograph below, an ulcerated mucosal lesion is shown at the anorectal junction. This lesion is

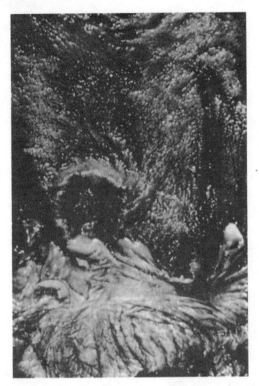

(A) a hemorrhoid
(B) a basaloid carcinoma
(C) a villous adenoma
(D) a polypoid adenoma
(E) a mesenteric thrombus

284. An 18-year-old woman presents with abdominal pain localized to the right lower quadrant, nausea and vomiting, mild fever, and an elevation of the peripheral leukocyte count to 17,000 cells per microliter. Examination of the surgically resected appendix is most likely to reveal

(A) an appendix with normal appearance
(B) neutrophils within the muscular wall
(C) lymphoid hyperplasia and multinucleated giant cells within the muscular wall
(D) a dilated lumen filled with mucus
(E) a yellow tumor nodule at the tip of the appendix

285. Finely nodular (micronodular) cirrhosis, as illustrated in the photomicrograph below, is seen in all the following conditions EXCEPT

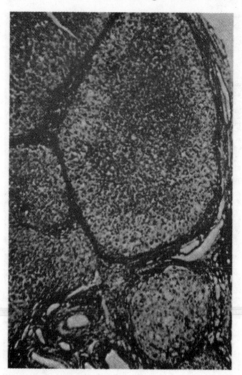

(A) postnecrotic cirrhosis
·(B) secondary biliary cirrhosis
(C) primary biliary cirrhosis
(D) alcoholic cirrhosis
(E) hemochromatosis

286. Which of the following cells found within the liver is the major source of the excess collagen deposited in cirrhosis?

(A) Hepatocytes
(B) Kupffer cells
(C) Ito cells
(D) Endothelial cells
(E) Bile duct epithelial cells

287. Which one of the following hepatitis profile patterns is most consistent with an asymptomatic hepatitis B carrier?

	HBsAg	HBeAg	anti-HBs	anti-HBc
(A)	+	−	−	−
(B)	+	+	−	−
(C)	+	+	−	+
(D)	+	−	−	+
(E)	−	−	+	+

288. A mononuclear portal inflammatory infiltrate that disrupts the limiting plate and surrounds individual hepatocytes (piecemeal necrosis), as shown in the photomicrograph below, is characteristic of

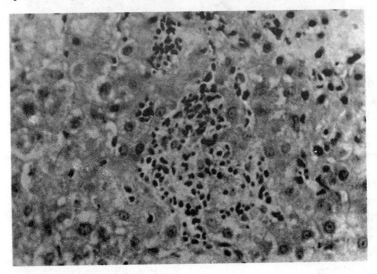

(A) ascending cholangitis
(B) chronic active hepatitis
(C) acute alcoholic hepatitis
(D) cholestatic jaundice
(E) nutritional cirrhosis

289. Which of the following statements regarding alcoholic steatosis and hepatitis is illustrated in the photomicrograph below is true?

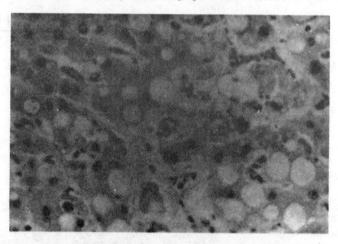

(A) Morphological changes of steatosis are irreversible
(B) Hepatocyte necrosis is most marked in the periportal area
(C) Perivenular and pericellular fibroses are precursors of cirrhosis
(D) Mallory's hyaline is pathognomonic of alcoholic liver damage
(E) The inflammatory infiltrate is chiefly lymphocytic

290. All the following produce a predominantly unconjugated hyper-bilirubinemia EXCEPT

(A) hemolytic anemias
(B) physiologic jaundice of the newborn
(C) Crigler-Najjar syndrome, type I
(D) Gilbert's syndrome
(E) Dubin-Johnson syndrome

291. Chronic hepatitis is most likely to develop in which one of the following clinical situations?

(A) Hepatitis A infection
(B) Hepatitis B infection
(C) Hepatitis C infection
(D) Hepatitis D and hepatitis B coinfection
(E) Hepatitis E infection

292. The photomicrograph below shows a section through the gallbladder wall. Which of the following statements regarding the condition illustrated is true?

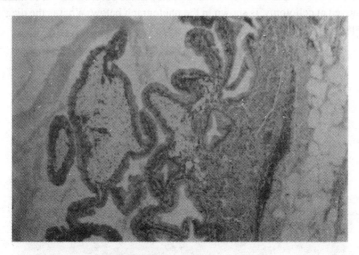

(A) It is known as cholesterolosis
(B) Changes often extend into the extrahepatic bile ducts
(C) It predisposes to acute cholecystitis
(D) It is strongly associated with pigment stones
(E) None of the above

---

293. Using an immunofluorescent procedure for detection of serum antibodies to mitochondria, one would expect a negative result in

(A) primary biliary cirrhosis
(B) chlorpromazine-induced jaundice
(C) acute viral hepatitis
(D) chronic active hepatitis
(E) systemic lupus erythematosus

294. Dilated sinusoids and irregular cystic spaces filled with blood within the liver, which may rupture leading to massive intraabdominal hemorrhage, are most commonly associated with

(A) salicylates
(B) estrogens
(C) anabolic steroids
(D) acetaminophen
(E) vinyl chloride

295. A middle-aged male alcoholic has had repeated bouts of pancreatitis following periods of binge drinking. In recent months he has had a low-grade fever, and on examination a mass is palpated in the epigastrium. This mass, removed at celiotomy, is shown in the photograph below. What is the diagnosis?

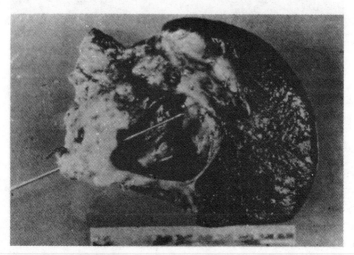

(A) Pancreatic carcinoma
(B) Mucinous cystadenoma
(C) Perforated ulcer
(D) Pancreatic pseudocyst
(E) Cystic hepatoma

296. The finding of multiple, pale yellow, hard, round stones within the gallbladder is associated with all the following EXCEPT

(A) oral contraceptives
(B) obesity
(C) biliary infection
(D) hyperlipidemia syndromes
(E) prevalence within the Native-American population

297. Which of the following statements regarding carcinoma of the exocrine pancreas is true?

(A) It arises from secretory cells of pancreatic acini
(B) It is decreasing in frequency
(C) It is most often located in the tail of the pancreas
(D) It is more common in diabetics than in nondiabetics
(E) It carries a 40 percent 5-year survival

298. Chronic pancreatitis is associated with all the following EXCEPT

(A) chronic alcoholism
(B) gallstones
(C) pancreatic pseudocyst
(D) pancreatic calcification
(E) fat malabsorption

299. A 38-year-old woman complains of fatigue and pruritus. She is found to have high serum alkaline phosphatase and slightly elevated serum bilirubin levels, and serum antimitochondrial antibodies are present. A liver biopsy reveals a marked lymphocytic infiltrate in the portal tracts along with occasional granulomas. The most likely diagnosis is

(A) impacted gallstone
(B) primary biliary cirrhosis
(C) primary sclerosing cholangitis
(D) von Meyenburg's complex
(E) Caroli's disease

300. A pancreatic islet cell tumor of the gastrin-secreting G cells will most likely produce

(A) hypoglycemia
(B) severe peptic ulceration of the duodenum
(C) mild diabetes
(D) steatorrhea
(E) profuse watery diarrhea

301. Diseases of the urinary tract occurring with increased frequency in patients with diabetes mellitus include all the following EXCEPT

(A) nodular or intercapillary glomerulosclerosis
(B) nephrotic syndrome
(C) atherosclerosis of the renal artery
(D) renal papillary necrosis
(E) uric acid stones

302. Components of diabetic glomerulopathy include all the following EXCEPT

(A) diffuse glomerulosclerosis
(B) nodular glomerulosclerosis
(C) thickening of capillary basement membranes
(D) mesangial proliferation
(E) fibrin thrombi

DIRECTIONS: Each group of questions below consists of lettered headings followed by a set of numbered items. For each numbered item select the **one** lettered heading with which it is **most** closely associated. Each lettered heading may be used **once, more than once, or not at all.**

Questions 303–305

Match each of the clinical and pathologic patterns of malabsorption syndrome with the appropriate cause.

(A) Abetalipoproteinemia
(B) Primary intestinal lymphoma
(C) Whipple's disease
(D) Disaccharidase deficiency
(E) Systemic mastocytosis

303. Recent viral infection, persistent diarrhea, normal bowel mucosa

304. Arthralgias, lymphadenopathy, blunted villi distended by macrophages

305. Failure to thrive, steatorrhea, lipid vacuolation of mucosal cells

Questions 306–308

For each patient below choose the most appropriate biochemical or serologic test.

(A) Serum alpha-fetoprotein
(B) Anti-hepatitis B surface antigen antibody (anti-HBsAg)
(C) Antimitochondrial antibody (AMA)
(D) Antineutrophil cytoplasmic antibody (ANCA)
(E) Serum ferritin

306. A 52-year-old woman with pruritus and markedly elevated serum alkaline phosphatase

307. A 65-year-old man with cardiomegaly and insulin-dependent diabetes mellitus of recent onset

308. A 43-year-old man with esophageal varices and rapidly increasing ascites

Gastrointestinal System
Answers

260. The answer is D. *(Robbins, 5/e, pp 751–752. Rubin, 2/e, pp 1252–1253.)* Warthin's tumors occur mainly in the lower regions of the parotid gland, especially near the angle of the mandible, and on rare occasion may be bilateral. They are completely benign neoplasms although they carry some undesirable synonyms: *adenolymphoma,* which is a misnomer, and *papillary cystadenoma lymphomatosum,* a term undesirable both for the *lymphomatosum* part as well as its length. For these reasons most workers prefer the term *Warthin's tumor.* The pattern is highly characteristic of an epithelial surface lining of acidophilic cells that overlay benign lymphoid tissue elements, including germinal centers. The epithelial portion probably arises from early duct cells that become entrapped within developing parotid lymph nodes during embryogenesis. Sebaceous lymphadenoma would have sebaceous cells within the lymphoid tissue. Thyroglossal duct cyst is located in the midline of the neck but may be found extending up to the base of the tongue, and there is a similarity between the lymphoid islands seen in thyroglossal duct cysts and in Warthin's tumor; however, thyroid follicles may lead to the correct diagnosis in the former. Lymphoepithelioma is a tumor that is recognized by hyperplastic duct epithelium surrounded by lymphoid tissue. Myoepithelial islands embedded in lymphoid tissue may be seen in the minor and major salivary glands in Sjögren's syndrome.

261. The answer is D. *(Robbins, 5/e, pp 738–741.)* Carcinoma of the oral cavity accounts for approximately 5 percent of all human malignancies. More than 90 percent are squamous cell type and precursor lesions include leukoplakia (dysplastic leukoplakia) and erythroplasia with transformation rates of approximately 15 and 50 percent, respectively. It is more common in males. Smoking, tobacco chewing, chronic irritation, heat exposure, and irradiation are all thought to contribute to carcinogenesis. The lower lip is the most common site followed by the floor of the mouth, anterior tongue, palate, and posterior tongue. Prognosis varies according to site but is best for lesions of the lip and worst for lesions in the floor of the mouth.

262. The answer is D. *(Robbins, 5/e, pp 762–764.)* The presence of columnar epithelium lining part or all of the distal esophagus is known as *Barrett's esophagus.* It is considered an acquired change resulting from reflux of acidic gastric contents with ulceration of the esophageal squamous epithelium and replacement by metaplastic, acid-resistant, columnar epithelium. Endoscopically it has a velvety-red appearance. Microscopically, intestinal-type epithelium is most common, but gastric-type epithelium is also seen. Varying degrees of dysplasia may be present. The risk of carcinoma is increased 30- to 40-fold. Virtually all of these tumors are of the adenocarcinoma type and they account for up to 10 percent of all esophageal cancers.

263. The answer is C. *(Robbins, 5/e, pp 749–753.)* The salivary glands give rise to a wide variety of tumors, the majority of which are of epithelial origin and benign. Most tumors occur in adults and have a slight female predominance. Approximately 75 to 85 percent occur in the parotids, 10 to 20 percent in the submandibular glands, and the remainder in the minor glands. In the parotid the vast majority are benign, whereas in the minor glands 35 to 50 percent are malignant. Mesenchymal tumors are rare. Clinically, most tumors of salivary glands present as palpable masses, regardless of histologic type. They occasionally present with symptoms related to local invasion, such as facial nerve palsy. Masses may be present for years before diagnosis, even when malignant. Carcinomas tend to run an indolent course, invade local structures slowly, recur locally after removal, and metastasize late. Prognosis is usually presented in 10- or 20-year survival rates.

264. The answer is E. *(Robbins, 5/e, pp 756–761.)* Most lesions of the esophagus present with similar symptoms, such as heartburn and dysphagia, but the most serious disease, which carries the risk of exsanguination, is bleeding esophageal varices. Varices occur in about two-thirds of all patients with cirrhosis, and in the majority of patients the etiology is alcoholic cirrhosis. The cirrhosis causes portal hypertension, which shunts blood into connecting channels between the portal and caval systems, such as the subepithelial plexus of veins in the lower esophagus. Varices produce no symptoms until they rupture and cause massive bleeding (hematemesis), which may lead to death. Other diseases may cause hematemesis such as gastritis, esophageal laceration (Mallory-Weiss tears), or peptic ulcer disease. Dysphagia (difficulty swallowing) is another esophageal symptom. It is seen in diseases with abnormal esophageal function, such as achalasia, and diseases that narrow the esophageal lumen, such as webs and rings. The characteristics of achalasia include aperistalsis, incomplete relaxation of the lower esophageal sphincter (LES) with swallowing, and increased resting tone of the LES, all of which lead to esophageal dilatation and symptoms of progressive dysphagia. Plummer-Vinson syndrome is the combination of esophageal webs in the upper esophagus and anemia. Outpouchings in the upper esophagus are called pharyngeal (Zenker's) diverticuli and may result in regurgitation and aspiration. Sliding hiatal hernias are associated with signs and symptoms of reflux esophagitis.

265. The answer is B. *(Robbins, 5/e, pp 770–778.)* *Helicobacter pylori* is a gram-negative, microaerophilic, curved bacillus found only on gastric-type epithelium. It is present in 10 percent of normal persons under 30 years of age with prevalence rising to 60 percent in those over 60 years of age. Virtually all patients with duodenal ulceration and 80 percent of those with gastric ulceration are infected by *H. pylori*. Many virulence factors aid the organism in colonization of the acid environment of the stomach, one of the most important of which is urease, which produces ammonia and buffers gastric acidity. The organism does not invade the tissues but induces surface epithelial cell damage and an inflammatory infiltrate in the lamina propria that is typically superficial and mixed granulocytic and lymphocytic.

266. The answer is E. *(Robbins, 5/e, pp 764–766.)* Carcinoma of the esophagus accounts for about 10 percent of malignancies of the GI tract, but for a disproportionate number of cancer deaths. Predisposing factors include smoking, esophagitis, and achalasia. Sixty to seventy percent are squamous cell carcinomas that characteristically begin as lesions in situ. Adenocarcinoma occurs mainly in the lower esophagus and may arise in up to 10 percent of cases of Barrett's esophagus. Anaplastic and small cell variants also occur. Polypoid lesions are most common, followed by malignant ulceration and diffusively infiltrative forms. Tumors tend to spread by direct invasion of adjacent structures, but lymphatic and hematogenous spread may occur. Distant metastases are, however, a late feature. Five-year survival is less than 10 percent.

267. The answer is B. *(Robbins, 5/e, pp 756, 769–770, 778, 786–787.)* Several congenital abnormalities of the gastrointestinal tract present with specific symptoms. Infants with congenital hypertrophic pyloric stenosis present in the second or third week of life with symptoms of regurgitation and persistent severe vomiting. Physical examination reveals a firm mass in the region of the pylorus. Surgical splitting of the muscle in the stenotic region is curative. Esophageal atresia is discovered soon after birth when feeding is attempted. Symptoms include regurgitation and possible aspiration, pneumonia, or suffocation. Diaphragmatic hernias, if large enough, may allow for abdominal contents—including portions of the stomach, intestines, or liver—to herniate into the thoracic cavity and cause respiratory compromise. Congenital aganglionic megacolon, Hirschsprung's disease, is caused by failure of the neural crest cells to migrate all the way to the anus, resulting in a portion of distal colon that lacks ganglion cells and both Meissner's submucosal and Auerbach's myenteric plexuses. This results in a functional obstruction and dilatation proximal to the affected portion of colon. Symptoms of Hirschsprung's disease include failure to pass meconium soon after birth followed by constipation and possible abdominal distention. Hypertrophic gastropathy refers to several diseases, such as Ménétrier's disease, which produce markedly enlarged gastric rugal folds secondary to hyperplasia of the mucosal epithelial cells. This lesion usually presents in older men with symptoms of epigastric pain, weight loss, and bleeding and may be mistaken radiographically for a gastric carcinoma or lymphoma.

268. The answer is D. *(Robbins, 5/e, pp 773–777. Rubin, 2/e, pp 637–643.)* Peptic ulceration may occur anywhere in the gastrointestinal tract exposed to acid-peptic activity. Over 98 percent of cases occur in the stomach or duodenum with duodenal cases outnumbering gastric by 4:1. Ulcers associated with the Zollinger-Ellison syndrome are typically multiple and frequently involve distal duodenum and jejunum. Duodenal ulceration appears to be related to hypersecretion of acid. Gastric ulceration typically occurs in a setting of normo- or hypochlorhydria with abnormality of mucosal defense mechanisms, back-diffusion of acid, and possibly local ischemia. *H. pylori* is associated with up to 100 percent of patients with duodenal ulcers, and about 75 percent of patients with gastric ulcers. Peptic ulcers are usually small but up to 10 percent of benign gastric ulcers are > 4 cm in diameter; malignant ulcers may be small.

269. The answer is A. *(Robbins, 5/e, pp 328–334, 790–794, 800, 804.)* The causes of diarrhea are immense and may be broadly classified into multiple categories including secretory diarrhea, osmotic diarrhea, and exudative diarrhea. Both secretory and exudative diarrhea may have infectious causes. Several viruses may cause secretory diarrhea. Rotavirus is a major cause of diarrhea in children between the ages of 6 and 24 months. Clinical symptoms consisting of vomiting and watery (secretory) diarrhea begin about 2 days after exposure. Bacterial enterocolitis may be related to either the production of preformed toxins, such as with *Vibrio cholerae* and enterotoxogenic *E. coli,* which is a major cause of "traveler's diarrhea," or it may be related to bacterial invasion of the colon, as seen with salmonella and shigella. *Entamoeba histolytica* is a cause of amebiasis and is endemic in underdeveloped countries. It characteristically produces flask-shaped ulcers in the colon and may embolize to the liver, where it produces amebic liver abscesses. Lactase deficiency, a cause of osmotic diarrhea, is very rarely a congenital disorder, but much more commonly is an acquired disorder seen in adults that results in malabsorption of milk and milk products. The onset of symptoms from ulcerative colitis are most commonly apparent between the ages of 20 and 25.

270. The answer is A. *(Robbins, 5/e, pp 797–798. Rubin, 2/e, pp 661–662.)* Celiac disease (gluten-sensitive enteropathy) is a disorder characterized by malabsorption induced by sensitivity to the gluten and gliadin in certain cereals, especially wheat, rye, and barley. Exposure to gluten results in a typical malabsorption syndrome of varying severity. There is a high incidence of HLA-B8 (over 85 percent of cases) and HLA-DQw2 (over 90 percent) antigens. Celiac disease and HLA-B8 are also associated with the skin disease dermatitis herpetiformis. Characteristic morphological changes include villus atrophy, crypt hypertrophy with increased mitotic activity in crypts, and chronic inflammatory infiltrate in the lamina propria of the duodenum and jejunum. The *proximal* small intestine shows the most severe and extensive involvement. Immunocytes express surface IgA antigliadin antibodies. Antigliadin antibodies are also present in the serum but the level correlates poorly with clinical status. Complications are numerous and, with disease lasting 10 years or more, include a 10 to 15 percent risk of malignancy. Half of these cancers are B-cell lymphomas; the remainder are carcinomas that may arise anywhere in the gastrointestinal tract, but occur frequently in the small bowel.

271. The answer is C. *(Robbins, 5/e, pp 779–783.)* "Signet-ring cell" carcinoma is a morphologic variant of adenocarcinoma most often seen in the stomach. In these tumors, intracellular mucin vacuoles coalesce and distend the cytoplasm of tumor cells, which compresses the nucleus toward the edge of the cell and creates a signet-ring appearance. Tumors of this type are usually deeply invasive and fall into the category of advanced gastric carcinoma. There is often a striking desmoplasia with thickening and rigidity of the gastric wall, which may result in the so-called linitis plastica appearance. Advanced gastric carcinoma is usually located in the pyloroantrum and the prognosis is poor with 5-year survival of only 5 to 15 percent.

272. The answer is B. *(Robbins, 5/e, pp 779–783.)* The death rate from gastric carcinoma has been decreasing for decades but still shows marked variations among countries; Japan, Chile, and Iceland have rates up to six times higher than those of the U.S. and Australia. First-generation migrants carry the risk of their country of origin, but subsequent generations assume the risk of their new country. The decreased rate is due to a decrease in the rate of one type of gastric cancer, the intestinal type. The incidence of the other type, diffuse gastric carcinoma, has not changed recently. *Early gastric carcinoma (EGC)* refers to a local neoplastic lesion limited to the mucosa and submucosa without penetration of the muscularis propria. Metastasis can occur, however, from EGC to local lymph nodes in up to 5 percent of cases. EGC is usually recognizable on radiographic or endoscopic examination, and so in most cases is potentially curable. It develops very slowly into a frankly invasive lesion and, if detected early and removed, allows a 5-year survival of up to 95 percent compared with 15 percent for gastric carcinoma overall. Of all gastric carcinomas, 50 to 60 percent arise in the pyloroantrum, 10 percent in the cardia, 10 percent in the whole organ, and the remainder in other sites. Diffusely infiltrative carcinoma extends widely through the stomach wall, often without producing an intraluminal mass, and incites a marked desmoplastic reaction that results in a thickened, inelastic stomach wall.

273. The answer is C. *(Robbins, 5/e, pp 797–799.)* Celiac disease, or gluten-sensitive enteropathy, is an inflammatory condition of the small intestinal mucosa related to dietary gluten. It is more common in females and shows familial clustering. Histologically it is characterized by villus atrophy with hyperplasia of underlying crypts and increased mitotic activity. The surface epithelium shows disarray of the columnar epithelial cells and increased intraepithelial lymphocytes. There is a chronic inflammatory infiltrate in the lamina propria. Definitive diagnosis in patients with these features on biopsy depends on response to a gluten-free diet and subsequent gluten challenge.

274. The answer is D. *(Robbins, 5/e, pp 329–334, 790–794, 804–806.)* Early stages of ulcerative colitis (UC) may be indistinguishable from gastroenteritis caused by *Salmonella choleraesuis* and *S. typhimurium.* In early stages, both diseases may show histologically a dense mononuclear inflammatory infiltrate in the lamina propria, occasional crypt abscesses, and mucosal edema and congestion. Even the respective clinical symptoms and colon x-ray changes may be similar, although marked vomiting should point to food poisoning. Salmonellae have been the cause of outbreaks and epidemics of acute gastroenteritis, and the cause has often been found to be contaminated fowl that has been insufficiently cooked to inactivate endotoxins.

275. The answer is D. *(Robbins, 5/e, pp 804–806. Silverberg, 2/e, pp 1166–1170.)* The condition illustrated is ulcerative colitis, an inflammatory disorder of unknown cause. It involves the distal colon with variable proximal extension; however, skip lesions are not present. Grossly there is ulceration with islands of residual mucosa present, which form pseudopolyps. The inflammation is predominantly superficial with an infiltrate of acute and chronic inflammatory cells in the lamina propria. Cryptitis and crypt abscesses are common. Many lymphoid follicles may be seen but epithelioid cells, giant cells, and granulomas, as may be seen in Crohn's disease, are absent. Cellular atypia is seen in regenerating mucosa. When ulcerative colitis is inactive, morphological abnormalities of glands, goblet cell depletion, and Paneth cell metaplasia indicate underlying disease.

276. The answer is D. *(Robbins, 5/e, pp 331–332, 801–806, 813–814.)* Hemorrhagic cobblestone appearance of the colon and small bowel may be seen in multiple states including inflammatory bowel disease, a term that can apply both to ulcerative colitis and regional enteritis (Crohn's disease). Other conditions that resemble cobblestoning of the mucosa of the bowel include multiple polyps such as occur in Gardner's syndrome, Turcot syndrome, familial polyposis, and multiple acquired polyps. Crohn's disease, however, differs from the others in that longitudinal ulcers may be present, yielding a long axis grooving, parallel to the long axis of the bowel. Such ulcers may also be seen in tuberculous enteritis; however, when inflammatory bowel disease is in the differential diagnosis, longitudinal ulcers are indicative of Crohn's disease.

277. The answer is D. *(Robbins, 5/e, pp 800–807.)* The two inflammatory bowel diseases (IBD), Crohn's disease (CD) and ulcerative colitis (UC), are both chronic, relapsing inflammatory disorders of unknown etiology. They both may show very similar morphologic features, such as mucosal inflammation, malignant transformation, and extragastrointestinal manifestations, such as erythema nodosum, arthritis, uveitis, pericholangitis, and ankylosing spondylitis. CD is a granulomatous disease; but granulomas are present in a minority of cases, so that the absence of granulomas does not rule out the diagnosis of CD. CD may involve any portion of the gastrointestinal tract and characteristically has skip lesions. In contrast, UC affects only the colon, and the disease involvement is continuous. Involvement of the intestines by CD is typically transmural, which leads to the formation of fistulas and sinuses. Since UC involves the mucosa and submucosa, fistula formation is absent. Additionally in Crohn's disease, the mesenteric fat wraps around the bowel surface, producing what is called "creeping fat," and the thickened wall narrows the lumen, producing a characteristic "string sign" on x-ray.

278. The answer is D. *(Robbins, 5/e, p 786.)* Meckel's diverticulum occurs in the ileum, usually within 30 cm of the ileocecal valve, and is present in approximately 2 percent of normal persons. It represents incomplete involution of the vitello-intestinal duct and always arises from the antimesenteric border of the intestine. Heterotopic gastric or pancreatic tissue may be present in about one-half of cases. Peptic ulceration, which occurs as a result of acid secretion by heterotopic gastric mucosa, is usually located in the adjacent ileum. Complications include perforation, ulceration, intestinal obstruction, intussusception, and neoplasms, including carcinoid tumors.

279. The answer is C. *(Robbins, 5/e, pp 300, 815–817.)* Ninety-five percent of all carcinomas of the colorectum are adenocarcinoma, and almost all begin as in situ lesions within adenomatous polyps. Many of the adenocarcinomas secrete mucin. When this secretion is extracellular, it dissects the gut wall cell planes and so aids extension of the malignancy. The gross pathology of left- and right-sided lesions differs; left-sided lesions tend to grow in an annular, "napkin-ring," encircling fashion, while right-sided lesions tend to be sessile or polypoid fungating masses. Carcinoembryonic antigen is the tumor marker longest used in diagnosis and follow-up of colorectal tumors. Its serum levels are directly related to both size and extent of spread of the primary tumor. Levels fall to zero with complete removal of tumor but rise again with recurrence at primary or secondary sites.

280. The answer is E. *(Robbins, 5/e, pp 818–820. Rubin, 2/e, pp 668–670.)* The patient shows two of the most common clinical manifestations of the carcinoid syndrome, which include flushing, diarrhea, bronchoconstriction, and right-sided cardiac valvular disease. The syndrome results from elaboration of serotonin (5-hydroxytryptamine) by a primary carcinoid tumor in the lungs or ovary, or from hepatic metastases from a primary carcinoid tumor in the gastrointestinal tract. Diagnosis is based on finding increased urinary 5-HIAA excretion from metabolism of excess serotonin and on histologic analysis of tumor tissue. Primary appendiceal carcinoid tumors, the most common gastrointestinal carcinoid tumors, very rarely metastasize and are virtually always asymptomatic.

281. The answer is D. *(Anderson, 9/e, p 1155. Robbins, 5/e, pp 806–808.)* Diverticula occur most frequently in men over the age of 50 and are most often located in the descending and sigmoid colon. The colon is the most commonly involved segment of the gastrointestinal tract. A majority of these lesions are not true diverticula since the mucosa and muscularis mucosae herniate through defects in the muscularis propria. Complications are not very common but include diverticulitis, hemorrhage, perforation, fistulas, intestinal obstruction, and, more commonly, bowel spasms or abnormal motility (irritable bowel syndrome).

282. The answer is C. *(Robbins, 5/e, pp 813–815.)* Although most colonic polyps occur sporadically, there are several conditions in which colonic polyposis is familial and sometimes associated with extraintestinal abnormalities. Familial polyposis coli is usually transmitted as an autosomal dominant condition and is characterized by multiple adenomatous colonic polyps with a minimum of 100 polyps necessary for diagnosis. As with sporadic adenomatous polyps, there is a risk of malignancy and this increases to 100 percent within 30 years of diagnosis. Panproctocolectomy is, therefore, usually recommended. Gardner's syndrome is the association of colonic polyposis with multiple osteomas, fibromatosis, and cutaneous cysts. The association of colonic polyposis with central nervous system tumors is known as Turcot's syndrome.

283. The answer is B. *(Rubin, 2/e, p 694. Silverberg, 2/e, pp 1225–1226.)* The lesion pictured is a basaloid, or cloacogenic, carcinoma that has the same gross appearance as the more common epidermoid carcinoma, although the lesion histologically resembles the basal cell carcinoma of the skin. The tumor arises from the anal canal within the transitional zone epithelium (anal columns). Some of these tumors resemble transitional epithelium, whereas others vary in their patterns, including one pattern similar to that of small cell (oat cell) carcinoma of the lung and other patterns that are totally undifferentiated. The prognosis for cloacogenic carcinoma is directly proportional to the degree of differentiation.

284. The answer is B. *(Robbins, 5/e, pp 818–820, 823–825. Rubin, 2/e, pp 343, 696–697.)* Acute appendicitis, a disease found predominantly in adolescents and young adults, is characterized histologically by acute inflammatory cells, neutrophils, within the mucosa and muscular wall. Clinically, acute appendicitis causes right lower quadrant pain, nausea, vomiting, a mild fever, and a leukocytosis in the peripheral blood. These symptoms may not occur in the very young or the elderly. The inflamed appendiceal wall may become gangrenous and perforate in 24 to 48 h. Even with classic symptoms, the appendix may be histologically unremarkable in up to 20 percent of the cases. False positive diagnoses are to be preferred to the possible severe or fatal complications of a false negative diagnosis of acute appendicitis that results in rupture. Lymphoid hyperplasia with multinucleated giant cells (Warthin-Finkeldey giant cells) is characteristic of measles (rubeola). These changes can be found in the appendix, but this is quite rare. Dilatation of the lumen of the appendix is called a *mucocele* and may be caused by mucosal hyperplasia, a benign cystadenoma, or a malignant mucinous cystadenocarcinoma. If the latter tumor ruptures, it may seed the entire peritoneal cavity, causing the condition called *pseudomyxoma peritonei*. The most common tumor of the appendix is the carcinoid tumor. Grossly it is yellow in color and is typically located at the tip of the appendix. Histologically, carcinoids are composed of nests or islands of monotonous cells. Appendiceal carcinoids rarely metastasize.

285. The answer is A. *(Robbins, 5/e, pp 834–835. Rubin, 2/e, pp 744–745.)* Cirrhosis is often subdivided into micronodular and macronodular types on the basis of the size of individual nodules within the cirrhotic liver. Although this division is entirely descriptive, most diseases that lead to cirrhosis result in one of these subtypes. Alcoholic liver damage, hemochromatosis, and biliary cirrhosis, both primary and secondary, typically result in a micronodular pattern with nodules < 3 mm in diameter. Postnecrotic cirrhosis is typically macronodular and a mixed or variable pattern may be seen in the cirrhosis of Wilson's disease and α_1-antitrypsin deficiency. It is also apparent that a micronodular pattern may convert over time to a macronodular pattern.

286. The answer is C. (*Fawcett, 12/e, pp 657–660. Robbins, 5/e, pp 832, 835.*) Ito cells are fat-containing lipocytes found within the space of Disse of the liver. They participate in the metabolism and storage of vitamin A and also secrete collagen in the normal and the fibrotic (cirrhotic) liver. In normal livers, types I and III collagens (interstitial types) are found in the portal areas and occasionally in the space of Disse or around central veins. In cirrhosis, types I and III collagens are deposited throughout the hepatic lobule. Endothelial cells normally line the sinusoids and demarcate the extrasinusoidal space of Disse. Attached to the endothelial cells are the phagocytic Kupffer cells, which are part of the monocyte-phagocyte system.

287. The answer is D. (*Robbins, 5/e, pp 844–846. Rubin, 2/e, pp 724–726.*) Hepatitis B virus (HBV) is a member of the DNA-containing hepadnaviruses. The mature HBV virion is called the "Dane particle." Products of the HBV genome include the nucleocapsid (hepatitis B core antigen, HBcAg), envelope lycoprotein (hepatitis B surface antigen, HBsAg), and DNA polymerase. After exposure to HBV, there is a relatively long asymptomatic incubation period, averaging 6 to 8 weeks, followed by an acute disease lasting several weeks to months. HBsAg is the first antigen to appear in the blood. It appears before symptoms begin, peaks during overt disease, and declines to undetectable levels in 3 to 6 months. HBeAg, HBV-DNA, and DNA polymerase appear soon after HBsAg. HBeAg peaks during acute disease and disappears before HBsAg is cleared. The presence of either HBsAg or HBeAg without antibodies to either is seen early in hepatitis B infection. Anti-HBsAg appears about the time of the disappearance of HBsAg and indicates complete recovery. Anti-HBc first appears much earlier, shortly after the appearance of HBsAg, and levels remain elevated for life. Its presence indicates previous HBV infection, but not necessarily that the hepatitis infection has been cleared. Persistence of HBeAg is an important indicator of continued viral replication with probable progression to chronic hepatitis. With normal recovery from hepatitis B, both HBsAg and HBeAg are absent from the blood, while anti-HBs and anti-HBc are present. If anti-HBs is never produced, then HBsAg may not be cleared. In this case, the patient may remove the HBeAg and be an asymptomatic carrier, or the HBeAg may persist and the patient could be a chronic carrier who has progressed to chronic active hepatitis. In both of these conditions, anti-HBc is still present.

288. The answer is B. *(Robbins, 5/e, pp 851–852.)* Chronic hepatitis has been defined as an inflammatory process of the liver that lasts longer than 1 year and lacks the nodular regeneration and architectural distortion of cirrhosis. In chronic active hepatitis, an intense inflammatory reaction with numerous plasma cells spreads from portal tracts into periportal areas. The reaction destroys the limiting plate and results in formation of periportal hepatocytic islets. Prognosis is poor, and the majority of patients develop cirrhosis. Chronic persistent hepatitis is usually a sequela of acute viral hepatitis and has a benign course, without progression to chronic active hepatitis or cirrhosis. The portal inflammation does not extend into the periportal areas, and this differentiates it from chronic active hepatitis.

289. The answer is C. *(Robbins, 5/e, pp 857–860.)* Alcoholic liver disease includes steatosis (fatty liver), hepatitis, and cirrhosis. Steatosis is the earliest hepatic consequence of excess alcohol intake and consists of cytoplasmic accumulation of lipid vacuoles that coalesce and distend the cells with ultrastructural evidence of cell injury. These changes are reversible. Alcoholic hepatitis is usually accompanied by some fatty changes and is characterized by hepatocellular swelling, necrosis, and neutrophil infiltration in the perivenular area, as well as the appearance of Mallory's hyaline—eosinophilic cytoplasmic inclusions composed of cytokeratin proteins. These inclusions may also, however, be seen in liver injury due to other causes. Pericellular fibrosis and fibrosis around the central vein are significant changes considered by some to indicate the possible development of cirrhosis.

290. The answer is E. *(Henry, 18/e, pp 232–234. Robbins, 5/e, pp 837–841.)* Jaundice is caused by increased blood levels of bilirubin, which result from abnormalities of bilirubin metabolism. Bilirubin, the end product of heme breakdown, is taken up by the liver, where it is conjugated with glucuronic acid by the enzyme bilirubin UDP-glucuronosyl transferase (UGT) and then secreted into the bile. Unconjugated bilirubin is not soluble in an aqueous solution, is complexed to albumin, and cannot be excreted in the urine. Unconjugated hyperbilirubinemia may result from excessive production of bilirubin, which occurs in hemolytic anemias. It can also result from reduced hepatic uptake of bilirubin, as occurs in Gilbert's syndrome, a mild disease associated with a subclinical hyperbilirubinemia. Finally, unconjugated hyperbilirubinemia may result from impaired conjugation of bilirubin. Examples of diseases resulting from impaired conjugation include physio-

logic jaundice of the newborn and the Crigler-Najjar syndrome, which result
from either decreased UGT activity (type II) or absent UGT activity (type I).
Conjugated bilirubin is water-soluble, nontoxic, and readily excreted in the
urine. Conjugated hyperbilirubinemia may result from either decreased hepatic excretion of conjugates of bilirubin, such as in the Dubin-Johnson syndrome, or impaired extrahepatic bile excretion, as occurs with extrahepatic
biliary obstruction.

291. The answer is C. *(Robbins, 5/e, pp 843–852.)* The hepatitis viruses
are responsible for most cases of chronic hepatitis, but the chance of developing chronic hepatitis varies considerably with the different types of hepatitis
viruses. Neither hepatitis A nor hepatitis E virus infection is associated with
the development of chronic hepatitis. About 5 percent of adults infected with
hepatitis B develop chronic hepatitis, and about one-half of these patients
progress to cirrhosis. In contrast to hepatitis B, chronic hepatitis develops in
about 50 percent of patients with hepatitis C. In the United States it is estimated that hepatitis B causes 30,000 new cases of chronic hepatitis each year,
but hepatitis C causes about 85,000 new cases annually. Hepatitis D infection
occurs in two clinical settings. There might be acute coinfection by hepatitis
D and hepatitis B, which results in chronic hepatitis in less than 5 percent of
cases. If instead hepatitis D is superinfected upon a chronic carrier of hepatitis
B virus, then about 80 percent of cases progress to chronic hepatitis.

292. The answer is A. *(Robbins, 5/e, p 893.)* Cholesterolosis of the gallbladder, also known as "strawberry gallbladder," is relatively common and,
although associated with cholesterol calculi, is not thought to predispose to
acute cholecystitis or malignancy. Lipid-laden macrophages accumulate
within the mucosal folds of the gallbladder and result in a yellow-flecked appearance. The pathophysiology is unclear but may be related to the presence
of supersaturated bile. Following acute or chronic cholecystitis there may be
diffuse calcium deposition in the gallbladder wall (calcified, or "porcelain,"
gallbladder), which is not associated with cholesterolosis. Pigment stones
may occur with increased concentration of unconjugated bilirubin in bile, as
in the hemolytic anemias.

293. The answer is C. *(Anderson, 9/e, pp 1255–1256.)* Antibodies to mitochondria are not present in the serum of patients who have acute viral hepatitis when immunofluorescent techniques are used. Serum antibodies to mitochondria are present, however, in 87 percent of patients who have primary
biliary cirrhosis, 69 percent of patients who have chlorpromazine-induced
jaundice, 66 percent of patients who have chronic active hepatitis, and 18 percent of patients who have systemic lupus erythematosus. Immunofluorescent

detection techniques for antibodies to mitochondria are not specific for one particular disease, but, when evaluated in conjunction with tests for antinuclear antibodies and antibodies to smooth muscle, they can be helpful in differential diagnosis.

294. The answer is C. *(Robbins, 5/e, pp 856–857, 865–866, 873.)* Hepatic injury can result from a wide range of drugs, chemicals, and toxins. Peliosis hepatis is an abnormality of the hepatic blood flow that results in sinusoidal dilatation and the formation of irregular blood-filled lakes, which may rupture and produce massive intraabdominal hemorrhage or hepatic failure. It is most often associated with the use of anabolic steroids, but more rarely it may be associated with oral contraceptives. Reye's syndrome, characterized by microvesicular fatty change in the liver and encephalopathy, has been related to the use of salicylates in children with a viral illness. Acetaminophen toxicity results in centrilobular liver necrosis, while estrogens may be related to thrombosis of the hepatic or portal veins. Several hepatic tumors are related to exposure to vinyl chloride, including angiosarcoma and hepatocellular carcinoma.

295. The answer is D. *(Robbins, 5/e, pp 904–905.)* Pseudocysts of the pancreas are so named because the cystic structure is essentially unlined by any type of epithelium. True cysts, wherever they are found in the body, are always lined by some type of epithelium, whether columnar cell, glandular, squamous, or flattened cuboidal cell. The pancreatic pseudocyst is most commonly found in a background of repeated episodes of pancreatitis. Eventual mechanical large duct obstruction by either an inflammatory process per se, periductal fibrosis, or an abscess along with inspissated duct fluid from secretions and enzymes leads to the expanding mass. The mass lesion may be located between the stomach and liver, between the stomach and colon or transverse mesocolon, or in the lesser sac. Drainage or excision is necessary for adequate treatment. Acute bacterial infection may complicate the course.

296. The answer is C. *(Robbins, 5/e, pp 884–888.)* Gallstones, which affect 10 to 20 percent of the adult population in developed countries, are divided into two main types. Cholesterol stones are pale yellow, hard, round, radiographically translucent stones that are most often multiple. Their formation is related to multiple factors including female sex hormones (such as with oral contraceptives), obesity, rapid weight reduction, and hyperlipidemic states. Their prevalence approaches 75 percent in some Native-American populations. The other main type of gallstones are pigment stones, which are brown or black in color and composed of bilirubin calcium salts. They are found more commonly in Asian populations and are related to chronic hemolytic states, diseases of the small intestines, and bacterial infections of the biliary tree.

297. The answer is D. *(Robbins, 5/e, pp 905–907.)* Carcinoma of the exocrine pancreas is a highly malignant tumor that accounts for 5 percent of cancer deaths in the U.S. Its occurrence has increased threefold in the past 40 years mainly as a result of smoking and exposure to chemical carcinogens. It is more frequent in diabetics than nondiabetics. Sixty percent of tumors are located in the head of the pancreas, 20 percent in the body, and 5 percent in the tail. The remainder are of indeterminate primary location. Growth is often insidious and presentation is often with jaundice due to compression of the extrahepatic bile ducts. The disease is rarely curable at presentation and prognosis is poor, with median survival from diagnosis of 6 months and 5-year survival of only 1 to 2 percent.

298. The answer is B. *(Robbins, 5/e, pp 899–904.)* Pancreatitis may be either acute or chronic. Acute pancreatitis may be clinically mild or severe. Acute hemorrhagic pancreatitis, which clinically is severe, is associated with alcoholism in men and chronic biliary disease in women. Chronic pancreatitis is characterized histologically by chronic inflammation and irregular fibrosis of the pancreas. The major cause of chronic pancreatitis is chronic alcoholism. Complications of chronic pancreatitis include pancreatic calcifications, pancreatic cysts and pseudocysts, stones within the pancreatic ducts, diabetes, and fat malabsorption, which results in steatorrhea and decreased vitamin K levels. Although gallstones are a common cause of acute pancreatitis, cholelithiasis is not an etiologic factor in chronic pancreatitis.

299. The answer is B. *(Robbins, 5/e, pp 867–871. Rubin, 2/e, pp 740–744.)* Diseases of the biliary tract may lead to manifestations of jaundice and if prolonged and severe may lead to cirrhosis. These diseases can be classified as either primary or secondary. Causes of secondary biliary cirrhosis include biliary atresia, gallstones, and carcinoma of the head of the pancreas. Histologic examination of the liver may reveal bile stasis in the interlobular bile ducts and bile duct proliferation in the portal areas. Primary biliary cirrhosis (PBC) is primarily a disease of middle-aged women and is characterized by pruritus, jaundice, and hypercholesterolemia. More than 90 percent of patients have antimitochondrial autoantibodies, particularly the "M2" antibody to mitochondrial pyruvate dehydrogenase. A characteristic lesion, called the florid duct lesion, is seen in portal areas and is composed of a marked lymphocytic infiltrate and occasional granulomas. Primary sclerosing cholangitis (PSC) is characterized by fibrosing cholangitis that produces concentric "onion-skin" fibrosis in portal areas. It is highly associated with chronic ulcerative colitis. Abnormal development of the biliary tract may lead to several abnormalities, including von Meyenburg's complex (small bile duct hamartomas near normal portal tracts) and Caroli's disease, which is characterized by segmental dilatation of the larger intrahepatic bile ducts.

300.   The answer is B. *(Robbins, 5/e, pp 922–924.)* Functional islet cell tumors of the pancreas secrete specific substances that result in several syndromes. Pancreatic gastrinomas, tumors of the G cells of the pancreas, secrete gastrin and are a cause of the Zollinger-Ellison syndrome. This syndrome consists of intractable gastric hypersecretion, severe peptic ulceration of the duodenum and jejunum, and high serum levels of gastrin. The majority of gastrinomas are malignant. Insulinomas, tumors of beta cells, are the most common islet cell neoplasm and are usually benign. Symptoms include low blood sugar, hunger, sweating, and nervousness. Glucagonomas, islet cell tumors of the alpha cells, secrete glucagon and are characterized by mild diabetes, anemia, venous thrombosis, severe infections, and a migratory, necrotizing, erythematous skin rash. Delta cell tumors, which secrete somatostatin, produce a syndrome associated with mild diabetes, gallstones, steatorrhea, and hypochlorhydria. The majority of delta cell tumors are malignant. D1 tumors (also called vasoactive intestinal peptide tumors, or VIPomas) produce the Verner-Morrison syndrome, which is characterized by explosive, profuse diarrhea with hypokalemia and hypochlorhydria. This combination of symptoms is referred to as *pancreatic cholera.*

301.   The answer is E. *(Robbins, 5/e, pp 920–921, 961–963, 985.)* Diabetes is a major cause of renal disease. It affects the glomeruli with resultant glomerulosclerosis, fibrin caps, and capsular drops. It also affects the renal vasculature, where it causes atheroma of the major renal arteries and hyaline arteriolosclerosis of both afferent and efferent arterioles. Acute infection of the renal pyramids occurs and in combination with impaired circulation to the papillae may lead to papillary necrosis. Uric acid stones are found in patients with hyperuricemia, such as patients with gout or leukemia.

302.   The answer is E. *(Robbins, 5/e, pp 920–921, 961–963.)* Thickening of the capillary basement membrane is a universal finding in diabetic kidney disease and consists of diffuse thickening as is seen in vasculopathy in other organ sites in diabetes. This has to be verified by ultrastructural examination by electron microscopy. Additionally, the mesangium widens and tubular basement membranes also thicken in diabetes. Thickening is produced by hyaline-like material, which reacts with the PAS stain. This may result from glycosylation of the proteins of the basement membrane. Thickening is probably also contributed by an increase in collagen type 4, as well as in the basement membrane glycoprotein laminen; however, the polyanionic proteoglycans are decreased. This may contribute to the increased permeability and consequent leakage of cationic proteins into the urine. Diffuse glomerulosclerosis results from an increase in the mesangial matrix as well as an increase in mesangial cells. This increase in matrix will also react with the PAS stain. Eventually, with continuing disease the glomerular tufts will become obliterated and yield a sclerosed, acidophilic tuft. At this stage the afferent and probably efferent arterioles will also be thickened and appear hyalinized.

Nodular glomerulosclerosis (Kimmelstiel-Wilson disease, intercapillary glomerulosclerosis) appears as laminated hyaline nodules at the peripheries of the glomerulus covered by what appears to be patent capillary loops. They may resemble amyloid and if they are present, amyloid stain should be done. Not always present, but highly characteristic of diabetic glomerulopathy are fibrin caps and capsular drops. The fibrin cap is a deposit that overlies a peripheral capillary within the glomerulus and consists of acidophilic deposits between the basement membrane and the endothelial cells. Capsular drops are PAS-positive proteinaceous foci that compose a thickening of the parietal layer of Bowman's capsule, giving the appearance of being free within the urinary ultrafiltrate.

303–305. The answers are 303-D, 304-C, 305-A. *(Robbins, 5/e, pp 799–800. Rubin, 2/e, pp 662–668.)* Malabsorption syndromes have protean causes and are broadly categorized on the basis of the underlying abnormality. Abetalipoproteinemia is a rare condition in which absence of lipoprotein B leads to inability to synthesize prebetalipoproteins (VLDL), betalipoproteins (LDL), and chylomicrons. Consequently, lipid accumulates in vacuoles in mucosal cells. Characteristic acanthocytic erythrocytes are seen in the peripheral blood.

Whipple's disease is a multisystem disorder of presumed infectious origin. The lamina propria of the small intestinal mucosa is distended by PA-positive macrophages containing bacillary bodies. The condition usually responds to broad-spectrum antibiotics.

Primary intestinal lymphoma usually arises in men under the age of 50 and may present with malabsorption. Malignant lymphoid cells infiltrate the lamina propria of the mucosa. Lymphadenopathy and hepatosplenomegaly are usually absent. Immunoproliferative small intestinal disease (IPSID) is a neoplastic proliferation of small intestinal B lymphocytes that secrete IgA (alpha-chain disease) and is seen in the Mediterranean region (Mediterranean lymphoma).

Disaccharidase (usually lactase) deficiency is most commonly secondary to infection, inflammation, celiac disease, or radiation enteritis; it is rarely inherited. Lactose cannot be broken down and the resulting osmotic load causes diarrhea. Morphology is normal and diagnosis is based on lactose challenge.

306–308. The answers are 306-C, 307-E, 308-A. *(Robbins, 5/e, pp 861–863, 868–869, 879–882.)* Primary biliary cirrhosis (PBC) is an idiopathic cholestatic condition that leads to cirrhosis. It is nine times more frequent in females and the average age of onset is 50 to 55 years. It is often insidious in onset; many patients are asymptomatic or have only pruritus despite a markedly increased serum alkaline phosphatase. Various autoantibodies may be present in the serum but the most sensitive and specific is antimitochondrial antibody, which is present in more than 90 percent of symptomatic patients. Diagnosis should be confirmed by liver biopsy.

Primary hemochromatosis is a genetic disorder that affects men five times more frequently than women. In this disease excessive amounts of iron are deposited in the parenchymal cells of various organs. Total body iron stores are grossly elevated. The organs chiefly affected are the liver, pancreas, myocardium, and endocrine glands; this may lead to cirrhosis, cardiomegaly and cardiac failure, and diabetes mellitus. In established cases serum iron is often > 250 μg/dL and serum ferritin > 500 ng/dL. There is also an increased risk of developing hepatocellular carcinoma.

Primary hepatocellular carcinoma represents 2 to 3 percent of all malignant neoplasms in the Western world and arises on a background of cirrhosis in 80 to 95 percent of these cases. Clinical presentation is often nonspecific, but hepatomegaly and ascites are usually present. Alpha$_1$-antitrypsin and alpha-fetoprotein may be demonstrated in the tumor cells by immunocytochemistry in up to 75 percent of cases, and 75 percent of cases also show elevated serum levels of alpha-fetoprotein, which is not seen in cirrhosis alone.

Endocrine System

309. A perimenopausal woman complains of slight swallowing difficulty, fatigue, and a change in bowel habits. The photomicrograph below is of her thyroid gland. This disorder is

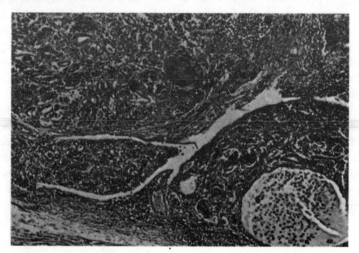

(A) subacute thyroiditis
(B) thyrotoxicosis
(C) autoimmune thyroiditis
(D) Riedel's thyroiditis
(E) conversion hysteria

310. Graves' disease is associated with all the following EXCEPT

(A) tachycardia
(B) anti-TSH receptor antibodies
(C) localized myxedema
(D) toxic nodular goiter
(E) exophthalmos

311. The section of tissue shown in the photomicrograph below (taken under low power) was probably removed from a patient who has

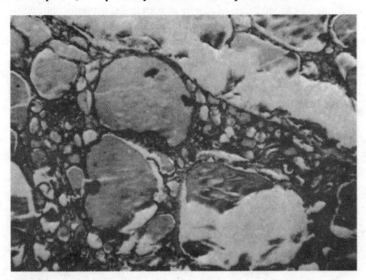

(A) a normal thyroid gland
(B) colloid storage goiter
(C) Graves' disease
(D) Riedel's struma
(E) Hashimoto's thyroiditis

312. Which of the following is physiologically the most active thyroid hormone?

(A) Thyroglobulin
(B) Monoiodotyrosine (MIT)
(C) Diiodotyrosine (DIT)
(D) Triiodothyronine (T_3)
(E) Thyroxine (T_4)

313. Follicular carcinoma of the thyroid may show all the following features EXCEPT

(A) vascular invasion and hematogenous metastasis
(B) multiple foci within the gland
(C) a clear cell variant that resembles renal carcinoma
(D) an insular type that is an aggressive form
(E) absence of ground-glass nuclei

314. A 37-year-old man presents with a single, firm mass within the thyroid gland. Histologic examination of this mass reveals organoid nests of tumor cells separated by broad bands of stroma as seen in the photomicrograph below. The stroma stained positively with the Congo red stain and demonstrated yellow-green birefringence. The most likely diagnosis of this lesion is

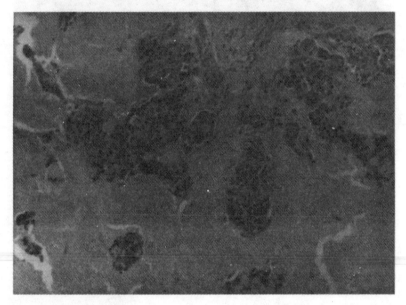

(A) follicular carcinoma
(B) papillary carcinoma
(C) squamous cell carcinoma
(D) medullary carcinoma
(E) anaplastic carcinoma

315. Bone lesions in association with hypocalcemia, hyperphosphatemia, and hypersecretion of parathyroid hormone may be seen in all of the following EXCEPT

(A) parathyroid hyperplasia
(B) parathyroid adenoma
(C) chronic renal failure
(D) intestinal malabsorption
(E) vitamin D deficiency

316. Signs and symptoms seen in patients with defects in parathyroid hormone interaction with G protein (Albright's hereditary osteodystrophy) include all the following EXCEPT

(A) short stature
(B) short fourth and fifth metacarpal bones
(C) mental retardation
(D) hypocalcemia
(E) decreased secretion of parathyroid hormone

317. The parathyroid glands can be described in terms of anatomic or developmental characteristics that include all the following EXCEPT

(A) embryonic development from the endodermal tissue of the third and fourth pharyngeal pouches
(B) the location of the superior glands normally at the lower border of the cricoid cartilage
(C) a spatial relationship with the thyroid and a temporal developmental relationship with the thymus
(D) usually four in number applied to the dorsum of the thyroid gland
(E) a constant location of the inferior glands

318. The most common etiologic factor in Cushing's syndrome is

(A) adrenal adenoma
(B) bilateral adrenal hyperplasia
(C) adrenal carcinoma
(D) ectopic adrenal tissue
(E) hypercorticism secondary to nonendocrine malignant tumors

319. Primary hyperaldosteronism is associated with all the following features EXCEPT

(A) carcinoma
(B) adenoma
(C) muscle weakness
(D) expansion of intravascular volume
(E) edema

320. A diagnosis of adrenogenital syndrome with demonstrable adrenal hyperplasia is consistent with

(A) generalized calcium oxalate deposition similar to that occurring in oxalosis
(B) accumulation of glycolipids in tissue
(C) salt loss similar to that of Addison's disease
(D) symptoms similar to those occurring in phenylketonuria
(E) severe acidosis

321. In type II polyglandular autoimmune syndrome (Schmidt's syndrome), autoimmune adrenocortical insufficiency may occur along with

(A) hypoparathyroidism
(B) mucocutaneous candidiasis
(C) Hashimoto's thyroiditis
(D) islet cell adenoma of the pancreas
(E) medullary carcinoma of the thyroid

322. Components of the normal thymus gland include all the following EXCEPT

(A) thymocytes
(B) epithelial cells
(C) neuroendocrine cells
(D) myoid cells
(E) germinal centers

323. All the following statements concerning thymomas are true EXCEPT

(A) they originate from epithelial cells
(B) they are most common in the anterosuperior mediastinum
(C) they are asymptomatic or cause local pressure effects
(D) neoplastic lymphocytes are a component
(E) most thymomas are benign

324. A 42-year-old man complains of recently having to change his shoe size from 9 to 10½, and he also says that his hands and jaw are now larger. The disorder is most likely mediated through

(A) prolactin
(B) ACTH
(C) somatomedin
(D) antidiuretic hormone
(E) thyrotropin

325. A 49-year-old man who smokes two packs of cigarettes a day presents with a lung mass on x-ray and recent weight gain. Laboratory examination shows hyponatremia with hyperosmolar urine. The patient probably has

(A) renal failure
(B) pituitary failure
(C) Conn's syndrome
(D) cardiac failure
(E) inappropriate ADH

DIRECTIONS: Each group of questions below consists of lettered headings followed by a set of numbered items. For each numbered item select the **one** lettered heading with which it is **most** closely associated. Each lettered heading may be used **once, more than once, or not at all.**

Questions 326–329

For each disorder listed, select the most appropriate feature or description.

(A) Panhypopituitarism in adults
(B) Cushing's syndrome in childhood
(C) Rare condition with very rare elaboration of hormones
(D) Postpartum pituitary necrosis
(E) Common cause of diabetes insipidus in children

326. Hand-Schüller-Christian disease

327. Sheehan's syndrome

328. Simmonds' disease

329. Adrenal cortical carcinoma

Questions 330–333

For each endocrinopathy, select the most appropriate condition.

(A) Empty sella syndrome
(B) Tumor of adrenal medulla
(C) Bilateral adrenalectomy
(D) Most common endocrinopathy caused by pituitary tumor
(E) Excess secretion of hormone in chronic renal insufficiency

330. Secondary hyperparathyroidism

331. Multiple endocrine neoplasia type 2 (MEN 2)

332. Nelson's syndrome

333. Hyperprolactinemia

Endocrine System
Answers

309. The answer is C. *(Robbins, 5/e, pp 1125–1128.)* Hashimoto's (autoimmune) thyroiditis is one of the conditions of chronic thyroiditis. It is not that uncommon in the United States. The stroma is permeated by a dense lymphoplasmacytic infiltrate with lymphoid follicles (germinal centers) that distorts and transforms thyroid follicles into collections of acidophilic cells (oncocytes, Hürthle-like cells). Not uncommonly, patients develop hypothyroidism as a result of follicle disruption, and the manifestations consist of fatigue, myxedema, cold intolerance, hair coarsening, and constipation. Whereas subacute (DeQuervain's) thyroiditis, Riedel's thyroiditis, and psychosomatic complaints may cause common symptoms, biopsy findings of these disorders are distinctly different from those of Hashimoto's disease.

310. The answer is D. *(Robbins, 5/e, pp 1129–1131.)* Graves' disease, or diffuse toxic goiter, is one of the three most common disorders associated with thyrotoxicosis or hyperthyroidism (the other two are toxic multinodular goiter and toxic adenoma). This hyperfunctioning and hyperplastic diffuse goiter is accompanied by infiltrative ophthalmopathy, including exophthalmos or proptosis—only seen in Graves' disease. Dermopathy or pretibial "myxedema" is present in up to 15 percent of cases. Graves' disease is an autoimmune form of goiter caused by thyroid-stimulating immunoglobulins or thyroid-stimulating hormone receptor antibodies. Autoantibodies to TSH receptor antigens are produced because of a defect in antigen-specific suppressor T cells. The antibodies bind to TSH receptors on thyroid follicular cells and function as TSH, with resultant thyroid growth and hyperfunction. Such antibodies can be identified in almost all cases of Graves' disease. Cardiac manifestations include tachycardia, cardiomegaly, and occasional arrhythmias (atrial fibrillation), and these are often early features. Diffuse toxic goiter is associated with HLA-DR3 genotype.

311. The answer is B. *(Anderson, 9/e, pp 1546–1549.)* The histologic appearance of colloid storage goiter generally includes abnormally large, colloid-filled follicles compressing the intervening small or normal-sized follicles that contain very little colloid. The epithelium of the follicles is predominantly flat cuboidal, with occasional epithelial papillary structures protruding into the follicles. In primary hyperplasia with Graves' disease, the follicular epithelium is tall, with papillary infoldings and peripheral vacuolation of the colloid. Riedel's struma appears histologically as a marked fibrous tissue replacement of the normal thyroid tissue. In Hashimoto's thyroiditis, only remnants of thyroid follicles and epithelial cells are found in sheets of lymphocytes with germinal centers.

312. The answer is D. *(Henry, 18/e, pp 314–317.)* Triiodothyronine (T_3) is the thyroid hormone with the greatest physiologic activity, although thyroxine (T_4) is present in greater quantities and thus is usually the best measure of thyroid activity. Monoiodotyrosine (MIT) and diiodotyrosine (DIT) are not released from the gland and have little activity. Thyroglobulin is the carrier protein for binding stored thyroid hormones.

313. The answer is B. *(Robbins, 5/e, pp 1136–1142.)* The four major histologic subtypes of thyroid carcinoma, in decreasing order of frequency, are papillary, follicular, medullary, and undifferentiated (anaplastic). Follicular carcinoma has a frequency of approximately 10 to 20 percent compared with papillary cancer at 60 to 70 percent. There are, of course, follicular variants of both papillary and medullary carcinoma, but these behave as papillary and medullary cancer, not as the follicular type. Other, much rarer variants of follicular cancer include the type resembling renal clear cell carcinoma and the insular type of thyroid cancer, which is an aggressive form of follicular carcinoma with a solid growth pattern. Vascular invasion and hematogenous metastasis are usual with follicular cancer, so that intrathyroidal foci from lymphatic spread would not occur, although they are very common with papillary cancer. Absence of ground-glass nuclei or well-formed papillae or psammoma bodies differentiates follicular from papillary carcinoma.

314. The answer is D. *(Robbins, 5/e, pp 1136–1142.)* The four major histologic subtypes of thyroid carcinoma are papillary, follicular, medullary, and undifferentiated (anaplastic). Medullary carcinoma, which originates from the parafollicular C cells, is characterized by its amyloid stroma, which classically has a yellow-green birefringence staining pattern with the Congo red stain; by its genetic (familial) associations with pheochromocytomas and parathyroid hyperplasia or adenomas (Sipple's syndrome, multiple endocrine neoplasia IIa); and by its elaboration of calcitonin and other substances. In contrast, papillary carcinomas are composed of papillary structures with fibrovascular cores, while follicular carcinomas typically have a microfollicular pattern. It is important prognostically to differentiate papillary carcinomas from follicular carcinomas, as papillary carcinomas tend to be indolent (up to 80 percent survival at 10 years), while follicular carcinomas are much more aggressive (5-year mortality up to 70 percent). Follicular areas may be present within a papillary carcinoma and in fact may be quite extensive. If present, these changes can make the diagnosis difficult. It is important to recognize this follicular variant of papillary carcinoma as its behavior remains similar to that of indolent papillary carcinoma. Features consistent with papillary carcinoma, even in predominantly follicular areas, include optically clear nuclei ("ground glass," "Orphan Annie eyes"), nuclear grooves, calcospherites (psammoma bodies), and intranuclear cytoplasmic pseudoinclusions.

315. The answer is B. *(Robbins, 5/e, pp 1144–1147. Rubin, 2/e, pp 1126–1128.)* It is important to distinguish primary from secondary hyperparathyroidism. Both forms may be associated with the development of bone lesions, but excess parathyroid hormone (PTH) production in primary hyperparathyroidism, which may be caused by a functioning parathyroid adenoma, leads to hypercalcemia and hypophosphatemia. In contrast, secondary hyperparathyroidism results from hypocalcemia, which causes secondary hypersecretion of PTH. It is principally found in patients with chronic renal failure, where phosphate retention is thought to cause hypocalcemia, but it can also be seen in vitamin D deficiency caused by intestinal malabsorption. Histologic hyperplasia of the parathyroid may be caused by either primary or secondary hyperparathyroidism, and therefore it can be seen with the changes of secondary hyperparathyroidism, namely hypocalcemia and hyperphosphatemia.

316. The answer is E. *(Robbins, 5/e, pp 1147–1148. Rubin, 2/e, pp 1125–1126.)* Hypoparathyroidism may be caused by either decreased secretion of parathyroid hormone (PTH) or end-organ insensitivity to PTH (pseudohypoparathyroidism), both of which are associated with hypocalcemia and hyperphosphatemia. Many patients with pseudohypoparathyroidism have a defect in binding of many hormones to guanine nucleotide–binding protein (G protein). These hormones include PTH, thyroid-stimulating hormone, glucagon, and the gonadotropins follicle-stimulating hormone and luteinizing hormone. These patients have characteristic signs and symptoms including short stature, round face, short neck, reduced intelligence, and abnormally short metacarpal and metatarsal bones. In contrast to patients with hypothyroidism caused by decreased levels of PTH, patients with pseudohypoparathyroidism (Albright's hereditary osteodystrophy) have normal or increased levels of circulating PTH and in fact have hyperparathyroidism.

317. The answer is E. *(Anderson, 9/e, p 1570.)* The parathyroid glands develop from the endodermal tissue of the dorsal diverticula of the third and fourth pharyngeal pouches and usually consist of four flattened, encapsulated, oval bodies that lie against the dorsum of the thyroid gland. The superior glands, derived from the fourth pharyngeal pouches, have an anatomic position that is more constant than that of the inferior pair. The inferior parathyroids, because they develop and move caudally with the thymus, sometimes become located below the thyroid level, and the inconstant location of these parathyroids is an important factor to consider in the search for pathologic parathyroid tissue during autopsy or surgery.

318. The answer is B. *(Henry, 18/e, pp 327–331. Rubin, 2/e, pp 1133–1138.)* Cushing's syndrome may be the result of bilateral adrenal hyperplasia, adrenal neoplasia, or excessive use of adrenocorticotropic hormone or glucocorticoids. However, bilateral adrenal hyperplasia is the most common etiologic factor. The clinical manifestations of the syndrome—whether it is induced by ectopic ACTH (small cell carcinoma of the lung), or exogenously, or endogenously by the adrenal—are similar. Levels of plasma and urinary cortisol and urinary 17-hydroxycorticoid are usually elevated.

319. The answer is E. *(Robbins, 5/e, pp 1153–1154.)* Edema is not a feature of primary hyperaldosteronism (Conn's syndrome), which is characterized by weakness, hypertension, polydipsia, and polyuria. The underlying physiologic abnormalities include alkaline urine, an elevated level of serum sodium, hypokalemic alkalosis, and excessive potassium loss by the kidneys. The level of serum aldosterone is elevated; that of plasma renin is suppressed. The elevated level of serum sodium causes expansion of the intravascular volume. A single adenoma has been described as the causative factor of primary hyperaldosteronism in the majority of patients, and carcinoma, multiple adenomas, and cortical hyperplasia have been cited occasionally as causes of this syndrome.

320. The answer is C. *(Robbins, 5/e, pp 1154–1157. Rubin, 2/e, pp 1129–1131.)* In the adrenal cortex, cholesterol is converted into either mineralocorticoids (aldosterone) in the zona glomerulosa, glucocorticoids (cortisol) in the zona fasciculata, or sex steroid precursors in the zona reticularis. Congenital adrenal hyperplasia (CAH) is a syndrome resulting from a defect in the synthesis of cortisol, which leads to excess ACTH production by the anterior pituitary. This in turn leads to adrenal hyperplasia. Most cases of CAH result from deficiency of 21-hydroxylase ($P450_{C21}$). Instead of forming cortisol, precursors are shunted into the pathway that forms androgens. This may cause virilism (pseudohermaphroditism) in female infants. Additionally, if the enzyme defect affects the zona glomerulosa, then aldosterone synthesis is also impaired, and this can lead to salt loss similar to that found in Addison's disease (primary chronic adrenal insufficiency).

321. The answer is C. *(Robbins, 5/e, pp 1158–1160. Rubin, 2/e, pp 1131–1133.)* In 1855, when Addison first described primary adrenal insufficiency, the most common cause was tuberculosis of the adrenal gland. Now the majority of patients have adrenal autoantibodies and are thought to have autoimmune Addison's disease. Half of these patients have other autoimmune endocrine diseases. Patients with type I polyglandular autoimmune syndrome have at least two of the following three diseases or abnormalities: Addison's disease, hypoparathyroidism, and mucocutaneous candidiasis. Type II polyglandular autoimmune syndrome, also called *Schmidt's syndrome,* lacks hypoparathyroidism and mucocutaneous candidiasis, and instead is associated with autoimmune thyroid disease (Hashimoto's thyroiditis) and insulin-dependent diabetes. Islet cell adenomas of the pancreas may be found in multiple endocrine neoplasia type 1 (MEN 1) syndrome along with pituitary adenomas and parathyroid hyperplasia or adenomas. Medullary carcinoma of the thyroid along with pheochromocytomas of the adrenal gland and parathyroid hyperplasia is seen in MEN 2A (Sipple's syndrome).

322. The answer is E. *(Robbins, 5/e, pp 1166–1167. Rubin, 2/e, pp 1144–1145.)* The thymus, derived from the third pair of pharyngeal pouches and inconsistently from the fourth pair, is divided into an outer cortex and an inner medulla and is composed of lymphocytes and epithelial cells. The lymphocytes are mainly T cells, which in the cortex are immature (thymocytes) and in the medulla are mature (having phenotypic characteristics of peripheral blood T lymphocytes). The epithelial cells are mainly located in the medulla, where they form Hassall's corpuscles. The thymus normally has a few neuroendocrine cells, which can give rise to carcinoid tumors or small cell carcinoma, and a few myoid cells, which are similar to striated muscle cells and may play a role in the autoimmune pathogenesis of myasthenia gravis. The appearance of lymphoid follicles with germinal centers is diagnostic of thymic hyperplasia and is not a normal component of the thymus gland.

323. The answer is D. *(Robbins, 5/e, pp 1167–1168.)* Thymomas are tumors arising from thymic epithelial cells and form one of the most common mediastinal neoplasms, especially in the anterosuperior mediastinum. There is a scant or rich lymphocytic infiltrate of T cells, which are not neoplastic, although their size and prominent nucleoli may cause histologic confusion with lymphoma. About 90 percent of thymomas are benign and occur at a mean age of 50 years. They are very rare in children. They may be asymptomatic or cause pressure effects of dysphagia, dyspnea, or vena cava compression. Associated systemic disorders include myasthenia gravis, hematologic cytopenias, collagen vascular disease (lupus), and hypogammaglobulinemia. Malignant thymomas show infiltration and capsular invasion plus pleural implants or distant metastasis.

324. The answer is C. *(Henry, 18/e, pp 310–311. Robbins, 5/e, p 1117.)* The constellation of cartilaginous-periosteal soft tissue growth of the distal extremities (acromegaly) and growth of the skull and face bones is characteristic of hypersecretion of growth hormone (GH) from an anterior pituitary adenoma. GH modulates the production of hepatic somatomedin (sulfation factor). Somatomedins are small peptides that act on the target organs after being synthesized under the influence of growth hormone. They have insulin-like properties but are immunologically distinct from insulin. In addition to acralskeletal expansion, patients with hyperpituitarism of the adult-onset variety (occurring after epiphyseal plate closure) have organomegaly, including increased size of the heart, kidneys, liver, and spleen. Cardiac failure is usually the mechanism of death.

325. The answer is E. *(Robbins, 5/e, p 1121.)* The syndrome of inappropriate antidiuretic hormone (SIADH) is an important cause of dilutional hyponatremia that has been identified in tumors of the thymus gland, malignant lymphoma, and pancreatic neoplasms. It occurs predominantly, however, as a result of ectopic secretion of ADH by oat cell carcinomas of the lung. Since the tumor cells per se are autonomously producing ADH, there is no feedback inhibition from the hypothalamic osmoreceptors, and the persistent ADH effect on the renal tubules causes water retention even with concentrated urine. Hence the term *inappropriate ADH* arises. Laboratory findings of the syndrome include low plasma sodium levels (dilutional hyponatremia), low plasma osmolality, and high urine osmolality caused by disproportionate solute excretion without water.

326–329. The answers are 326-E, 327-D, 328-A, 329-B. *(Anderson, 9/e, pp 1526–1527, 1529, 1599–1605.)* Panhypopituitarism results from destruction of at least 75 percent of the anterior pituitary. This destruction usually is caused by tumors (e.g., metastatic carcinoma of the breast or lung) and infarction, but destruction can also be caused by inflammatory disorders, abscesses, granulomas (giant cell granulomas of older women), and histiocytic infiltrates. *Simmonds' disease*—the eponym for the classic clinical syndrome caused by panhypopituitarism in the adult—involves insufficiency of the gonads, thyroid, and adrenals and is secondary to the absence of stimulation by the respective trophic hormones.

Sheehan's syndrome consists of symptoms of pituitary failure that occur as the result of infarction of the pituitary because of postpartum hemorrhage or other types of massive hemorrhage. In Sheehan's syndrome the pituitary infarction frequently occurs in the presence of intravascular coagulopathy of pregnancy.

Hand-Schüller-Christian disease (HSC) features histiocytic infiltrates in the pituitary and xanthomatous deposits in the skull and dura. Because the infundibular portion of the pituitary may be involved in HSC, the disease may cause diabetes insipidus in children as the pituitary is subjected to bony encasement with destruction of the nerve tracts in the neurohypophysis.

Before the age of 10, Cushing's syndrome is probably most often related to adrenal carcinoma, a tumor present in at least 50 percent of cases, while most of the remaining cases are associated with adrenocortical hyperplasia. After the age of 10, zona fasciculata hyperplasia accounts for approximately 70 percent of cases. In the adult, adrenocortical carcinoma is responsible for only 10 percent of the cases of Cushing's syndrome. Adrenal carcinomas are differentiated from adenomas by capsular or vascular invasion and metastasis.

Primary carcinoma of the anterior pituitary is not only rare but is rather undifferentiated, so that the cell type cannot be identified. However, most cases are of chromophobe origin; therefore, hormonal elaboration is very rare. It is difficult to differentiate the carcinoma from an adenoma and very local invasion is also unreliable; thus, metastasis is the only valid criterion of malignancy.

330–333. The answers are 330-E, 331-B, 332-C, 333-D. *(Robbins, 5/e, pp 1117, 1146–1147, 1162–1164, 1169–1170. Rubin, 2/e, pp 1104–1106.)* In secondary hyperparathyroidism, the excess secretion of parathormone (PTH) in chronic renal insufficiency is characterized by high serum phosphate and low, normal, or subnormal calcium values. Since the failing kidney is not able to synthesize 1α,25-dihydroxycholecalciferol, the most active form of vitamin D, this deficiency leads to poor absorption of calcium from the gut and relative hypocalcemia, which stimulates PTH oversecretion. Chronic renal failure is the most important cause, but secondary hyperparathyroidism also occurs in vitamin D deficiency, malabsorption syndromes, and pseudohypoparathyroidism.

Tumors of the adrenal medulla include pheochromocytoma, neuroblastoma, and ganglioneuroma. Pheochromocytoma usually occurs sporadically, but also in familial syndromes, two of which are part of MEN 2. It comprises tumors of thyroid (medullary carcinoma) and of adrenal medulla (pheochromocytoma) and chief cell hyperplasia of the parathyroids. The familial form is Sipple's syndrome (MEN 2A) in which pheochromocytomas are bilateral in 60 to 100 percent of cases. MEN 2B includes thyroid carcinoma (medullary), pheochromocytoma, and associated neurologic abnormalities and mucosal neuromas.

Nelson's syndrome occurs following bilateral adrenalectomy for Cushing's disease; it is marked by an invasive, inoperable, hormone-secreting pituitary corticotroph adenoma. With lack of adrenal feedback control, the adenoma may release large amounts of ACTH and melanocyte-stimulating peptides into the blood, resulting in marked brown melanin pigmentation in the skin.

Hyperprolactinemia is the most common hypersecretory endocrinopathy caused by a pituitary tumor—a prolactin-producing eosinophilic adenoma. In women, an amenorrhea-glactorrhea syndrome results; in men, there may be loss of libido because of mass effect with inhibition of gonadotropin secretion or effects. Since other causes of hyperprolactinemia exist, including lesions in the hypothalamus, estrogen therapy, and drugs such as methyldopa, diagnosis of a prolactinoma requires evidence of an anterior lobe mass and elevated plasma levels of prolactin.

Genitourinary System

DIRECTIONS: Each question below contains five suggested responses. Select the **one best** response to each question.

334. All the following characteristics are associated with the disorder depicted in the photograph below EXCEPT

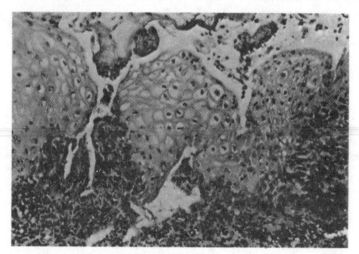

(A) massive unilateral enlargement
(B) autosomal dominant inheritance in adult form
(C) autosomal recessive inheritance in childhood form
(D) hepatic cysts in childhood form
(E) possible association with berry aneurysms

335. A major role in the exclusion of albumin from the ultrafiltrate in the normal human glomerulus is played by

(A) sodium-potassium ATPase
(B) parietal epithelium
(C) endothelial fenestrations
(D) proteoglycans
(E) podocytes

336. A patient being investigated for hematuria and proteinuria has a renal biopsy that shows changes in the glomeruli as depicted below. All the following diseases can be associated with changes seen in this biopsy EXCEPT

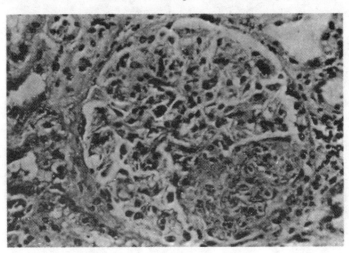

(A) bacterial endocarditis
(B) anaphylactoid purpura
(C) systemic lupus erythematosus
(D) hereditary nephritis (Alport's syndrome)
(E) diabetes mellitus

---

337. A significant role in vascular permeability, particularly in the renal glomerulus, is played by

(A) collagen type IV
(B) desmin
(C) fibronectin
(D) podocytes
(E) polyanions

338. Acute poststreptococcal glomerulonephritis usually does all the following EXCEPT

(A) follow infection with group A beta-hemolytic streptococci
(B) follow a streptococcal infection in less than 5 days
(C) have a better prognosis in children than in adults
(D) show low serum complement levels (hypocomplementemia)
(E) exhibit elevation of antistreptolysin O (ASO) titer

339. Marked thickening of the glomerular basement membrane, as shown in the photomicrograph below, may be seen in

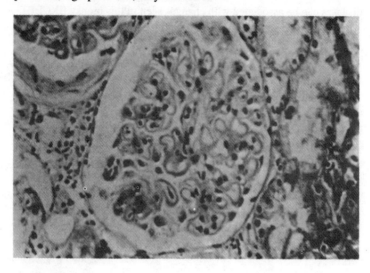

(A) lipoid nephrosis
(B) membranous glomerulonephritis
(C) Goodpasture's syndrome
(D) acute pyelonephritis
(E) chronic glomerulonephritis

340. All the following renal disorders are associated with the nephrotic syndrome EXCEPT

(A) membranous glomerulonephritis
(B) lipoid nephrosis
(C) membranoproliferative glomerulonephritis
(D) acute tubular necrosis
(E) focal segmental glomerulosclerosis

341. A linear pattern of immunoglobulin deposition along the glomerular basement membrane that can be demonstrated by immunofluorescence is typical of

(A) lupus nephritis
(B) diabetic glomerulopathy
(C) Goodpasture's syndrome
(D) Goldblatt's kidney
(E) renal vein thrombosis

342. An 18-month-old infant is evaluated for generalized tissue edema and ascites. Urinalysis shows numerous hyaline casts and lipid droplets. Total plasma protein and albumin are markedly decreased, whereas total lipids are increased. A light micrograph of a renal biopsy glomerulus is shown below. Statements applicable to this disorder include that

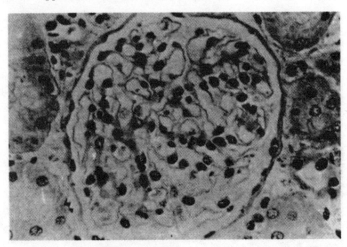

(A) the problem is hepatic, not renal
(B) electron microscopy is diagnostic
(C) light microscopy is diagnostic
(D) exacerbations are uncommon
(E) response to steroid therapy is poor

343. A 10-year-old boy has a bout of ordinary upper respiratory infection followed within 36 h by an episode of hematuria. There are no joint symptoms, gastrointestinal symptoms, petechiae, or rashes. To confirm the suspicion of Berger's disease, which of the following is indicated?

(A) Examination of urinary sediment
(B) Renal scan
(C) Renal biopsy immunofluorescence
(D) Creatinine clearance
(E) Intravenous pyelogram

344. The photomicrograph below shows evidence of glomerular fibrin deposition. This histopathology is a supplemental finding in a 2-year-old child who has a history of abdominal pain and bloody diarrhea, followed by acute glomerulonephritis, Coombs'-negative severe hemolytic anemia, and renal failure. The likely diagnoses might include

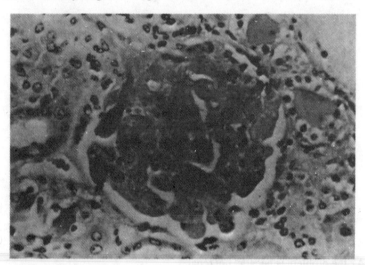

(A) lupus erythematosus
(B) acute poststreptococcal glomerulonephritis
(C) lipoid nephrosis
(D) hemolytic-uremic syndrome
(E) bacterial endocarditis

345. An adult medical laboratory technician recovering from hepatitis B develops hematuria, proteinuria, and red cell casts in the urine. Which of the following would best describe the changes within the kidney in this patient?

(A) Plasma cell interstitial nephritis
(B) IgG linear fluorescence along the glomerular basement membrane
(C) Granular deposits of antibodies in the glomerular basement membrane
(D) Diffuse thickening of the glomerular basement membrane by subepithelial immune deposits
(E) Nodular hyaline glomerulosclerosis

346. The gross appearance of the kidney shown is most compatible with which of the following conditions?

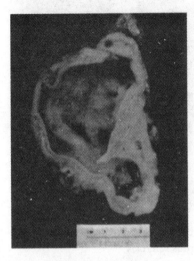

(A) Cystic renal dysplasia
(B) Acute pyelonephritis
(C) Chronic pyelonephritis
(D) Acute glomerulonephritis
(E) Chronic glomerulonephritis

347. Acute tubular necrosis (ATN) is a fairly common renal lesion and is associated with all the following EXCEPT

(A) red cell casts in the urine
(B) proteinuria
(C) proximal tubular damage in toxic ATN
(D) oliguria
(E) acute renal failure

348. What is the correct treatment for a patient who has hypertension secondary to unilateral renal artery stenosis when the contralateral kidney shows severe arteriolonephrosclerosis?

(A) Ureteral reimplantation
(B) Removal of the kidney supplied by the stenotic artery
(C) Repair of the renal artery stenosis and ipsilateral nephrectomy
(D) Repair of the renal artery stenosis and contralateral nephrectomy
(E) Nonsurgical management

349. All the following renal diseases cause hypertension EXCEPT

(A) small, bilateral renal infarcts
(B) renal artery arteriosclerosis
(C) fibromuscular dysplasia of the renal artery
(D) hydronephrosis
(E) pyelonephritis

350. All the following statements are true of urinary calculi EXCEPT that

(A) they are more common in males
(B) they are bilateral in 40 percent of cases
(C) they are radiopaque in about 90 percent of cases
(D) they may be associated with *Pseudomonas* infections
(E) the incidence is increased in leukemia

351. The kidney shown in the photomicrograph below exhibits a tumor that has originated in the upper pole. Correct statements about this tumor include all the following EXCEPT that

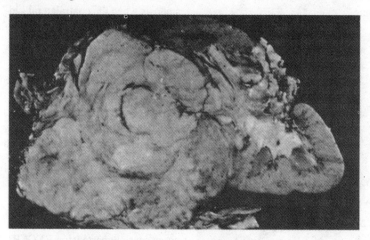

(A) it is sometimes associated with polycythemia
(B) it is sometimes associated with tuberous sclerosis
(C) it may produce glucocorticoids
(D) it originates from proximal convoluted tubular cells
(E) it occurs predominantly in the sixth decade

352. A middle-aged man comes to you with the single presenting symptom of occasional hematuria of very recent onset. The most probable cause is

(A) acute pyelonephritis
(B) nephroblastoma
(C) renal cell carcinoma
(D) mesoblastic nephroma
(E) renal pelvic urothelial tumor

353. All the following abnormalities are associated with an increased incidence of Wilms' tumor EXCEPT

(A) aniridia
(B) male pseudohermaphroditism
(C) hemihypertrophy
(D) renal medullary cysts
(E) hypoplasia of radii

354. The condition shown in the photomicrograph, malacoplakia of the urinary bladder, is considered to be associated with

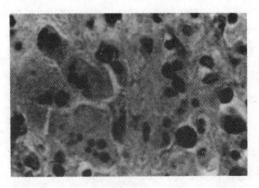

(A) tuberculosis
(B) urothelial carcinoma
(C) schistosomiasis
(D) staphylococcal infections
(E) defects in phagocytosis

---

355. A sexually active man who has had a negative evaluation for gonococcal infection and who complains of persistent dysuria but no other symptoms should be considered to have

(A) prostatic hypertrophy
(B) epididymitis
(C) orchitis
(D) nonspecific urethritis
(E) renal stones

356. All the following statements are true regarding transitional cell carcinoma of the bladder EXCEPT that

(A) it is more common in men than in women
(B) it is associated with infection by *Schistosoma haematobium*
(C) it is associated with cigarette smoking
(D) it shows increased incidence in aniline dye workers
(E) it tends to recur after excision, regardless of grade

357. The photomicrograph below shows an abnormal renal tubular epithelial cell with a large, intranuclear inclusion surrounded by a clear halo. It was found in a urinary specimen from a very ill renal transplant patient. The disease diagnosed is associated with all the following EXCEPT

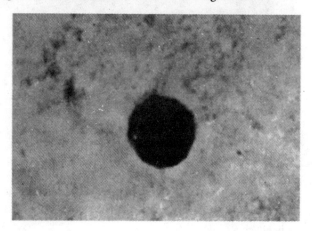

(A) interstitial pneumonitis
(B) hepatitis
(C) a herpesvirus
(D) gastrointestinal ulcers
(E) detection of antigen in 1 to 3 weeks

---

358. Primary germ cell tumors of the testis occur predominantly in the younger male with the exception of

(A) embryonal carcinoma
(B) spermatocytic seminoma
(C) polyembryoma
(D) choriocarcinoma
(E) teratocarcinoma

359. A small, palpable, well-circumscribed nodule in the epididymis is most likely to be

(A) androblastoma
(B) tuberculous granuloma
(C) carcinoma
(D) adenomatoid tumor
(E) adrenocortical rest

360. The photomicrograph below is of a section from a testis removed from the inguinal region of a man aged 25. Which of the following statements is true regarding the condition illustrated?

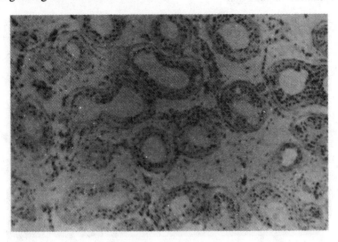

(A) It is bilateral in the majority of cases
(B) Teratoma is the most common malignancy to arise
(C) Risk of associated malignancy is reduced by orchiopexy
(D) There is increased risk of malignancy in the contralateral testis
(E) Both Leydig and Sertoli cells are reduced in number

---

361. Which of the following testicular tumors is most radiosensitive?

(A) Seminoma
(B) Embryonal carcinoma
(C) Choriocarcinoma
(D) Yolk sac tumor
(E) Immature teratoma

362. Within prostatic glands, features consistent with prostatic intraepithelial neoplasia (PIN) include all the following EXCEPT

(A) cellular crowding
(B) absence of a basal cell layer
(C) variation in nuclear size
(D) nucleoli
(E) hyperchromatism

363. The photomicrograph below shows a section through a testis removed from a 30-year-old man with acute scrotal pain. True statements regarding this condition include that

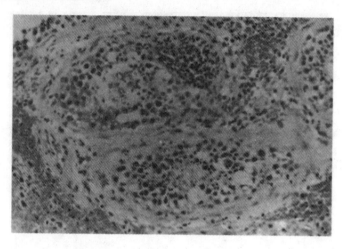

(A) infection is usually by the hematogenous route
(B) sterility is a rare condition
(C) the epididymis is usually spared
(D) *Chlamydia trachomatis* is a common pathogen
(E) interstitial cells of Leydig are destroyed

---

364. Histologic examination of an excision specimen from a lesion on the dorsal surface of the penis reveals a papillary lesion with clear vacuolization of epithelial cells on the surface and extension of the hyperplastic epithelium into the underlying tissue along a broad front. The most likely diagnosis of this lesion is

(A) condyloma acuminatum
(B) Bowen's disease
(C) erythroplasia of Queyrat
(D) verrucous carcinoma
(E) squamous cell carcinoma

365. Carcinoma of the prostate tends to do all the following EXCEPT

(A) be adenocarcinoma
(B) arise in the posterior lobe
(C) cause elevation of serum acid phosphatase
(D) be estrogen-dependent
(E) form osteoblastic metastases

366. The photomicrograph below depicts a biopsy of the uterine cervix that was done following an abnormal Pap smear report. This histologic section shows

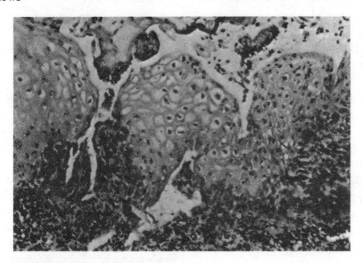

(A) condyloma acuminatum
(B) carcinoma in situ
(C) dysplasia
(D) cervical intraepithelial neoplasia
(E) squamous metaplasia

367. Vaginal adenosis precedes the development of which of the following?

(A) Condyloma acuminatum
(B) Cervical carcinoma
(C) Clear cell carcinoma
(D) Carcincoma of the endometrium
(E) Squamous carcinoma of the vagina

368. Primary malignant neoplasms of the vagina include all the following EXCEPT

(A) sarcoma botryoides
(B) clear cell carcinoma
(C) squamous carcinoma
(D) vaginal adenosis
(E) rhabdomyosarcoma

369. Which of the following is sufficiently different from the others to be discriminated by histologic examination only?

(A) Bowen's disease
(B) Squamous cell carcinoma in situ
(C) Erythroplasia of Queyrat
(D) Bowenoid papulosis
(E) Human papillomavirus (HPV) condyloma

370. A major risk factor for squamous carcinoma of the cervix is now considered to be

(A) early sexual activity
(B) multiple sexual partners
(C) human papillomavirus types 16/18
(D) herpes simplex virus type 2
(E) *Chlamydia trachomatis*

371. All the following endometrial changes are consistent with secretory endometrium EXCEPT

(A) basal cytoplasmic vacuoles
(B) secretions within glandular lumen
(C) predecidual reaction within stroma
(D) neutrophil infiltrate
(E) plasma cell infiltrate

372. A woman harboring endometrial adenocarcinoma nearly always has antecedent

(A) obesity
(B) diabetes mellitus
(C) endometrial polyps
(D) endometrial hyperplasia
(E) systemic hypertension

373. Cystic hyperplasia of the endometrium is associated with all the following EXCEPT

(A) occurrence at or just before menopause
(B) increased estrogen administration or production
(C) excessive uterine bleeding
(D) secretory cells lining the cystically dilated glands
(E) functioning granulosa-theca cell tumors

374. A 46-year-old woman undergoes an abdominal hysterectomy for a "fibroid" uterus. The surgeon requests a frozen section on the tumor, which is deferred because of the lesion's degree of cellularity. Which of the following criteria will be used by the pathologist in determining benignancy versus malignancy in permanent sections?

(A) Mitotic rate
(B) Cell pleomorphism
(C) Cell necrosis
(D) Nucleocytoplasmic (NC) ratio
(E) Tumor size

375. True statements about endometrial adenocarcinoma include all the following EXCEPT

(A) it is more common than invasive squamous cervical cancer
(B) it causes fewer deaths than invasive cervical cancer
(C) the peak incidence is at age 55 to 65 years
(D) the major symptom is pain
(E) abnormal glucose tolerance is a risk factor

376. Common outcomes of the uterine abnormality illustrated below include all the following EXCEPT

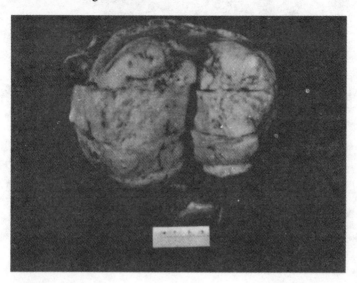

(A) malignant change
(B) cystic degeneration
(C) calcification
(D) rapid enlargement during pregnancy
(E) atrophy after menopause

377. A female patient is being treated with penicillin for acute salpingitis and pelvic inflammatory disease without benefit. Which of the following organisms should now be considered in the differential diagnosis?

(A) *Treponema pallidum*
(B) *Neisseria gonorrhoeae*
(C) *Chlamydia trachomatis*
(D) Adenoviruses
(E) Herpesviruses

378. Ovarian cystadenomas or cystadenocarcinomas (serous or mucinous)

(A) always produce androgens
(B) seldom are bilateral
(C) can be papillary
(D) usually occur during pregnancy
(E) are extremely rare

379. The ovarian lesion in the photomicrograph below is

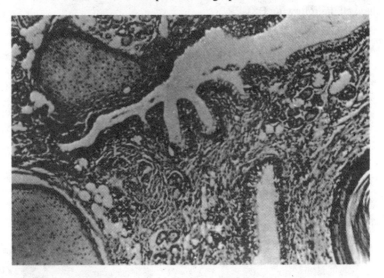

(A) chronic salpingitis
(B) an ectopic pregnancy
(C) a granulosa cell tumor
(D) a cystic teratoma
(E) metastatic squamous cell carcinoma

---

380. In the list below, the ovarian tumor with the highest degree of bilateral involvement is

(A) endometrioid carcinoma
(B) serous cystadenoma
(C) mucinous cystadenoma
(D) mucinous cystadenocarcinoma
(E) serous cystadenocarcinoma

381. The majority of malignant tumors of the ovary take their origin from

(A) surface epithelium
(B) urogenital stem cells
(C) ovarian germ cells
(D) stromal cells
(E) hilar cells

382. A 25-year-old woman in her 15th week of pregnancy presented with uterine bleeding and passage of a small amount of watery fluid and tissue. She is found to have a uterus that is much larger than estimated by her gestational dates. Her uterus is found to be filled with cystic, avascular, grapelike structures that do not penetrate the uterine wall. No fetal parts are found. The most likely diagnosis for this abnormality is

(A) partial hydatidiform mole
(B) complete hydatidiform mole
(C) invasive mole
(D) placental site trophoblastic tumor
(E) choriocarcinoma

383. A young woman with lower pelvic pain, menometrorrhagia, and a negative β-hCG test undergoes uterine dilatation and curettage. The pathology report on the endometrial sample states, "Compatible with decidualized gestational hyperplasia, no chorionic villi present." The next step would be to

(A) repeat the β-hCG test
(B) discharge the patient
(C) consider ectopic pregnancy
(D) consider appendicitis
(E) consider pelvic inflammatory disease

DIRECTIONS: Each group of questions below consists of lettered headings followed by a set of numbered items. For each numbered item select the **one** lettered heading with which it is **most** closely associated. Each lettered heading may be used **once, more than once, or not at all.**

Questions 384–387

Match the listed clinical or pathologic characteristics with the appropriate ovarian tumor.

    (A) Benign ovarian fibroma
    (B) Endometrioid tumor
    (C) Brenner tumor
    (D) Granulosa-theca cell tumor
    (E) Metastatic signet-ring cancer

384. Approximately 20 percent of all ovarian cancers

385. Endometrial hyperplasia

386. Ascites and pleural effusion

387. Gastrointestinal carcinoma

Questions 388–391

Match each disease with the pathologic finding that is most characteristic.

    (A) Malignant nephrosclerosis
    (B) Benign nephrosclerosis
    (C) Preeclampsia
    (D) Analgesic abuse nephropathy
    (E) Systemic lupus erythematosus

388. Hyaline arteriolosclerosis

389. Swollen glomerular endothelial cells

390. Papillary necrosis

391. Arteriolar fibrinoid necrosis

Questions 392–395

Match the renal disorders with the pathologic findings with which they are most likely to be associated.

    (A) Hyalinzed glomeruli
    (B) Splitting of the glomerular basement membranes
    (C) Diffuse thickening of capillary walls
    (D) Mesangial deposits and subepithelial "humps"
    (E) Linear IgG deposits

392. Membranoproliferative glomerulonephritis

393. Membranous glomerulonephritis

394. Poststreptococcal glomerulonephritis (PSGN)

395. Goodpasture's syndrome

Genitourinary System
Answers

334. The answer is A. *(Robbins, 5/e, pp 934–937.)* Polycystic kidney disease is a serious renal disorder that is inherited in two forms. The adult form is autosomal dominant with high penetrance of nearly 100 percent involvement of progeny who live to be older. The childhood polycystic form is autosomal recessive in inheritance. In the adult form one-third of the patients have cysts within the liver, while nearly all the childhood cases have hepatic cysts. Congenital hepatic fibrosis is associated with childhood polycystic kidney disease. In the adult form bilateral renal involvement is nearly invariable. One-third of patients with the adult form of polycystic kidney disease succumb to renal failure, while death occurs in another third as a consequence of hypertension.

335. The answer is D. *(Robbins, 5/e, pp 929–931. Rubin, 2/e, pp 806–809.)* The unique structure and composition of the glomerular basement membrane and associated cells account for the formation of the plasma ultrafiltrate referred to as *urine*. The glomerular basement membrane is approximately 320 nm wide in the normal human with a central electron-dense lamina densa and electron-lucent lamina rara interna and externa with fenestrated endothelial cells immediately adjacent to the capillaries and the visceral epithelial cells (podocytes). Glomerular basement membrane is made up of collagen type 4, with laminen especially concentrated on both laminae rarae. Clustered also on both laminae rarae are polyanionic proteoglycans (especially heparan sulfate), which are thought to play a major role in the exclusion of albumin in the urinary filtrate by a mechanism of charge dependence restriction. This is based on the electronegative charge of the proteoglycans and the anionic charges of albumin. The mechanism is based on different isoelectric points. Thus it is felt that the glomerulus, because of these proteoglycans, may be able to discriminate materials passing through it according to electronegative charge. Glomerular basement membrane does function by exclusion of materials based on size. Mesangial cells, by nature of their contractility, are thought to control intraglomerular blood flow under neurohormonal stimulation. Mesangial cells are not thought to function in filtration per se. The parietal cells lining the Bowman's membrane may function as a barrier but do not participate in the ultrafiltration. The fenestrated endothelial cells and podocytes are part of the filtering membranes but probably play a minor role compared with the glomerular polyanion barrier.

336. The answer is E. *(Anderson, 9/e, p 815. Robbins, 5/e, pp 947–948, 952–954, 956–958.)* The photomicrograph shows focal glomerulonephritis with crescent formation and focal hypercellularity involving only one portion of the glomerulus. Focal glomerulonephritis involves some glomeruli, but not all, and may involve the entire glomerulus (global) or only parts of the glomerulus (segmental). The photomicrograph demonstrates focal segmental glomerulonephritis, which may be seen in systemic diseases as well as disorders affecting only the kidney. Hypercellularity involved several mesangia with proliferation of epithelial cells lining Bowman's capsule near the damaged capillary loops. This process is referred to as *crescent formation*. The disease may be seen in bacterial endocarditis and other systemic infections. Immunologic disorders causing focal segmental glomerulonephritis may include IgA focal glomerulonephritis, systemic lupus erythematosus, polyarteritis nodosa, and Schönlein-Henoch purpura (anaphylactoid purpura). IgA focal glomerulonephritis, also known as Berger's disease, has deposits of IgA and some IgG in the involved mesangium as demonstrated by immunofluorescence. Alport's syndrome is a hereditary form of chronic renal disease that may be associated with neural deafness and death at an early age, usually less than 30. Large collections of foam cells are also seen in the renal cortex in these patients. Electron microscopy shows splitting of the glomerular basements accompanied by small, electron-dense granules. Diabetes mellitus is associated with nodular glomerulosclerosis (Kimmelstiel-Wilson disease).

337. The answer is E. *(Robbins, 5/e, pp 929–931. Rubin, 2/e, pp 806–809.)* It has been recently shown that polyanionic molecules at sites on the luminal endothelial cells retard anions by electronegativity forces, which aids the transport of cationic proteins. They may greatly increase vascular permeability, especially in the renal glomerulus. The glomerular basement membrane contains the glycoprotein entactin, fibronectin, collagen type IV, laminen, and polyanionic proteoglycans (heparan sulfate) found at sites on both laminae rarae. The glomerular filtration barrier is made possible by these polyanions. The podocyte is attached to the lamina rara externa on the epithelial (urine filtrate) side of the glomerular basement membrane. Desmin is an intermediate filament protein found in fibroblasts and muscle cells. Bowman's capsule epithelial cells line the inner side of the glomerulus and are bathed in urinary ultrafiltrate. Fibronectin—a connective tissue protein formed by endothelial cells, fibroblasts, and macrophages—stabilizes endothelial cell attachments and functions in wound healing.

338. The answer is B. *(Robbins, 5/e, pp 945–947. Rubin, 2/e, pp 828–831.)* The acute nephritic syndrome (hematuria, red cell casts, proteinuria, and edema) may follow either pharyngitis or pyoderma (impetigo) in children or, less often, in adults. The latent period from onset of infection to evidence of renal disease averages 10 days with pharyngitis and 21 days with pyoderma; latency of less than 5 days suggests IgA nephropathy, benign hematuria, or exacerbation by infection of a chronic glomerulonephritis (GN). Clinically, 95 percent of children recover, but only about 60 percent of adults with the sporadic form recover promptly; some develop rapidly progressive GN and some of these develop chronic GN.

339. The answer is B. *(Robbins, 5/e, pp 949–950, 954–956, 958–960.)* The thickening of the basement membrane in systemic lupus erythematosus and membranous glomerulonephritis is thought to result from deposition of immune complexes. The pathogenesis of this same lesion in diabetes mellitus and renal vein thrombosis is unknown. Electron-dense deposits are classically seen in a subendothelial position on the glomerular basement membrane but may be subepithelial as well in some cases.

340. The answer is D. *(Robbins, 5/e, pp 948–958.)* While many varieties of glomerulonephritis can produce the nephrotic syndrome, a few disorders will virtually always produce it. Included in the latter group are focal (segmental) glomerulosclerosis, membranous glomerulonephritis (GN), lipoid nephrosis, membranoproliferative glomerulonephritis, systemic diseases (such as amyloidosis and systemic lupus erythematosus), some tumors, hepatitis B, syphilis, drugs such as penicillamine, and certain allergies. Light microscopy shows very little change in glomeruli in lipoid nephrosis, and a diffuse absence of glomerular epithelial foot processes is noted with electron microscopy. Membranoproliferative GN is characterized by an increase in mesangial cellularity accompanied by splitting of the glomerular basement membranes ("double contour"). Membranous GN shows electron-dense deposits of immunoglobulin in the subepithelial portion of the basement membrane. The nephrotic syndrome includes massive albuminuria with significant loss of protein (more than 3 to 5 g of protein) in 24 h, consequent reduced plasma albumin (less than 3 g/dL), hyperlipidemia, and anasarca (generalized edema).

341. The answer is C. *(Robbins, 5/e, pp 717–718, 940.)* In Goodpasture's syndrome, circulating antibodies reactive with the glomerular basement membrane will bind in a linear pattern along the entire length of the glomerular basement membrane, which is their specific antigen. IgG is deposited in the basement membrane, along with complement. There are focal interruptions of the glomerular basement membrane as well, along with deposits of fibrin, as seen with electron microscopy.

342. The answer is B. *(Anderson, 9/e, pp 808, 818–819. Robbins, 5/e, pp 950–952.)* There are numerous causes of nephrotic syndrome (NS), including immune complex diseases, diabetes, amyloidosis, toxemia of pregnancy, and such circulating disturbances as bilateral renal vein thrombosis, but NS in small children (under 3 years of age) should suggest the possibility of the renal disease known as *minimal change nephropathy,* which is synonymous with *foot process disease,* or *nil disease.* This peculiar entity presents clinically as insidious nephrotic syndrome, characteristically occurring in younger children, but also seen in adults (rarely), with hypoalbuminemia, edema, hyperlipidemia, massive proteinuria, and lipiduria. The glomeruli are known for their rather normal appearance on light microscopy—at worst, there is mild and focal sclerosis. Electron microscopy is necessary for demonstrating characteristic attenuation and flattening of the foot processes of the podocytes attached to the Bowman's space side of the glomerular basement membrane. The podocytes may revert to normal (with steroid immunosuppressive therapy), or the foot-process attenuation may persist to some extent, in which case the proteinuria also persists. To date, no immune complex deposits or abnormalities of the glomerular basement membrane or mesangium have been demonstrated ultrastructurally.

343. The answer is C. *(Robbins, 5/e, pp 956–957.)* Many diseases involve hematuria, and a few diseases occur in the setting of an upper respiratory infection or of upper respiratory signs and symptoms (streptococcal glomerulonephritis, Henoch-Schönlein purpura, Wegener's granulomatosis, and bacterial endocarditis with embolism), but when the hematuria follows within 1 to 1½ days of onset of an upper respiratory infection without skin lesions in a young patient, IgA nephropathy (Berger's disease) should be considered. This disease involves the deposition of IgA in the mesangium of the glomeruli. Light microscopic examination may suggest the disease, but renal biopsy immunofluorescence must be performed to confirm it. This disorder is not at all uncommon and may become recurrent, with proteinuria that may approach nephrotic syndrome proportions. Serum levels of IgA may be elevated. A small percentage of patients may progress to renal failure over a period of years.

344. The answer is D. *(Robbins, 5/e, pp 979–981.)* The group of renal diseases associated with microangiopathic hemolytic anemia includes both childhood and adult hemolytic-uremic syndrome (HUS), thrombotic thrombocytopenic purpura, and scleroderma. Endothelial injury and intravascular coagulation occur in all. HUS is characterized by acute renal failure, microangiopathic hemolytic anemia, and thrombocytopenia and is one of the main causes of acute renal failure in children. Prodromal features in children include a gastrointestinal or respiratory tract infection. Lupus erythematosus does not occur in very young children. Acute poststreptococcal glomerulonephritis occurs in older children, is a proliferative lesion, and is not usually associated with hemolytic anemia or fibrin deposition. Lipoid nephrosis shows no glomerular changes with light microscopy.

345. The answer is C. *(Robbins, 5/e, pp 939–945, 949–950.)* Glomerular injury caused by circulating antigen-antibody complexes is a secondary effect from a nonprimary renal source. Numerous clinical examples exist of a serum sickness-like nephritis as a consequence of systemic infection, with classic clinical models such as syphilis, hepatitis B, malaria, and bacterial endocarditis leading to renal disease. Immune complexes to antigens from any of these sources are circulating within the vascular system and become entrapped within the filtration system of the glomerular basement membranes. This can be seen as granular, bumpy deposits by immunofluorescence within the basement membranes of the glomeruli. Linear fluorescence, on the other hand, is seen in primary antiglomerular basement membrane disease, wherein antibodies are directed against the glomerular basement membrane itself. Plasma cell interstitial nephritis is seen in immunologic rejection of transplanted kidneys. Nodular glomerulosclerosis is an effect of diabetes mellitus. The presence of red blood cell casts in the urine nearly always indicates that there has been glomerular injury but is not specific for any given cause. Thickening of the glomerular basement membrane caused by subepithelial immune deposits is seen in membranous glomerulonephritis. While the morphology of membranous glomerulonephritis is different from that of nephritis caused by circulating antigen-antibody complexes (immune complexes), there are similarities in the pathogenesis in that both disorders may be a consequence of or in association with infections such as hepatitis B, syphilis, and malaria. Other causes for membranous glomerulonephritis include reactions to penicillamine, gold, and certain malignancies such as malignant melanoma.

346. The answer is C. *(Robbins, 5/e, pp 934–935, 958–959, 971–972.)* The kidney shown is typical of chronic pyelonephritis with dilatation of the renal pelvis, clubbing of the calyces, and irregular reduction in parenchymal mass. Chronic pyelonephritis is an asymmetric, irregularly scarring process that may be unilateral or bilateral. Microscopically, there is atrophy and dilatation of tubules with colloid in some tubules. Chronic inflammation and fibrosis occur in the cortex and medulla. Chronic glomerulonephritis causes bilateral, symmetrically shrunken and scarred kidneys. Histologic changes depend on the stage of the disease. Cystic dysplasia is characterized by undifferentiated mesenchyme and immature cartilage and collecting ductules.

347. The answer is A. *(Robbins, 5/e, pp 964–967.)* In ATN, renal tubular damage follows toxic or ischemic injury and is the commonest cause of acute renal failure (ARF). Red blood cells and proteinaceous casts are usually present, but red cell casts are not associated and would suggest nephritis. Toxic ATN is caused by drugs, toxins, heavy metals (Hg), and organic solvents, and the tubular injury is predominant in proximal convoluted tubules, probably because this is the major site of nephrotoxin reabsorption. Ischemic ATN occurs after shock caused by severe infections, burns, or crush injuries with peripheral circulatory collapse. In ischemic ATN there is multiple focal tubular necrosis along the nephron often with rupture of basement membranes. Although urinary output in ATN often decreases to less than 400 mL per day (oliguria), up to 50 percent of patients with ATN may not have oliguria but may have increased urinary volumes.

348. The answer is D. *(Robbins, 5/e, pp 978–979.)* In a patient with a surgically correctable lesion of the renal artery, the corresponding kidney, which is potentially the less damaged one, should be saved. The contralateral kidney may be severely affected with arteriolonephrosclerosis and could perpetuate the hypertension if not removed. In a patient with parenchymal renal disease leading to hypertension, such as pyelonephritis, removal of the affected kidney may relieve the hypertension.

349. The answer is A. *(Robbins, 5/e, pp 484–489, 976–978, 982.)* Many pathologic processes affecting the kidney can lead to hypertension. The three main categories are renovascular, renal parenchymal, and urinary tract obstruction. The renin-angiotensin system has been implicated in renovascular hypertension but has not been proved to be of etiologic importance in the other two categories. The most common parenchymal diseases leading to hypertension are pyelonephritis and hydronephrosis. Large infarcts of one kidney can cause hypertension, but many small infarcts are clinically silent.

350. The answer is B. *(Robbins, 5/e, pp 984–985.)* Urinary calculi are a common problem and may arise at any level of the urinary tract, but mainly in the kidney. They are more common in males and most patients are over 30 years of age. Urinary calculi are unilateral in 80 percent of cases, and 90 percent are radiopaque since most contain calcium oxalate or calcium phosphate. Other constituents include magnesium ammonium phosphate, cystine, and uric acid. Urate stones are radiolucent and are increased in hyperuricemia due to gout and in conditions with rapid cell turnover such as leukemia. Urea-splitting organisms such as *Pseudomonas* predispose to calculi.

351. The answer is B. *(Robbins, 5/e, pp 986–987.)* Renal cell carcinoma (renal adenocarcinoma) accounts for 85 percent of primary renal tumors and usually occurs in the sixth decade, although sometimes at a much younger age. These tumors may produce hormones or hormonelike substances, for example, renin (hypertension), glucocorticoids (Cushing's syndrome), and gonadotropins (feminization and masculinization). More frequently, though in only 5 to 10 percent of patients, polycythemia or erythrocytosis occurs owing to production of erythropoietin. Renal cell carcinoma is not associated with tuberous sclerosis in which the common renal lesion is angiomyolipoma (hamartoma). It is associated with the von Hippel–Lindau syndrome in which many patients develop bilateral renal cell carcinomas. Translocations between chromosomes 3 and 8 and between 3 and 11 have been found in some cases of familial renal cancer and in a few sporadic cases. Hematuria is often the first symptom but often occurs late, after invasion of the renal vein or widespread metastases frequently to lung, bone, or brain. Renal cell carcinoma is predominantly of clear cell type with intracytoplasmic glycogen and lipid, but less often granular cells with numerous mitochondria or spindle cells occur. Diagnosis requires IVP, CT, and ultrasound to differentiate benign cysts, as well as percutaneous needle aspiration for cytology.

352. The answer is E. *(Robbins, 5/e, pp 462–465, 986–988.)* A middle-aged patient is highly unlikely to have either of the predominantly childhood tumors nephroblastoma (Wilms' tumor) or mesoblastic nephroma (benign hamartoma). Mesoblastic nephroma, which may be seen in the first year of life, caused difficulty in differential diagnosis from Wilms' tumor in children. Acute pyelonephritis features signs of acute infection with flank pain, pyuria, fever, and a high bacterial colony count in urine. Renal cell carcinoma is unlikely to cause hematuria until far advanced with invasion of the collecting system. Urothelial renal pelvis tumors cause hematuria early, even when quite small. They form 5 to 10 percent of primary renal tumors and range from apparently benign papillomas to papillary or anaplastic carcinomas. There may be multicentric involvement of ureters or bladder. Diagnosis is by x-ray and cytologic examination of at least three voided urine specimens; malignant cells are not found if the ureter is obstructed by tumor, or if the cells are degenerate or mildly atypical, as in papilloma. Prognosis is not very good for high-grade infiltrating tumors and is very poor for the squamous cell variant (about 15 percent of pelvic tumors); therefore, early diagnosis is paramount.

353. The answer is E. *(Robbins, 5/e, pp 462, 614.)* Wilms' tumor is the most common primary tumor of children, and its incidence is increased in several syndromes involving distinct chromosomal loci and congenital malformations. Patients with the WAGR syndrome, which is characterized by aniridia, genital abnormalities, and mental retardation, have a one-third chance of developing Wilms' tumor. The majority of patients with the Denys-Drash syndrome, characterized by gonadal dysgenesis (male pseudohermaphroditism) and nephropathy, develop Wilms' tumor. Both of these syndromes involve the Wilms' tumor–associated gene *WT1,* located at band p13 on chromosome 11. A second Wilms' tumor gene, *WT2,* located on chromosome 11 distal to *WT1,* is associated with the Beckwith-Wiedemann syndrome, which is characterized by enlargement of body organs, hemihypertrophy, renal medullary cysts, and adrenal cytomegaly. These patients are also at an increased risk for developing Wilms' tumor. Hypoplasia of the radii, along with hypoplasia of the kidney and spleen, is associated with Fanconi's anemia, an autosomal recessive disorder of defective DNA repair.

354. The answer is E. *(Anderson, 9/e, pp 856–857. Robbins, 5/e, pp 996–997.)* Malacoplakia is an uncommon chronic inflammatory disease of unknown cause, characterized by soft yellow mucosal plaques, infiltration of large histiocytes containing phagolysosomes, and intracytoplasmic and extracellular laminated calcospherules, Michaelis-Gutmann (MG) bodies. While malacoplakia usually involves the mucosa of the urinary bladder, it occurs also in extravesical sites such as the colon, lungs, kidneys, prostate, and brain. It occurs with greater frequency in the immunosuppressed. Histologically, the plaques contain numerous, large, foamy or granular macrophages that are PAS-positive and often include bacterial debris. Laminated, mineralized MG bodies are also numerous in and between macrophages. The cause of malacoplakia is not clear, but it has been associated with *E. coli* infections and is thought to be due to defective removal by macrophages of phagocytosed bacteria with overloaded phagosomes and MG bodies resulting from calcium deposition on the phagosomes. In recent reports, however, cerebral malacoplakia was not associated with bacterial infection.

355. The answer is D. *(Robbins, 5/e, p 1004.)* Nonspecific urethritis may actually be the most common cause of dysuria in sexually active males, although gonorrhea should always be excluded by laboratory examination. Causes of nonspecific urethritis include some bacteria, such as *Escherichia coli* and streptococci, but recent evidence implicates chlamydiae of the TRIC group as being perhaps the most common offending agents. The organism may take up residence in the prostate, producing chronic and active prostatitis. Prostatic hypertrophy, epididymitis, orchitis, and renal stones may cause urinary symptoms but also produce other signs and symptoms that distinguish them from nonspecific urethritis.

356. The answer is B. *(Robbins, 5/e, pp 997–1002.)* Approximately 90 percent of carcinomas of the bladder are of transitional cell type. They are more common in men. Known etiologic factors include cigarette smoking, persistent mucosal inflammation, exposure to certain chemicals (notably beta-naphthylamine), and administration of the immunosuppressive agent cyclophosphamide (Cytoxan). Infection by *Schistosoma haematobium* is associated with squamous cell cancer. All transitional cell cancers, regardless of grade, tend to recur; the frequency of recurrence increases with the tumor grade.

357. The answer is E. *(Anderson, 9/e, pp 379–382.)* Cytomegalic inclusion disease is diagnosed in the immunosuppressed or AIDS patient by finding large intranuclear inclusions surrounded by a clear halo in enlarged cells in urinary sediment, in sputum or bronchial lavage, in spinal fluid specimens, or in liver biopsy. Small intracytoplasmic inclusions may be found. Cytomegalovirus (CMV) is a DNA member of the herpesvirus group that causes disseminated disease, including interstitial pneumonitis in the debilitated or immunosuppressed adult. Disseminated infection with CMV in AIDS is associated with pneumonitis, heptitis, idiopathic ulcerative colitis, encephalitis, and retinitis. Rising antibody titers may not be detectable for up to 4 weeks after primary infection and early diagnosis may be achieved by finding typical inclusion bodies in cytologic or biopsy specimens. However, the shell vial technique has revolutionized detection of CMV in cell culture with detection of early antigen in 24 h instead of 1 to 3 weeks.

358. The answer is B. *(Anderson, 9/e, pp 882–886.)* Most malignant germ cell tumors of the gonads, specifically the testis, typically occur in the younger man between the ages of 22 and 35. The seminoma has several types, most of which are found also in younger persons. The classic seminoma is populated by differentiated seminiferous tubule–type epithelium with intervening lymphocytes, while the anaplastic seminoma contains an increase in mitoses and a moderate degree of anaplasia. The spermatocytic seminoma, however, occurs in older patients, often between ages 55 and 65, and is a soft, yellowish, sometimes mucoid tumor that microscopically has several cell types: classic intermediate-sized germ cells; smaller, secondary spermatocytic-type cells; and large mononuclear and multinuclear giant cells. Polyembryoma and embryonal carcinoma are related, occur in the younger patient, and are less common than the seminomas. The most malignant germ cell tumor of the testis is the choriocarcinoma, which is characterized by large cytotrophoblastic and syncytiotrophoblastic cells. Teratocarcinomas are tumors of more than one histologic type that may contain seminomatous or embryonal components, or both.

359. The answer is D. *(Anderson, 9/e, p 891.)* The adenomatoid tumor is benign and is the most common tumor of the epididymis. Its origin is probably the mesothelium. It presents as a small, firm, gray-white nodule less than 5 cm in diameter; similar tumors occur in the fallopian tube, ovary, and posterior uterus. Histology reveals glandlike, mesothelium-lined, spaced and fibrous connective tissue stroma with smooth muscle fibers. Androblastoma, or Sertoli cell tumor, is a sex cord testicular tumor, often benign; tuberculous epididymitis presents multiple confluent tubercles with caseation. Carcinomas of the epididymis and adjacent structures occur but are very rare. Adrenocortical rests are common but usually too small for clinical detection.

360. The answer is D. *(Robbins, 5/e, pp 1011–1013.)* The condition illustrated is cryptorchidism, failure of the testis to descend into the scrotum. It is present in up to 1 percent of males after puberty and is unilateral in the majority of cases. The testis is small, brown, and atrophic grossly. Microscopically, the tubules are atrophic with thickened basement membranes. The interstitial cells are usually prominent and occasional focal proliferations of Sertoli cells may be seen. The incidence of malignancy is increased 7- to 11-fold, and this risk is greater for abdominal than for inguinal location. Seminoma is the most common malignancy. The risk of malignancy is not reduced by orchiopexy. There is a smaller but definite risk of malignancy in the contralateral, correctly placed testis.

361. The answer is A. *(Robbins, 5/e, pp 1015–1022.)* Germ cell tumors of the testis are clinically divided into two categories, seminomas and nonseminomatous germ cell tumors (NSGCTs), because of their differences in presentation, metastasis, prognosis, and therapy. The NSGCTs include embryonal carcinoma, yolk sac tumor (also called *infantile embryonal carcinoma* or *endodermal sinus tumor*), choriocarcinoma, and immature teratoma. When compared with NSGCTs, seminomas are extremely radiosensitive, and they are more commonly present with stage I disease. NSGCTs are relatively radioresistant, are more aggressive, and have a worse prognosis. Seminomas typically spread by lymphatics after having remained localized for a long time. Embryonal carcinoma, choriocarcinoma, and mixed tumors with an element of choriocarcinoma tend to metastasize early via the blood. Choriocarcinomas are the most aggressive variant.

362. The answer is B. *(Brawer, Hum Pathol 23:242–248, 1992. Robbins, 5/e, pp 1028–1029.)* Premalignant, intraepithelial abnormalities are found within several organ systems, including the endometrium, cervix, urothelium, respiratory tract, and prostate. Within the prostate these changes, which are referred to as prostatic intraepithelial neoplasia (PIN), consist of proliferation and dysplastic changes of the normal epithelial cells of the prostatic ducts and acini. Histologic features of PIN include cellular crowding and stratification, variation in cellular and nuclear size, hyperchromasia, and nucleoli. One of the major distinguishing features between PIN and carcinoma is that in PIN there remains the normal two distinct epithelial cell layers: the basal layer and the luminal layer. Prostatic carcinoma is characterized instead by a single layer of neoplastic, atypical epithelial cells, and stromal infiltration is present.

363. The answer is D. *(Robbins, 5/e, p 1013.)* The condition illustrated is acute orchitis. There is hemorrhage and inflammation in and between tubules with disruption of spermatogenesis. Bacteria are present in the tubules. Orchitis is somewhat less common than epididymitis and, when present, is usually due to extension of infection from the urinary tract via epididymal lymphatics or the vas deferens. Infection is rarely blood-borne. *E. coli* and *C. trachomatis* are the most common pathogens. Sequelae include tubular atrophy and excretory duct obstruction, both of which may cause sterility. Chronic infection may occur. Interstitial cells are more likely to survive or regenerate, so sexual function is often retained.

364. The answer is D. *(Robbins, 5/e, pp 1008–1010.)* Clear vacuolization of the superficial layers of the epithelial cells, koilocytosis, is characteristic of infection by human papillomavirus (HPV). These changes are found in both condyloma acuminatum and verrucous carcinoma, but condyloma is a benign papillary lesion that does not grow into the underlying tissue, while verrucous carcinoma, also known as *giant condyloma* or *Buschke-Löwenstein tumor,* invades into the underlying tissue along a broad front. This type of invasion is in contrast to squamous cell carcinomas, which invade tissue as fingerlike projections of atypical squamous epithelial cells. Three dysplastic, precancerous intraepithelial lesions of the penis that do not invade into the underlying tissue are Bowen's disease, erythroplasia of Queyrat, and bowenoid papulosis.

365. The answer is D. *(Robbins, 5/e, pp 1026–1031.)* Over 95 percent of prostatic cancers are adenocarcinomas. In nearly 75 percent of cases adenocarcinoma of the prostate arises in the posterior lobe, usually in a subcapsular location. The lateral lobes are the next, much less frequent site. Nodular hyperplasia occurs in the periurethral region. When prostatic cancer is extracapsular or metastatic (commonly osteoblastic metastases to pelvis and lumbar vertebrae), serum tumor markers such as prostatic acid phosphatase (PAP) or prostatic-specific antigen (PSA) are detectable by standard assays. Tumor growth may be inhibited by estrogen therapy; it is not estrogen-dependent. Invasion of capsule, blood vessels, and perineural spaces is useful in diagnosis of well-differentiated tumor. Diagnosis may include needle biopsy or fine needle aspiration (80 percent accuracy).

366. The answer is A. *(Robbins, 5/e, pp 1041–1043, 1047–1053.)* Cervical condylomata, particularly flat condylomata, although benign are considered to be precursors of cervical intraepithelial neoplasia (CIN), which comprises both dysplasia and carcinoma in situ (CIS). Histologically, these condylomata consist of connective tissue stroma covered by hyperplastic epithelium with prominent perinuclear cytoplasmic vacuolization (koilocytosis). Koilocytotic cells are characteristic of human papillomavirus (HPV) infection. More than 50 genotypes of HPV are known at present, and condylomata acuminata are associated with types 6/11 while HPV types 16/18 are usually present in CIN. Following an abnormal Pap smear report suggesting condyloma, CIN, or possible invasive carcinoma, workup of the patient should include colposcopy, multiple cervical punch biopsies, and endocervical curettage to distinguish patients who have invasive cancer, CIN, or flat condylomata.

367. The answer is C. (*Robbins, 5/e, pp 1044–1045. Rubin, 2/e, pp 920–921.*) Adenocarcinomas of the vagina and cervix have existed for years but increased in young women whose mothers received diethylstilbestrol (DES) while they were pregnant. DES was used in the past to terminate an attack of threatened abortion and thereby stabilize the pregnancy. However, a side effect of this therapy proved to be a particular form of adenocarcinoma, clear cell carcinoma. This phenomenon was elucidated by Herpses and Scully in 1970. This unique adenocarcinoma was discovered in daughters between the ages of 15 and 20 of those women who had received DES. The tumor, which carries a poor prognosis, has at least three histologic patterns. One is a tubulopapillary configuration, followed by sheets of clear cells and glands lined by clear cells, and solid areas of relatively undifferentiated cells. Many of the cells have cytoplasm that protrudes into the lumen and produces a "hobnail" (nodular) appearance. Prior to the development of adenocarcinoma, a form of adenosis consisting of glands with clear cytoplasm that resembles that of the endocervix can be seen. This has been termed *vaginal adenosis* and may be a precursor of clear cell carcinoma. Clinically adenosis of the vagina is manifested by red, moist granules superimposed on the pink-white vaginal mucosa.

368. The answer is D. (*Robbins, 5/e, pp 1044–1045. Rubin, 2/e, pp 920–922.*) Neoplasms of the vagina are rare, but of these squamous cell carcinoma is the most common. Vaginal clear cell adenocarcinoma occurs occasionally (1 or less per 1000) in girls in their late teens whose mothers had received diethylstilbestrol during pregnancy. In about one-third of cases, such cancers arise in the cervix. More frequently, in about half of the population at risk, small glandular or microcystic lesions appear in the mucosa—vaginal adenosis. These benign lesions appear as red, velvety foci and are lined by mucus-secreting or ciliated columnar cells. From these areas the rarer clear cell adenocarcinoma arises. Sarcoma botryoides, which produces soft, polypoid, grapelike masses, is another rare primary vaginal cancer found usually in infants and children under age 5. It is a rhabdomyosarcoma that can also occur in the urinary bladder.

369. The answer is E. *(Robbins, 5/e, pp 1008–1010, 1045–1052.)* Of all the choices given, human papillomavirus (HPV) condyloma without dysplasia is the only lesion that can be histologically discriminated from the others. The typical HPV condyloma has hyperplastic squamous mucosa that shows progressive maturation from the stratum germinativum to the surface that is often parakeratotic, without cells of dysplasia or malignancy. There often are vacuolated squamous cells in several layers of the mucosa. However, condylomas, whether arising in the female or the male genital areas, may have atypia or dysplasia or even be associated histologically with carcinoma. If present, these features must be commented upon in a pathology report. Condyloma not otherwise specified indicates that none of these disorders of growth are present along with it. Bowen's disease and erythroplasia of Queyrat are different clinical forms of squamous cell carcinoma in situ. Erythroplasia of Queyrat is a specialized form of squamous carcinoma in situ or severe dysplasia occurring on the glans penis mainly. It is characterized by a moist, macular, spreading red surface. It usually occurs in males of advanced age. Bowen's disease is also squamous carcinoma in situ but may have an association with malignancies of the viscera. Bowenoid papulosis refers to multiple, small, banal-appearing clinical papules on the vulvar or penile surfaces; it histologically shows features of Bowen's disease, and for all practical purposes cannot be distinguished from that disease on histologic grounds only. It is a rather new entity, histologically similar to carcinoma in situ, and it behaves as a self-healing and reversible lesion. Bowenoid papulosis usually occurs in young patients and is often associated with condylomas.

370. The answer is C. *(Robbins, 5/e, pp 1047–1053. Rubin, 2/e, pp 926–931.)* Cervical squamous cell cancer and its precursors (dysplasia) are considered to be sexually transmitted diseases. Women having sexual intercourse at an early age or with multiple male partners, particularly those with penile condylomas, are at risk for development of genital tract squamous neoplasms. Herpes simplex virus (HSV) type 2 was considered an important cause, but now the major risk factor is human papillomavirus (HPV) types 16/18. Existence of the genome of HPV types 6, 11, 16, 18, 31, and 33 has been documented by DNA hybridization methods in several genital lesions including condylomas, cervical intraepithelial neoplasia (CIN) carcinoma in situ, and invasive cervical cancer. In most studies HPV 6 and 11 were confined to lesions with a good prognosis such as condylomas and mild dysplasia (CIN I), whereas HPV 16 and 18 were found predominantly in CIN III (severe dysplasia and carcinoma in situ) and in invasive carcinoma.

371. The answer is E. *(Fawcett, 12/e, pp 840–843. Robbins, 5/e, pp 1035–1037, 1053–1054.)* Histologic examination of the endometrium is important clinically to determine hormonal status, document ovulation, and evaluate the causes of dysfunctional uterine bleeding. After menses, under the influence of estrogen, the basal third of the endometrium proliferates rapidly (proliferative phase) to form straight, tubular glands lined by pseudostratified columnar cells. Characteristically, mitoses are numerous. Following ovulation the endometrium changes to a secretory-type endometrium, which is characterized by secretory vacuoles that form first in the basal parts of the cells, glandular secretions, stromal cell hypertrophy with abundant eosinophilic cytoplasm (predecidual change), and lack of glandular mitoses. Throughout the cycle lymphocytes may be found in the endometrium, but toward the end of the secretory phase there is a marked infiltrate of neutrophils. In contrast, the presence of any plasma cells within the endometrium is diagnostic of chronic endometritis.

372. The answer is D. *(Robbins, 5/e, pp 1060–1062.)* Endometrial adenocarcinoma appears to be increasing in frequency in the United States, especially in younger women. It is now accepted that a high estrogen-to-progestin ratio predisposes to the development of this tumor. At menopause, estrogen in the form of estrone continues to be produced in the adrenal glands, and the amounts are directly proportional to body fat. This continues in a milieu in which progesterone is at a minimum because of noncycling. These factors explain why obese women are at an increased risk during and after menopause. Diabetes and hypertension are also associated factors, but they are more likely to be effects of obesity than isolated risk factors for developing cancer. Endometrial adenocarcinoma is nearly always preceded by endometrial hyperplasia in some form. This, of course, is not documented in every case because not every patient has had a diagnostic dilatation and curettage of the endometrium prior to development of the carcinoma. Furthermore, endometrial hyperplasia does not always lead to adenocarcinoma.

373. The answer is D. *(Robbins, 5/e, pp 1057–1058). Cystic endometrial hyperplasia* refers to the abnormal growth of endometrium associated with either an absolute or a relative estrogen excess. These are common findings at the time of menopause and in conditions causing an absolute excess of estrogen—e.g., Stein-Leventhal syndrome, functioning granulosa and thecal cell ovarian tumors, and the exogenous administration of estrogenic substances. The microscopic findings in an endometrial biopsy are dominated by the marked dilatation of the endometrial glands, which gives the tissue section the appearance of Swiss cheese. The glands are lined by benign columnar epithelium that is nonsecretory.

374. The answer is A. *(Anderson, 9/e, pp 1860–1864. Rubin, 2/e, p 946.)* "Fibroids" of the uterus are among the most common abnormalities seen in uteri surgically removed in the United States in women of reproductive age. They arise in the myometrium, submucosally, subserosally, and midwall, both singly and several at a time. Sharply circumscribed, they are benign, smooth muscle tumors that are firm, gray-white, and whorled on cut section. Their malignant counterpart, leiomyosarcoma of the uterus, is quite rare in the de novo state and arises even more rarely from an antecedent leiomyoma. Whereas cell pleomorphism, tissue necrosis, and cytologic atypia per se are established criteria in assessing malignancy in tumors generally, they are important to the pathologist in uterine fibroids only if mitoses are also present. Regardless of cellularity or atypicality, if 10 or more mitoses are present in 10 separate high-power microscopic fields, the lesion is leiomyosarcoma. If 5 or fewer mitoses are present in 10 fields with bland morphology, the leiomyoma will behave in a benign fashion. Problems arise when the mitotic counts range between 3 and 7 per 10 fields with varying degrees of cell and tissue atypicality. These equivocal lesions should be regarded by both pathologist and clinician as "gray-area" smooth muscle tumors of unpredictable biologic behavior. Fortunately, the "gray-area" leiomyoma of the uterus is rarely seen. Thus mitoses are the most important criteria in assessing malignancy in smooth muscle tumors of the uterus.

375. The answer is D. *(Anderson, 9/e, pp 1659–1661.)* Endometrial carcinoma affects menopausal and postmenopausal women, with the peak incidence at 55 to 65 years of age. Although it was much less common than squamous cervical cancer several decades ago, it has not been controlled as effectively as cervical cancer by the Papanicolaou smear technique and therapy, so that it is now more common than invasive cervical cancer. However, the major symptom of endometrial carcinoma, postmenopausal bleeding, results in diagnosis while the tumor is still confined to the uterus (stage I or II), which permits cure by surgery or radiotherapy. The annual death rate in the U.S. from endometrial cancer is 3000, while more than 6000 deaths result from squamous cervical cancer. Risk factors for endometrial cancer include obesity and glucose intolerance or diabetes.

376. The answer is A. *(Robbins, 5/e, pp 1059–1060. Rubin, 2/e, p 945.)* The condition illustrated is a uterine leiomyoma (fibroid). This is an extremely common tumor occurring in up to 25 percent of women of reproductive age. The cause is unknown, but the growth is estrogen-dependent and for this reason the tumor may enlarge rapidly during pregnancy. If the tumor becomes very large, areas within it may undergo softening followed by liquefaction and cystic degeneration. Fibroids tend to regress in the postmenopausal period; with atrophy they become collagenous and calcification often occurs.

377. The answer is C. *(Anderson, 9/e, pp 1667–1668. Robbins, 5/e, pp 1038–1039, 1063.)* *Neisseria gonorrhoeae* is a very common bacterium that causes acute pelvic inflammatory disease with salpingitis in this country as a result of venereal infection. Tuboovarian abscesses may develop from this bacterium, as well as other bacteria, but these organisms are susceptible to penicillin therapy. In the presence of unresponsiveness to penicillin, consideration should be given to *Bacteroides* species, which are important anaerobic gram-negative bacilli and are generally refractory to penicillin. These anaerobic bacteria may produce serious infections if uncontrolled. Chlamydiae, while considered to be nongonococcal in origin, are nevertheless important agents in venereal transmission and often are contracted at the same time as *Neisseria* species. When the gonococcus is adequately treated with penicillin, and symptoms continue, there may have been concurrent infection with chlamydia that is not responsive to penicillin but is sensitive to tetracycline. Adenoviruses are responsible for keratoconjunctivitis, tracheobronchitis, pneumonia in children, acute gastroenteritis, and occasionally hemorrhagic cystitis, but are not ordinarily causative in pelvic inflammatory disease.

378. The answer is C. *(Robbins, 5/e, pp 1067–1077.)* Ovarian cystadenomas are common neoplasms that are bilateral in 15 to 40 percent of patients and are frequently papillary. The less malignant lesions tend to be more papillary. Ovarian cystadenomas originate in surface epithelial cells from the müllerian system. The papillae may show complex arborization with an increase in cell layers without stromal invasion; in such cases, the tumors are classified as borderline malignant because of their less aggressive clinical course. Unlike true cystadenocarcinomas, the presence of peritoneal dissemination in cystadenomas of borderline malignancy does not appear to influence the clinical course.

379. The answer is D. *(Anderson, 9/e, pp 1688–1690. Robbins, 5/e, pp 1072–1073.)* Benign cystic teratomas constitute about 10 percent of cystic ovarian tumors. The cysts contain greasy sebaceous material mixed with a variable amount of hair. The cysts' walls contain skin and skin appendages, including sebaceous glands and hair follicles. A variety of other tissues—such as cartilage, bone, tooth, thyroid, respiratory tract epithelium, and intestinal tissue—may be found. The presence of skin and skin appendages gives the tumor its other name, "dermoid cyst." Dermoid cysts are benign, but in less than 2 percent, one element may become malignant, most frequently the squamous epithelium.

380. The answer is E. *(Robbins, 5/e, pp 1065–1071.)* Primary ovarian tumors have a rather high degree of bilateral involvement compared with tumors of other bilateral organs. Bilaterality could reflect either concurrent simultaneous primary tumors or vascular and lymphatic spread from one side to the other. The ovarian tumor with the highest rate of bilaterality (65 percent) is the serous cystadenocarcinoma. Serous cystadenomas have a 20 to 25 percent rate of bilaterality, while mucinous cystadenomas are bilateral in about 5 percent of cases. In contrast, mucinous cystadenocarcinomas are bilateral in 20 percent of cases, and endometrioid carcinoma is higher at about 45 percent. There is a higher probability of extension of endometrioid carcinoma outside the ovaries when it presents with bilaterality.

381. The answer is A. *(Robbins, 5/e, pp 1065–1077.)* Malignant tumors of the ovary most commonly occur between the ages of 40 and 64. These, in the main, arise from the surface epithelium, which takes its origin from cells of the müllerian system. These cells are also referred to as *surface,* or *coelomic, epithelium.* The müllerian system has the ability to form lining cells of the fallopian tubes, endometrium, and endocervical gland epithelium. Hence, many malignant tumors that take their origin from the surface coelomic epithelium of the ovary resemble these structures. Examples include the borderline serous tumor, serous cystadenocarcinoma, serous cystadenofibrocarcinoma, borderline mucinous tumor, mucinous cystadenocarcinoma, endometrioid carcinoma, undifferentiated carcinoma, malignant Brenner tumor, and clear cell adenocarcinoma. Stem cells from the urogenital ridge can give rise to any genitourinary structure. Hilar cells represent small clusters and cords of androgen-producing cells. These presumably give rise to sex cord and Sertoli-Leydig cell tumors. Stromal cell tumors include granulosa cell tumors, theca cell tumors, thecomas, and fibromas. Germ cell tumors give rise to malignant and benign teratomas, including the cystic form (dermoid cyst), dysgerminoma, endodermal sinus tumor, choriocarcinoma, and mixed germ cell tumors.

382. The answer is B. *(Robbins, 5/e, pp 1081–1086.)* Gestational trophoblastic diseases include the benign hydatidiform mole (partial and complete), the invasive mole (chorioadenoma destruens), placental site trophoblastic tumor, and choriocarcinoma. Hydatidiform moles are composed of avascular, grapelike structures that do not invade the myometrium. In complete (classic) moles, all the chorionic villi are abnormal and fetal parts are not found. They have a 46,XX diploid pattern and arise from the paternal chromosomes of a single sperm by a process called *androgenesis.* In partial moles, only some of the villi are abnormal and fetal parts may be seen. These moles have a triploid or a tetraploid karyotype and arise from the fertilization of a single egg by two sperm. About 2 percent of complete moles may develop into choriocarcinoma, but partial moles are rarely followed by malignancy. The invasive mole penetrates the myometrium and may even embolize to distant sites. A similar lesion is the placental site trophoblastic tumor, which is characterized by invasion of the myometrium by intermediate trophoblasts. Gestational choriocarcinomas, composed of malignant proliferations of both cytotrophoblasts and syncytiotrophoblasts without the formation of villi, can arise from either normal or abnormal pregnancies; 50 percent arise in hydatidiform moles, 25 percent in previous abortions, 22 percent in normal pregnancies, and the rest in ectopic pregnancies or teratomas. Both hydatidiform moles and choriocarcinomas have high levels of human chorionic gonadotropin (hCG); the levels are extremely high in choriocarcinoma unless considerable tumor necrosis is present.

383. The answer is A. *(Robbins, 5/e, p 1079.)* Ectopic pregnancy is a potentially life-threatening condition if it is not treated by removal before rupture and hemorrhage with fatal exsanguination. The most common location for extrauterine implantation is the fallopian tube (more than 85 percent of cases), with rare implantation in the ovary or abdomen. If the tubal implantation has existed from 1 to 4 weeks, the β-hCG test result is likely to be negative; thus a negative result does *not* exclude pregnancy. It is always worthwhile to repeat a laboratory test when the result is unexpected. Tubal pregnancy is not uncommon and should always be considered if endometrial samples suggest gestational change without chorionic villi.

384–387. The answers are 384-B, 385-D, 386-A, 387-E. *(Robbins, 5/e, pp 1070, 1074–1077.)* The Krukenberg tumor is usually a bilateral ovarian tumor. It practically always metastasizes from the gastrointestinal tract and most frequently arises from a gastric adenocarcinoma. Histologically, there is diffuse infiltration of mucinous signet-ring cells.

The ovarian fibroma is a relatively common, benign ovarian tumor (about 4 percent of all types) that may be accompanied by ascites in about 40 percent of all cases. Less common is pleural effusion, often right-sided. The combination of ovarian fibroma, ascites, and hydrothorax is known as Meigs' syndrome. Rarely, the basal cell nevus syndrome is associated.

The granulosa-theca cell tumors are sex cord–stromal in origin and account for 5 percent of all ovarian tumors. They range from almost pure granulosa cell tumors to pure thecomas. These tumors may occur at any age, but about two-thirds occur in postmenopausal women and, because of estrogen production, may be associated with endometrial hyperplasia, endometrial carcinoma, or cystic breast disease. Tumors with a large thecal component may cause precocious sexual development in prepubertal girls. Granulosa-theca cell tumors are potentially malignant (5 to 25 percent), but pure thecomas are not.

Endometrioid tumors are approximately 20 percent of all ovarian cancers; they may be carcinomas, borderline lesions, or benign. Up to 30 percent of the carcinomas are associated with endometrial carcinoma or endometriosis. They are solid and cystic tumors containing tubular glands similar to those of benign or malignant endometrium. About 40 percent are bilateral and the 5-year survival rate is 40 to 50 percent.

Brenner tumors, 2 percent of ovarian neoplasms, are usually benign, solid, often small, unilateral tumors. Their dense, fibrous stroma has nests of transitional cells like urothelium.

388–391. The answers are 388-B, 389-C, 390-D, 391-A. *(Robbins, 5/e, pp 875, 973–974, 976–978, 1079–1081.)* Benign nephrosclerosis, renal disease occurring in benign hypertension, is characterized by hyaline arteriolosclerosis with thickened hyalinized arteriolar walls and narrowed lumina. Fibroelastic hyperplasia occurs in the larger muscular arteries. Small kidneys with granular surfaces often result because of ischemic atrophy of nephrons.

Renal arteriolar changes in malignant nephrosclerosis (malignant hypertension) include fibrinoid necrosis of arterioles (necrotizing arteriolitis), hyperplastic arteriolosclerosis (onion-skinning), necrotizing glomerulitis, and often a thrombotic microangiopathy. The clinical course is often downhill with only 50 percent of patients surviving 5 years; marked proteinuria, hematuria, cardiovascular problems, and finally renal failure contribute to death. The disease is often associated with accelerated preexisting benign essential hypertension, chronic renal disease (glomerulonephritis), or scleroderma.

Preeclampsia is characterized by hypertension, proteinuria, and edema that begins after 20 weeks of gestation but is obvious clinically after 32 weeks. Most common in the last trimester of a first pregnancy, it occurs in about 6 percent of all pregnancies. It may progress to eclampsia with convulsions and coma. Renal involvement involves the glomeruli with narrowing or obliteration of capillary lumina due to swelling of endothelial and mesangial cells (glomerular endotheliosis). Electron microscopy shows widening of the subendothelial region between basement membrane and endothelial cell by electron-lucent and dense material (fibrin); this change is similar to that in HUS. Pathogenesis includes placental ischemia with decreased production of vasodilator prostaglandins (PGI_2, PGE_2) and increased release of vasoconstrictors.

Analgesic abuse nephropathy (analgesic nephritis) occurs because of excessive intake of *mixtures* of aspirin and phenacetin. It requires the synergistic action of these drugs, and cases due to aspirin, or phenacetin, or acetaminophen alone are rare. Analgesic abuse nephropathy eventually results in papillary necrosis (necrotizing papillitis) with secondary chronic tubulointerstitial nephritis. Clinical findings include sterile pyuria, anemia, GI symptoms, urinary tract infections, and hypertension. Chronic renal failure may occur, but drug withdrawal often stabilizes kidney function. There is, however, an increased incidence of urothelial carcinoma of the renal pelvis.

392–395. The answers are 392-B, 393-C, 394-D, 395-E. *(Robbins, 5/e, pp 717–718, 940, 945–947, 949–950, 954–956.)* Membranoproliferative glomerulonephritis occurs in two types. Type I, which is associated with nephrotic syndrome, is driven by immune complexes; type II is associated with hematuria and chronic renal failure and, in addition to immune complexes, involves alternate complement activation. In either type there is mesangial proliferation accompanied by thickening of the glomerular basement membranes, and a special finding that often supports the diagnosis of membranoproliferative glomerulonephritis is the presence of actual splitting of the glomerular basement membranes. In type I there are subendothelial deposits of IgG, C3, C1, and C4. In type II there are dense deposits of C3 (dense-deposit disease) with or without IgG and no C1.

Membranous glomerulonephritis, rather than being driven by an immune complex, is antibody-mediated and results in diffuse thickening of glomerular capillary walls by subepithelial deposits of IgG and C3 in a diffuse involvement of the glomeruli. These deposits are seen by fluorescence as granular deposits. Membranous glomerulonephritis is also associated with the nephrotic syndrome.

In PSGN the light microscopy reveals diffuse endothelial and mesangial cell proliferation with neutrophil infiltration, so that narrowing of capillary lumens and enlargement of the glomerular tuft to fill Bowman's space occur. Electron microscopy reveals the mesangial deposits and hump-shaped subepithelial deposits in peripheral capillary loops that are so characteristic of PSGN. Immunofluorescence shows granular deposits containing IgG, C3, and often fibrin in glomerular capillary walls and mesangium.

Goodpasture's syndrome is an acute, serious disease often heralded by pulmonary hemorrhages and remarkable hemoptysis accompanied by acute glomerulonephritis that often is of the rapidly progressive form. Antiglomerular basement membrane antibodies are seen in Goodpasture's syndrome and result in linear IgG deposits along the glomerular basement membranes. Also seen are marked and dramatic formations of epithelial cell crescents accompanied by infiltrates of monocytes and neutrophils with fibrin deposition and necrosis of epithelial and endothelial cells. There is no accompanying fragmentation of glomerular basement membranes as there is in membranoproliferative glomerulonephritis.

Hyalinized glomeruli may be seen in any terminal glomerulonephritis (GN) but are best seen in chronic renal failure caused by chronic GN.

Nervous System

DIRECTIONS: Each question below contains five suggested responses. Select the **one best** response to each question.

396. True statements regarding neuroglial cells include all the following EXCEPT

(A) they include astrocytes
(B) they include oligodendrocytes
(C) they include ependymal cells and microglial cells
(D) all function to shelter and maintain neurons
(E) all function as macrophages, when activated

397. A known alcoholic is brought to the emergency room following an altercation in a local bar. The intern observes respiratory irregularity, coma, and papilledema. Emergency surgery is planned in order to prevent all the following EXCEPT

(A) brainstem herniation
(B) cerebellar herniation
(C) Duret hemorrhages
(D) ruptured aneurysm
(E) death of the patient

398. Subdural hematomas occur most frequently in the

(A) supracerebellar region
(B) infracerebellar region
(C) cerebellopontine angle
(D) pituitary region
(E) cerebral hemisphere convexities

399. Which of the following conditions is the most frequent cause of intracerebral hemorrhage?

(A) Ruptured aneurysm
(B) Trauma
(C) Blood dyscrasias
(D) Angiomas
(E) Hypertensive vascular disease

400. Hypertension is most closely related to the formation of which one of the following types of aneurysms?

(A) Berry aneurysm
(B) Atherosclerotic aneurysm
(C) Mycotic aneurysm
(D) Charcot-Bouchard aneurysm
(E) Saccular aneurysm

401. The majority of cases of subarachnoid hemorrhage result from

(A) transection of a branch of the middle meningeal artery
(B) bleeding from torn bridging veins
(C) rupture of a preexisting aneurysm
(D) rupture of an arteriovenous malformation
(E) cortical bleeding occurring opposite the point of a traumatic injury

402. Cerebral embolism occurs frequently in association with all the following conditions EXCEPT

(A) cardiac mural thrombi
(B) left-sided endocarditis
(C) right-sided endocarditis
(D) cardiac catheterization
(E) prosthetic cardiac valves

403. Syringomyelia is characterized by all the following EXCEPT

(A) segmental loss of pain and temperature sensation
(B) segmental loss of touch sensation
(C) loss of tissue (cavitation) within the cervical spinal cord
(D) small muscle atrophy of the hands
(E) kyphoscoliosis

404. Laminar necrosis and watershed infarcts are most suggestive of

(A) shock
(B) hypertension
(C) fat emboli
(D) vascular thrombosis
(E) venous sinus thrombosis

405. Tabes dorsalis is characterized by

(A) hydrophobia
(B) increased neutrophils in the cerebrospinal fluid (CSF)
(C) involvement of the motor neurons of the spinal cord
(D) degeneration of posterior columns of the spinal cord
(E) infection of oligodendrocytes

406. Creutzfeldt-Jakob disease displays all the following characteristics EXCEPT

(A) spongiform encephalopathy
(B) rapidly progressive dementia
(C) worldwide incidence of 1 case per 100,000 population
(D) absence of an inflammatory infiltrate
(E) inactivation by hypochlorite solution

407. Characteristics of AIDS-related neurologic abnormalities include all the following EXCEPT

(A) areas of demyelination
(B) preferential infection of cortical neurons
(C) multinucleated giant cells
(D) vacuolar myelopathy
(E) increased incidence of progressive multifocal leukoencephalopathy (PML)

408. An elevated IgG level in cerebrospinal fluid and an abnormal band on agar gel electrophoresis of cerebrospinal fluid are findings consistent with the diagnosis of

(A) secondary stage of syphilis
(B) muscular dystrophy
(C) tumor involvement of the spinal cord
(D) meningeal involvement by leukemia
(E) multiple sclerosis

409. All the following have been commonly associated with pyogenic brain abscesses EXCEPT

(A) congenital heart disease
(B) sinusitis
(C) lung abscess
(D) liver abscess
(E) mastoiditis

410. Alzheimer's disease is characterized by all the following EXCEPT

(A) cerebral atrophy in superior temporal and frontal lobes
(B) neuritic or senile plaques
(C) amyloid β-protein deposits
(D) Lewy bodies
(E) granulovacuolar degeneration

411. In subacute combined degeneration (SCD) there is

(A) association with hemolytic anemia
(B) usually involvement of gray matter of the spinal cord
(C) usually no motor impairment
(D) failure of the enzyme methylmalonic CoA mutase
(E) dermatitis, enteritis, and dementia

412. Select the disorder below that has the most clinicopathologic features in common with postvaccinal encephalomyelitis.

(A) Metachromatic leukodystrophy
(B) Multifocal leukoencephalopathy
(C) Guillain-Barré syndrome
(D) Hypoxic encephalopathy
(E) Hypertensive encephalopathy

413. Clinicopathologic features of amyotrophic lateral sclerosis (ALS) include all the following EXCEPT

(A) degeneration in the pyramidal motor system
(B) sensory loss secondary to involvement of dorsal nerve roots
(C) loss of anterior horn neurons
(D) loss of myelinated fibers in corticospinal tracts
(E) dysphagia

414. Diseases that are classified as slow viral infections or unconventional agent (spongiform) encephalopathies include all the following EXCEPT

(A) Reye's syndrome
(B) subacute sclerosing panencephalitis
(C) Creutzfeldt-Jakob disease
(D) progressive multifocal leukoencephalopathy
(E) kuru

415. A 9-year-old boy who had been suffering from a gait disturbance for several weeks was found to have a posterior fossa mass on CT scan. The most likely cause for these findings is

(A) a berry aneurysm
(B) astrocytoma
(C) medulloblastoma
(D) oligodendroglioma
(E) pseudotumor cerebri

416. A 55-year-old woman is suspected of having a brain tumor because of the onset of seizure activity. Computerized tomograms (CT scans) and skull x-rays demonstrate a mass in the right cerebral hemisphere that is markedly calcific. A high index of suspicion should exist for

(A) oligodendroglioma
(B) astrocytoma
(C) cerebral lymphoma
(D) metastatic carcinoma
(E) brown tumor

417. Retinoblastoma, the most common intraocular tumor of children, is associated with all the following EXCEPT

(A) occurrence in both familial and sporadic patterns
(B) unilateral and unifocal sporadic tumors
(C) inactivation of cancer suppressor genes
(D) poor prognosis even with treatment
(E) frequent histologic occurrence of rosettes

418. Which of the following tumors is characterized by pseudopalisading, necrosis, endoneurial proliferation, hypercellularity, and atypical nuclei?

(A) Schwannoma
(B) Medulloblastoma
(C) Oligodendroglioma
(D) Glioblastoma multiforme
(E) Ependymoma

419. All the following statements apply to ependymomas EXCEPT that

(A) they are the most common type of intraspinal glioma
(B) they are most commonly located in the lateral ventricles
(C) patients may present with headache and papilledema
(D) they may require differentiation from choroid plexus papilloma
(E) histologic sections display rosettes

420. True statements about meningiomas include all the following EXCEPT

(A) they usually present clinically with headaches or seizures
(B) they constitute about 20 percent of primary brain tumors
(C) they usually display rapid growth
(D) they arise from arachnoid cap cells
(E) they may be multiple in neurofibromatosis type 2

421. The Arnold-Chiari malformation is characterized by

(A) hypoplasia of the cerebellar vermis
(B) herniation of the cerebellum and the fourth ventricle into the foramen magnum
(C) facial angiofibromata and tubers of the cerebral cortex
(D) hemangioblastomas of the retina and brain
(E) facial port-wine stains

422. The lesion shown in the photomicrograph below was removed from a patient's nasal cavity. With no age given and at this low magnification, the most likely diagnosis is

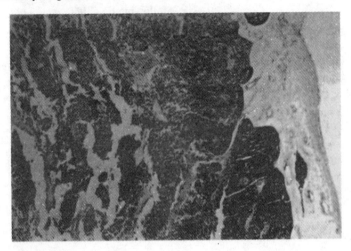

(A) adenocarcinoma
(B) nasal glioma
(C) olfactory neuroblastoma
(D) nasopharyngeal angiofibroma
(E) multiple myeloma

423. Intracerebral calcification is associated with all the following EXCEPT

(A) glioblastoma multiforme
(B) tuberous sclerosis
(C) oligodendroglioma
(D) craniopharyngioma
(E) hypoparathyroidism

424. The most frequent of all the following intracranial tumors in adults is

(A) ependymoma
(B) medulloblastoma
(C) meningioma
(D) glioma
(E) metastasis

425. Transection of a peripheral nerve will result in all the following EXCEPT

(A) dissolution of the Nissl substance in the nerve cell body
(B) degeneration of the nerve fiber distal to the cut
(C) proliferation of the Schwann sheath from the proximal nerve segment
(D) loss of the entire Schwann sheath proximal to the cut
(E) degeneration of the axons from 1 to 3 nodes of Ranvier proximal to the cut

426. All the following tumors may be found arising within the pineal gland EXCEPT

(A) teratoma
(B) pineoblastoma
(C) embryonal carcinoma
(D) choriocarcinoma
(E) craniopharyngioma

427. True statements about classic neurofibromatosis (von Recklinghausen's disease) include all the following EXCEPT

(A) malignant degeneration may occur
(B) hamartomas of the iris are very common
(C) hemangioblastomas of the brain are associated
(D) acoustic neuroma is associated
(E) pheochromocytomas and meningiomas are associated

DIRECTIONS: Each group of questions below consists of lettered headings followed by a set of numbered items. For each numbered item select the **one** lettered heading with which it is **most** closely associated. Each lettered heading may be used **once, more than once, or not at all.**

Questions 428–431

For each disease, choose the sign with which it is most likely to be associated.

(A) Neurofibrillary tangles
(B) Cowdry A intranuclear inclusions
(C) Optic nerve demyelination
(D) Hepatolenticular degeneration
(E) Verocay bodies
(F) Lewy bodies

428. Idiopathic parkinsonism

429. Herpes simplex encephalitis

430. Wilson's disease

431. Schwannoma

Questions 432–434

For each of the conditions below, choose the most appropriate description.

(A) Herniation of the meninges alone
(B) Herniation of meninges and brain parenchyma
(C) Developmental bone defect
(D) Herniation of meninges and a portion of the spinal cord
(E) Herniation at the roof of the mouth

432. Meningocele

433. Meningoencephalocele

434. Spina bifida

Questions 435–439

For each disease, choose the sign with which it is most likely to be associated.

(A) Accumulation of GM_2 ganglioside
(B) Genetic defect involving gene for amyloid precursor protein
(C) Primary CNS demyelination
(D) Abnormal or defective myelin metabolism
(E) Loss of striatal neurons in the caudate nucleus

435. Familial Alzheimer's disease

436. Huntington's disease

437. Multiple sclerosis

438. Metachromatic leukodystrophy

439. Postinfectious encephalomyelitis

Nervous System
Answers

396. The answer is E. *(Fawcett, 12/e, pp 354–357. Robbins, 5/e, pp 1296–1298.)* The neuroglial cells—astrocytes, oligodendrocytes, ependymal cells, and microglial cells—provide supportive and protective functions for neurons. However, only microglial cells are phagocytic and, in response to injury or destruction of the brain, become activated as macrophages (gitter cells, compound granular corpuscles). Astrocytes support neurons and react to CNS injury by formation of glial scars (gliosis). Oligodendrocytes produce and maintain CNS myelin, and diseases affecting them include multiple sclerosis and the leukodystrophies. The lining ependymal cells do not produce or absorb cerebrospinal fluid. Cell processes of astrocytes, or "glial" fibers, contain vimentin and glial fibrillary acidic protein (GFAP).

397. The answer is D. *(Robbins, 5/e, pp 1298–1300. Rubin, 2/e, p 1439.)* The clinical constellation of altered sensorium and papilledema should call to mind the presence of intracranial pressure, regardless of the cause, which can be due to cerebral edema, tumor mass, or, more commonly, intracranial bleeding with hematoma formation. If the pressure is severe enough, downward displacement of the cerebellar tonsils into the foramen magnum may occur, producing further compression on the brainstem with consequent hemorrhage into the pons and midbrain (Duret hemorrhages). This is nearly always associated with death, since the vital centers, including respiratory control, are located in these regions. Subdural as well as epidural hemorrhages are sufficient to cause critical downward displacement of the cerebellar tonsils. The situation can be remedied with appropriate neurosurgical intervention. In this situation, the downward displacement could be due to hemorrhage-hematoma formation into the posterior intracranial fossa, caused by either a direct (coup) or an indirect (contracoup) blow to the occiput.

398. The answer is E. *(Anderson, 9/e, pp 2187–2188.)* When blood enters the potential space between the arachnoid and dura, a subdural hematoma forms. Subdural hematomas are most commonly located over the cerebral hemisphere convexities. The traditional explanation for the formation of subdural hematomas has been tearing of the bridging veins that pass from the cortical surface to the superior sagittal sinus. Blood may also leak from lacerated cortical vessels or arachnoidal vessels ruptured by a meningeal tear.

399. The answer is E. *(Robbins, 5/e, pp 1311–1312.)* Hypertension is 10 to 20 times more frequent than all the other causes of intracerebral hemorrhage and is also the most common cause of death from cerebrovascular disease. Major sites of hemorrhage are the putamen (more than 50 percent); the cortex and subcortex (15 percent); and the thalamus, the pons, and the cerebellum (each approximately 10 percent). Hypertensive hemorrhage shows a predilection for the distribution of the lenticulostriate arteries with small (lacunar) hemorrhages, or large hemorrhages obliterating the corpus striatum, including the putamen and internal capsule. It is possible that development of microaneurysms (Charcot-Bouchard aneurysms) with subsequent rupture is a precipitating factor.

400. The answer is D. *(Robbins, 5/e, pp 1311–1314. Rubin, 2/e, pp 1393–1399.)* Hypertension results in the deposition of lipid and hyaline material in the walls of cerebral arterioles, which is called *lipohyalinosis*. This weakens the wall and forms small Charcot-Bouchard aneurysms, which may eventually rupture. Berry aneurysms (small saccular aneurysms) are the result of congenital defects of the media of blood vessels and are located at the bifurcation of arteries. Atherosclerotic aneurysms are fusiform (spindle-shaped) aneurysms, usually located in the major cerebral vessels. They rarely rupture, but may become thrombosed. Mycotic (septic) aneurysms result from septic emboli, most commonly from subacute bacterial endocarditis.

401. The answer is C. *(Robbins, 5/e, pp 1304–1308.)* Trauma may cause bleeding within the brain parenchyma, on the surface of the brain, or within spaces overlying the brain. Epidural hemorrhages result from the rupture of one of the meningeal arteries, usually the middle meningeal artery, which run between the dura and the skull. Subdural hemorrhages result from bleeding of torn bridging veins, which connect the venous system of the brain with the large venous sinuses within the dura. About two-thirds of the cases of subarachnoid hemorrhage are the result of rupture of a preexisting arterial aneurysm rather than trauma, while in about 10 percent of cases, an arteriovenous malformation (AVM) is found. AVMs more commly bleed into *both* the subarachnoid space and the brain parenchyma. Traumatic head injury may produce contusions (bruises) at the point of impact ("coup"), or if the head is in motion, such as in a backward fall, contusions may occur on the surface of the brain opposite the point of impact ("contracoup").

402. The answer is C. *(Robbins, 5/e, pp 111–112, 1309–1310. Rubin, 2/e, pp 539–540.)* Cerebral embolism is probably the most common cause of stroke and most cerebral emboli arise in the heart. Myocardial infarction with mural thrombi, atrial fibrillation thrombi, and left-sided bacterial endocarditis are frequent sources, but in right-sided bacterial endocarditis (drug addicts, patients with gonococcal endocarditis or ventricular septal defect) emboli to organs other than the lungs are very rare, except in paradoxical embolism of septal defect. Endocarditis must be excluded when cerebral embolism is suspected. Thromboembolism from prosthetic heart valves has not been unusual. Cardiac catheterization and other invasive procedures involving an atherosclerotic aorta or femoral or iliac arteries may cause atheroemboli (cholesterol emboli) with resultant small infarcts of brain, kidney, gut, skin, or other organs. At least 35 to 40 percent of all strokes are embolic, and emboli are the predominant cause of infarction in the area supplied by the middle cerebral artery.

403. The answer is B. *(Robbins, 5/e, p 1303. Rubin, 2/e, p 1382.)* Syringomyelia is a chronic myelopathy. There is cavitation involving the central gray matter of the spinal cord where pain fibers cross to join the contralateral spinothalamic tract. Interruption of the lateral spinothalamic tracts results in segmental sensory dissociation, with loss of pain and temperature sense, but preservation of the sense of touch and pressure, or vibration, usually over the neck, shoulders, and arms. Characteristic features also include wasting of the small intrinsic hand muscles (clawhand) and thoracic scoliosis. The cause of syringomyelia is unknown, although one type is associated with a Chiari malformation with obstruction at the foramen magnum.

404. The answer is A. *(Robbins, 5/e, pp 1308–1309, 1311. Rubin, 2/e, pp 1397–1403.)* Decreased brain perfusion may be generalized (global) or localized. Global ischemia results from generalized decreased blood flow, such as with shock, cardiac arrest, or hypoxic episodes (e.g., near-drowning or carbon monoxide poisoning). Global hypoxia results in watershed (border-zone) infarcts, which typically occur at the border of areas supplied by the anterior and middle cerebral arteries, and laminar necrosis, which is related to the short, penetrating vessels originating from pial arteries. The Purkinje cells of the cerebellum and the pyramidal neurons of Sommer's sector in the hippocampus are particularly sensitive to hypoxic episodes. Atherosclerosis, which predisposes to vascular thrombi and emboli, is related to regional ischemia. Hypertension damages parenchymal arteries and arterioles, producing small ischemic lesions (lacunar infarcts). Fat emboli, related to trauma of long bones, lodge in small capillaries to form petechiae. Venous sinus thrombosis is related to systemic dehydration, phlebitis, and sickle cell disease.

405. The answer is D. *(Robbins, 5/e, pp 1317–1318, 1320, 1322–1323.)* Neurosyphilis, a tertiary stage of syphilis, includes syphilitic meningitis, paretic neurosyphilis, and tabes dorsalis. Syphilitic meningitis is character-ized by perivascular infiltrates of lymphocytes and plasma cells that cause obliterative endarteritis and meningeal fibrosis. Tabes dorsalis is the result of degeneration of the posterior columns of the spinal cord. This is caused by compression atrophy of the posterior spinal sensory nerves, which produces impaired joint position sensation, ataxia, loss of pain sensation (leading to joint damage, Charcot joints), and Argyll Robertson pupils (pupils that react to accommodation but not to light). Rabies, caused by a single-stranded RNA rhabdovirus, is transmitted by the bite of a rabid animal, usually a dog. The virus is transmitted through peripheral nerves to the brain, where it forms characteristic inclusions within neurons (Negri bodies). Symptoms related to destruction of neurons in the brainstem include irritability, difficulty in swal-lowing and spasms of the throat (these two resulting in "hydrophobia"), seizures, and delirium. The illness is almost uniformly fatal. Poliomyelitis is caused by an enterovirus that produces a nonspecific gastroenteritis and then secondarily invades the anterior horn motor neurons of the spinal cord, where it causes muscular paralysis. Progressive multifocal leukoencephalopathy (PML) is a viral infection of oligodendrocytes that causes demyelination and symptoms of dementia and ataxia. The causative agents of PML are two closely related papovaviruses, JC virus and SV40. The pathognomonic fea-ture of PML is oligodendrocytes in areas of demyelination with a "ground-glass" appearance of their nuclei. PML typically occurs as a terminal compli-cation in immunosuppressed patients.

406. The answer is C. *(Robbins, 5/e, pp 1323–1324.)* In Creutzfeldt-Jakob disease there is a spongiform change in the cortical gray matter and, some-times, the basal ganglia are affected. There is little, or no, gross atrophy of the brain and no inflammatory response in brain tissue. The disease is similar to kuru in humans and scrapie in sheep and goats. Rapidly progressive dementia occurs. Worldwide incidence is about one case per million population. The disease is caused by transmissible agents, or prions, which are proteinaceous infective particles, resistant to formalin and ionizing radiation, but inactivated by autoclaving, hypochlorite solutions (bleach), and alcoholic iodine.

407. The answer is B. *(Robbins, 5/e, pp 225–227. Rubin, 2/e, pp 1419–1420.)* The nervous system is frequently affected in patients with AIDS. Opportunistic infections, such as toxoplasmosis, CMV, and PML, are in-creased in incidence, but in most patients the encephalopathy is the result of direct action of the virus itself. HIV-1 preferentially infects macrophages and microglial cells in the CNS, resulting in multinucleated giant cells, microglial nodules, and secondary loss of neurons and areas of demyelination. About one-third of patients have a vacuolar myelopathy marked by vacuolation of the posterior and lateral columns of the spinal cord, which is similar to the changes produced by decreased vitamin B_{12}. This abnormality causes ataxia and spastic paraparesis.

408. The answer is E. *(Henry, 18/e, pp 452–454. Robbins, 5/e, p 1326.)* Elevations in cerebrospinal fluid globulins often occur in multiple sclerosis (MS) and other demyelinating diseases. Most patients with MS have oliclonal bands, which are the result of B-cell proliferation in the central nervous system. Late tertiary syphilis may cause these findings, but they would not occur in the secondary stage. Tumor or meningeal leukemia can also produce elevated levels of globulin in cerebrospinal fluid, but the presence of tumor cells and absence of an electrophoretic band would lead to the proper diagnosis.

409. The answer is D. *(Anderson, 9/e, p 2158.)* Pyogenic brain abscesses may have a number of possible sources, but the origin can often be determined from the location and number of abscesses in the brain parenchyma. Isolated lesions in the frontal lobes often arise from extension of sinus infections. In the temporal lobe or cerebellum, an isolated lesion may have the middle ear or mastoid as the primary site. Multiple lesions, especially in the superior aspects of the cerebrum, are seen with hematogenous dissemination, often from lung infection or in association with the lesions of congenital heart disease.

410. The answer is D. *(Robbins, 5/e, pp 1329–1331.)* Alzheimer's disease (AD) is characterized by numerous neurofibrillary tangles and senile plaques with a central core of amyloid β-protein. Both tangles and plaques are found to a lesser extent in other conditions, e.g., neurofibrillary tangles in Down's syndrome. Silver stains demonstrate tangles and plaques and Congo red shows amyloid deposition in plaques and vascular walls (amyloid angiopathy). In AD there are also numerous Hirano bodies, and granulovacuolar degeneration is found in more than 10 percent of the neurons of the hippocampus. AD often begins insidiously with impairment of memory and progresses to dementia. Grossly, brain atrophy (narrowed gyri and widened sulci) is predominant in frontal and superior temporal lobes. Lewy bodies are found in idiopathic parkinsonism and in diffuse Lewy body disease.

411. The answer is D. *(Robbins, 5/e, pp 605–608, 1339–1340.)* Chronic deficiency of cobalamin (vitamin B_{12}) has two major effects: a macrocytic megaloblastic anemia and a spinal cord degeneration, which may precede the anemia by months. The posterior columns and lateral corticospinal tracts undergo myelin degeneration, but the gray matter is rarely affected. Motor weakness with spasticity is the characteristic result, preceded by persistent paresthesias of the feet and hands. SCD is due to failure of the cobalamin-dependent enzyme methylmalonic CoA mutase, which is essential for maintenance of myelinated fibers. The classic triad of dermatitis, diarrhea, and dementia occurs in pellagra, which is due to niacin/nicotinic acid (vitamin B_5) deficiency.

412. The answer is C. *(Robbins, 5/e, p 1279. Rubin, 2/e, p 1425.)* Guillain-Barré (GB) syndrome (acute inflammatory polyradiculoneuropathy) is similar to postinfectious (or postvaccinal) encephalomyelitis in that both cause a process of demyelination and show perivascular infiltrates of lymphoid cells (in the brain and brainstem in encephalomyelitis and in the craniospinal nerve, roots, and ganglia in GB syndrome). In addition, the anterior horn cells in GB syndrome may be degenerative. GB syndrome manifests clinically as lower limb weakness and paralysis with varying sensory disturbances, such as hypesthesia of the lower limbs. The disease is characterized by an ascending paralysis, which may progress to involvement of the musculature of the upper body, including the muscles of respiration, which in turn can lead to respiratory arrest in the absence of mechanical ventilatory assistance. GB syndrome was identified in some persons who were vaccinated with influenza vaccines during the late 1970s.

413. The answer is B. *(Robbins, 5/e, pp 1336–1337.)* ALS, which is a disease of unknown cause with no effective treatment, is fatal in 2 to 6 years. It results in progressive loss of upper and lower motor neuron function. Early symptoms include limb weakness and cramping, then muscle atrophy and fasciculations, often in the hands and arms, but also in a leg (loss of lower motor neurons). Reflexes are hyperactive in upper and lower extremities, and a positive extensor plantar (Babinski) reflex occurs (loss of upper motor neurons). Early in the disease, upper motor neuron signs may predominate, with resultant spasticity of some muscles. The triad of atrophic weakness of hands and forearms, slight spasticity of the legs, and generalized hyperreflexia—in the absence of sensory changes—suggests the diagnosis. There is atrophy and loss of cells in the anterior gray horns and of motor nuclei of the lower brainstem, with bilateral degeneration of the pyramidal tracts that results in mixed upper and lower motor neuron disease. Symptoms of brainstem involvement include dysarthria and dysphagia. Variants of motor neuron disease include progressive muscular atrophy with only lower motor neuron signs and primary lateral sclerosis with only upper motor neuron signs and symptoms.

414. The answer is A. *(Adams, 5/e, pp 656–657. Robbins, 5/e, pp 865–866, 1322–1324.)* Subacute sclerosing panencephalitis (SSPE) is caused by the measles virus following infection early in life. There is a long latent period, protracted course, and high mortality. Histopathologic and electron-microscopic changes include perivascular mononuclear cell infiltrates, extensive neuronal loss, and intranuclear inclusions containing paramyxovirus particles in oligodendrocytes and neurons. The CSF contains oligoclonal immunoglobulins against viral components.

Progressive multifocal leukoencephalopathy (PML) is a viral infection of myelin-producing oligodendrocytes and causes primary demyelination. Oligodendroglial nuclei are enlarged and contain inclusion bodies, and bizarre giant astrocytes and foamy macrophages with myelin debris are seen in lesions. Electron microscopy reveals papovavirus particles in oligodendrocyte nuclei. Reye's syndrome occurs within 3 to 5 days of viral infection (influenza, chickenpox) treated with aspirin and is associated with severe or fatal brain edema. Creutzfeldt-Jakob disease, a spongiform encephalopathy, and kuru are probably transmitted by unconventional agents, or prions, that do not appear to be conventional viruses.

415. The answer is C. *(Robbins, 5/e, p 1347).* Astrocytomas are not at all uncommon in the younger age group, but when a child presents with clinical symptoms pointing to the intracranial posterior fossa, a cerebellar medulloblastoma should be suspected, especially if the child has no prior history of leukemia or neuroblastoma. Medulloblastomas occur predominantly in childhood and usually arise in the midline of the cerebellum (the vermis). They do occur (less commonly) in adults, in whom they are more apt to arise in the cerebellar hemispheres in a lateral position. They grow by local invasive growth and may block cerebrospinal fluid circulation (CSF block) by compression of the fourth ventricle. Recent aggressive treatment with the combined modalities of excision, radiotherapy, and chemotherapy have improved survival.

416. The answer is A. *(Robbins, 5/e, pp 1343–1345. Rubin, 2/e, pp 1440–1441.)* Although several lesions within the brain may be associated with dystrophic or metaplastic calcification, the presence of a calcified tumorlike mass lesion in the cerebral hemispheres should arouse suspicion of oligodendroglioma. Oligodendrogliomas are often slowly growing gliomas composed of round cells with clear cytoplasm ("fried-egg" appearance); they generally occur in the fourth and fifth decades of life. However, some oligodendrogliomas do proliferate in a rapid and aggressive fashion and may be associated with a malignant astrocytoma component. The brown tumor associated with hypercalcemia of hyperparathyroidism is associated with osteitis fibrosa cystica of bone. Some metastatic carcinomas may show microcalcifications in the form of psammoma bodies, as do some meningiomas. Papillary carcinomas of the thyroid and ovary are the best examples of such lesions, but the calcifications found in papillary carcinomas are rarely of the degree and magnitude of those found in some oligodendrogliomas.

417. The answer is D. *(Robbins, 5/e, pp 265–268, 461–462.)* Familial cases of retinoblastoma are frequently multiple and bilateral, although like all the sporadic, nonheritable tumors they can also be unifocal and unilateral. Histologically, rosettes of various types are frequent (similar to neuroblastoma and medulloblastoma). There is a good prognosis with early detection and treatment; spontaneous regression occurs rarely. Retinoblastoma belongs to a group of cancers (osteosarcoma, Wilms' tumor, meningioma, rhabdomyosarcoma, uveal melanoma) in which the normal cancer suppressor gene (antioncogene) is inactivated or lost, with resultant malignant change. Retinoblastoma and osteosarcoma arise after loss of the same genetic locus—hereditary mutation in the q14 band of chromosome 13.

418. The answer is D. *(Robbins, 5/e, pp 1342–1349.)* The features listed in the question are characteristic of a glioblastoma multiforme. Schwannomas generally appear as extremely cellular, spindle cell neoplasms, sometimes with metaplastic elements of bone, cartilage, and skeletal muscle. Medulloblastomas occur exclusively in the cerebellum and microscopically are highly cellular with uniform nuclei, scant cytoplasm, and, in about one-third of cases, rosette formation centered by neurofibrillary material. Oligodendrogliomas, which are marked by foci of calcification in 70 percent of cases, commonly show a pattern of uniform cellularity and are composed of round cells with small dark nuclei, clear cytoplasm, and a clearly defined cell membrane. Ependymomas are distinguished by ependymal rosettes, which are ductlike structures with a central lumen around which columnar tumor cells are arranged in a concentric fashion.

419. The answer is B. *(Robbins, 5/e, pp 1345–1346. Rubin, 2/e, pp 1438, 1441–1442.)* Ependymomas often occur in childhood and adolescence but have been noted at all ages. They form more than 60 percent of intraspinal gliomas, but only about 5 percent of intracranial gliomas. They are most commonly found in the fourth ventricle, not the lateral ventricles, which have a larger ependymal surface. Hydrocephalus can be a complication of intraventricular ependymoma. The papillary intraventricular ependymoma is similar grossly to the choroid plexus papilloma. Microscopically, the diagnostic rosette and pseudorosette formations are seen in the ependymoma, with tumor cells arranged around a central space (rosette) or around a blood vessel (pseudorosette). Blepharoplasts, the basal bodies of cilia, are pathognomonic if present.

420. The answer is C. *(Robbins, 5/e, p 1349. Rubin, 2/e, pp 1442–1443.)* Meningiomas arise from arachnoid villi of brain or spinal cord and have a female:male ratio of 3:2. Although they are usually tumors of middle or later life, a small number occur in persons 20 to 40 years of age. They commonly arise along the venous sinuses (parasagittal, sphenoid wings, and olfactory groove). Although benign and usually slow-growing, some meningiomas have progesterone receptors and rapid growth in pregnancy occurs occasionally. The rare malignant meningioma may invade or even metastasize. The typical case, however, does not invade the brain, but displaces it, causing headaches and seizures. Histologically, syncytial, transitional, and fibroblastic forms occur; psammoma bodies are found, particularly in the transitional pattern. The cut surface often has a whorled appearance. Meningioma is usually solitary, but multiple meningiomas occur, especially in neurofibromatosis type 2. Orbital meningiomas (female:male ratio of 5:1) may cause unilateral exophthalmos and often occur in patients under 20 years of age.

421. The answer is B. *(Robbins, 5/e, pp 509, 1302–1303, 1354. Rubin, 2/e, pp 1446–1447.)* Developmental abnormalities of the brain include the Arnold-Chiari malformation, the Dandy-Walker malformation, and the phakomatoses, which include tuberous sclerosis, neurofibromatosis, von Hippel–Lindau disease, and Sturge-Weber syndrome. The Arnold-Chiari malformation consists of herniation of the cerebellum and fourth ventricle into the foramen magnum, flattening of the base of the skull, hydrocephalus secondary to the cerebral aqueduct, and spina bifida with meningomyelocele. Severe hypoplasia or absence of the cerebellar vermis occurs in the Dandy-Walker malformation. There is cystic distention of the roof of the fourth ventricle, hydrocephalus, and possibly agenesis of the corpus callosum. Tuberous sclerosis may show characteristic firm, white nodules (tubers) in the cortex and subependymal nodules of gliosis protruding into the ventricles ("candle drippings"). Other signs of tuberous sclerosis include a triad of seizures, mental retardation, and congenital white spots or macules (leukoderma). Facial angiofibromata (adenoma sebaceum) also occur. In von Hippel–Lindau disease, multiple benign and malignant neoplasms occur including hemangioblastomas of the retina, cerebellum, and medulla oblongata, angiomas of the kidney and liver, and renal cell carcinoma. Patients with Sturge-Weber syndrome, a nonfamilial congenital disorder, have angiomas of the brain, leptomeninges, and ipsilateral face, which are called *port-wine stains (nevus flammeus).*

422. The answer is C. *(Anderson, 9/e, pp 1082, 1089.)* The photomicrograph (at low magnification) shows an intact overlying mucosa with a subjacent highly cellular neoplasm composed of small, dark-staining cells ("tumor of small blue cells"). In the child, small, blue cell tumors comprise lymphoma, neuroblastoma, cerebellar medulloblastoma, undifferentiated nephroblastoma (Wilms' tumor), retinoblastoma, embryonal rhabdomyosarcoma, and Ewing's sarcoma. In the adult, anaplastic, small cell carcinomas of the lung, pancreas, uterine cervix, and anorectum (cloacogenic carcinoma); plasmacytomas; and neuroectodermal tumors of thoracopulmonary origin are also included. In addition to the age of the patient and the organ site, certain structures visible at higher magnification, such as rosettes (retinoblastoma) and pseudorosettes (anaplastic small cell carcinoma, neuroblastoma) aid in the differential diagnosis. In the example given, the lesion is too cellular to be either nasal glioma (large, pale glial cells) or nasopharyngeal angiofibroma (vascular structures). The olfactory neuroblastoma (the tumor depicted in the photomicrograph) arises from the olfactory placode of the stem cell referred to as the *esthesioneuroblast.* The cells populating the tumor are round or oval neuroepithelial cells occurring in clusters and associated with a fibrillary intercellular matrix.

423. The answer is A. *(Robbins, 5/e, pp 1120–1121, 1147–1148, 1342–1345, 1354.)* Glioblastoma multiforme is a rapidly growing cerebral tumor in which calcification does not develop, but in which necrosis and hemorrhage are frequent. Both oligodendroglioma and craniopharyngioma show fairly frequent calcification; oligodendroglioma is often located in the frontal lobe, whereas craniopharyngioma occurs in the third ventricle. CT scan and particularly MRI are essential in diagnosis. Patchy intracerebral calcification may develop in tuberous sclerosis, an autosomal dominant disease characterized by the triad of epilepsy, mental retardation, and facial skin lesions (multiple angiofibromas). In addition, subependymal gliosis, cardiac rhabdomyoma, renal angiomyolipoma, and periungal fibroma occur. Calcification of the basal ganglia occurs in about 20 percent of patients with chronic hypoparathyroidism, which sometimes leads to a parkinsonian syndrome.

424. The answer is D. *(Robbins, 5/e, pp 1342–1349. Silverberg, 2/e, pp 2093–2102.)* Gliomas are the most frequent intracranial tumors of adults; they constitute 40 to 50 percent of such tumors, with glioblastoma multiforme making up 25 to 30 percent. Gliomas at the opposite end of the spectrum include ependymoma and oligodendroglioma, each constituting only 2 to 3 percent. Medulloblastoma also forms 2 to 3 percent of intracranial tumors in adults. Astrocytomas have an 8 to 12 percent and meningiomas a 12 to 15 percent intracranial incidence. Metastatic tumors have an intracranial incidence of 25 to 30 percent; metastatic carcinoma (lung, breast, kidney, GI)

and melanoma are predominant. Metastases are often multiple and demar-
cated from surrounding brain tissue.

425. The answer is D. *(Robbins, 5/e, pp 1277–1278.)* The axonal reaction
that occurs when a peripheral nerve is cut includes a number of striking
changes. In the cell body, swelling and dissolution of the Nissl substance are
apparent within 24 to 48 h after transection. The axon and covering myelin or
Schwann sheath distal to the lesion first degenerate and undergo resorption.
In addition, the axis cylinder and Schwann sheath degenerate proximal to the
cut over the distance of a few nodal segments. Regeneration occurs when the
Schwann cells proliferate from the proximal portion to form a hollow myelin
sheath through which the axons grow again.

426. The answer is E. *(Robbins, 5/e, pp 1168–1169. Rubin, 2/e, pp 1146–
1147.)* Primary tumors of the pineal gland are very uncommon but are of interest, especially in view of the mysterious and relatively unknown functions
of the pineal gland itself. The gland secretes neurotransmitter substances such
as serotonin and dopamine, with the major product being melatonin. Tumors
of the pineal gland include germ cell tumors of all types including embryonal
carcinoma, choriocarcinoma, teratoma, and various combinations of germino-
mas. Germ cell tumors may arise extragonadally within the retroperitoneal
space and the pineal gland, with the only commonality being that these structures are in the midline. Primary tumors of the pineal gland occur in two
forms: the pineoblastoma and the pineocytoma. Pineoblastomas occur in
young patients and consist of small tumors having areas of hemorrhage and
necrosis with pleomorphic nuclei and frequent mitoses. Pineocytomas occur
in older adults and are slow-growing; they are better differentiated and have
large rosettes. Craniopharyngiomas occur not in the pineal gland but above
the pituitary gland in the hypothalamus and are thought to arise from structures related to Rathke's pouch.

427. The answer is C. *(Robbins, 5/e, pp 148–149, 1354. Rubin, 2/e, pp
228–230.)* In von Hippel–Lindau disease, a rare autosomal dominant disorder,
multiple benign and malignant neoplasms occur. These include hemangioblastomas of retina and brain (cerebellum and medulla oblongata), angiomas of
kidney and liver, and renal cell carcinoma in 25 to 50 percent of cases. Classic
neurofibromatosis (NF-1) is characterized by café-au-lait skin macules, axillary freckling, multiple neurofibromas, plexiform neurofibromas, and Lisch
nodules (pigmented iris hamartomas). Lisch nodules are found in 95 percent of
patients after age 6. Hamartomas of the iris are not present in central or
acoustic neurofibromatosis (NF-2), though both types of neurofibromatosis

have café-au-lait macules and neurofibromas. Only the central, or acoustic, form has bilateral acoustic neuromas; the classic form may have unilateral acoustic neuroma. There is increased risk of developing meningiomas or even pheochromocytoma. A major complication of NF-1 is the malignant transformation of a neurofibroma to a neurofibrosarcoma. The gene for the classic form (NF-1) is located on chromosome 17. It encodes for a protein, neurofibromin, which regulates the function of p21 *ras* oncoprotein.

428–431. The answers are 428-F, 429-B, 430-D, 431-E. *(Robbins, 5/e, pp 863–864, 1319, 1332–1333, 1351–1352.)* In classic, or idiopathic, parkinsonism (Parkinson's disease) there is degeneration and loss of pigmented cells in the substantia nigra. With less than 25 percent of nigral cells remaining, there is a deficiency of dopamine in the nigral cells, where dopamine is synthesized, and at the synaptic endings of nigral fibers in the striatum. The severity of the motor syndrome correlates with the degree of dopamine deficiency. Lewy bodies, eosinophilic intracytoplasmic inclusions, are found in remaining neurons of the substantia nigra and are largely localized there in classic Parkinson's disease, unlike diffuse Lewy body disease.

Postencephalitic parkinsonism (von Economo's disease), one of the complications of encephalitis lethargica, is similar to classic Parkinson's disease in degeneration of the striatonigral pathway with diminished dopamine and depigmentation in the corpus striatum. However, it occurs earlier and is not progressive. In postencephalitic parkinsonism, neurofibrillary tangles, which are thickened and tortuous neurofilaments stainable by silver, form within neurons.

In Pick's disease, a presenile dementia, neurofibrillary tangles are also demonstrable, but they are fewer than in either Alzheimer's disease or postencephalitic parkinsonism. Pick's disease is a major cortical degenerative disease associated with marked atrophy of frontal lobes and partial temporal lobe atrophy.

Herpes simplex encephalitis causes necrotizing lesions with Cowdry A intranuclear inclusions in oligodendroglia and occasional neurons. Perivascular mononuclear infiltrates occur and hemorrhagic necrosis is present in the temporal and frontal lobes, especially the orbital gyri.

Wilson's disease (hepatolenticular degeneration) is inherited as a primary defect in copper metabolism with increased copper in liver (cirrhosis) and brain (cavitation). Degenerative cavitation or brown discoloration occurs mainly in the lenticular nucleus and thalamus, and copper pigmentation in the cornea (Kayser-Fleischer rings) is distinctive.

Schwannomas (neurilemmomas) are single, encapsulated tumors of nerve sheaths, usually benign, occurring on peripheral, spinal, or cranial nerves. The acoustic neuroma is one example. Microscopically, Verocay bodies, which are foci of palisaded nuclei, may be found in the more cellular (Antoni A) tissue.

Devic's syndrome (neuromyelitis optica) is a variant of multiple sclerosis with rapid onset of demyelination of the optic nerve and of the spinal cord with paraplegia. A pleocytosis with polymorphonuclear cells and a protein content higher than is usual in multiple sclerosis may be seen in cerebrospinal fluid.

432–434. The answers are 432-A, 433-B, 434-C. *(Robbins, 5/e, pp 1300–1303.)* Developmental anomalies of the central nervous system occur under genetic and environmental influences or sporadically during a critical phase in gestation. Various trisomies are examples of genetic mishaps. Environmental factors include drugs (both therapeutic and illegal), ionizing radiation, infections (rubella, syphilis, toxoplasmosis), malnutrition, and circulatory insufficiency.

When the bony spinal cord fails to close, multiple errors, occurring sporadically as single entities or in association with other central nervous system anomalies, are possible. Spina bifida, the most common developmental defect that occurs in the neural tube, involves the failure of the vertebral arches to close completely. Meningomyelocele is herniation of part of the spinal cord tissue and the meninges through such a defect. In spina bifida occulta the defect in the closure of the neural tube is covered by skin and dermis, with only a pinpoint sinus or hair-covered depression marking the site. Bacterial meningitis, or meningomyelitis, is the major potential risk in these patients.

A developmental defect in the skull bones similar to spina bifida is cranium bifidum, which is regarded as a congenital cranial cleft. Meningocele is herniation of the meninges alone through a cranium bifidum.

Meningoencephalocele includes herniation of meninges and brain substance in the region of the occipital bone. Meningoencephalocystocele, a herniation at the roof of the mouth, together with cranial meningocele and cranial meningoencephalocele, occurs less frequently than the herniations associated with spina bifida.

The Arnold-Chiari malformation consists of herniation of the cerebellum and fourth ventricle into the foramen magnum, skull base flattening, and cerebral aqueduct stenosis with hydrocephalus and meningomyelocele. Various combinations of the above abnormalities exist, and it is not necessary for all of them to be uniformly present for the disease to qualify as Arnold-Chiari malformation. In all cases, however, the clinical course is reflected by the degree of hydrocephalus.

435–439. The answers are 435-B, 436-E, 437-C, 438-D, 439-C. *(Robbins, 5/e, pp 1326–1331, 1334, 1337–1338, 1434–1436.)* Tay-Sachs disease (GM_2 gangliosidosis type I) is one of the lysosomal storage diseases and, more specifically, is one of the sphingolipidoses. Absence of hexosaminidase A leads to accumulation of ganglioside in neurons of the central and autonomic nervous systems and retina. Neurons appear swollen and vacuolated with lysosomes filled with gangliosides. The characteristic cherry-red spot in the macula (due to contrasting gangliosidic retinal pallor) may also be seen in up to 50 percent of cases of Niemann-Pick disease, in which sphingomyelin accumulates.

Major histologic features of Alzheimer's disease include neurofibrillary tangles, neuritic (senile) plaques, amyloid angiopathy, granulovacuolar degeneration, and Hirano bodies. Genetic studies have revealed a genetic defect in familial Alzheimer's disease with the gene that codes for the amyloid precursor protein (APP).

In primary CNS demyelination there is loss of myelin sheaths but relative preservation of axons. This type of demyelination is seen predominantly in multiple sclerosis, in the perivenous encephalomyelopathies (acute disseminated encephalomyelitis and acute hemorrhagic leukoencephalitis), and in progressive multifocal leukoencephalopathy. Secondary CNS demyelination occurs because of destruction of the axons themselves.

Multiple sclerosis of unknown etiology causes disseminated but focal plaques of primary demyelination in gray and white matter anywhere in the CNS, but often near the angles of the lateral ventricles. It affects adults between 20 and 40 years of age who may have nystagmus, tremor, dysarthria, paresthesias, and incoordination. A relapsing and remitting course is usual.

In acute disseminated encephalomyelitis (postinfectious or postvaccinal) there are many foci of perivenous demyelination. It occurs, rarely, after a viral infection (measles, mumps, chickenpox) but is not a slow viral infection. Although the disease is fatal in up to 20 percent of cases, prognosis in survivors is quite good.

Abnormal or defective myelin metabolism is characteristic of Krabbe's disease (globoid cell leukodystrophy) and metachromatic leukodystrophy. These leukodystrophies or inborn errors of metabolism usually appear in early childhood. Metachromatic leukodystrophy is an autosomal recessive disorder of sphingomyelin metabolism and results from deficiency of cerebroside sulfatase (aryl-sulfatase A). Sulfatides accumulate in lysosomes and stain metachromatically with cresyl violet. Diagnostic measures include amniocentesis, enzyme analysis, and measuring decreased urinary aryl-sulfatase A. Demyelination is widespread in the cerebrum and peripheral nervous system. Krabbe's disease, also autosomal recessive, is marked by accumulation of galactocerebroside, demyelination, and multinucleate histiocytes (globoid cells) in the white matter.

Huntington's disease is autosomal dominant with its defective gene on chromosome 4. It involves the extrapyramidal system and causes loss of striatal neurons in the caudate nuclei and putamen. Choreiform movements and progressive dementia seldom appear before age 30.

Musculoskeletal System

DIRECTIONS: Each question below contains five suggested responses. Select the **one best** response to each question.

440. Characteristics of normal striated muscle include

(A) hypercontraction bands
(B) central location of majority of nuclei
(C) angulated fibers
(D) ring fibers
(E) "checkerboard" ATPase staining pattern

441. Elevated levels of serum creatine kinase (CK) are seen in all the following EXCEPT

(A) muscular dystrophy
(B) polymyositis
(C) myasthenia gravis
(D) myocardial infarction
(E) hypothyroidism

442. A pathognomonic feature of denervation followed by reinnervation is the histologic finding of

(A) atrophic fibers
(B) angular fibers
(C) type-specific grouping of fibers
(D) eosinophilic infiltrates
(E) lymphohistiocytic infiltrates

443. A section of bone shows prominent osteoid seams, very large osteoclasts with more than 12 hyperchromatic nuclei, and viral-type inclusion particles. This is most characteristic of

(A) Paget's disease
(B) Gaucher's disease
(C) fibrous dysplasia
(D) giant cell tumors of bone
(E) brown tumor of bone

444. A 59-year-old woman presents with difficulty swallowing, ptosis, and diplopia. Which of the following is most consistent with these symptoms?

(A) Antibodies to the acetylcholine receptor
(B) Antibodies to the microvasculature of skeletal muscle
(C) Lack of lactate production during ischemic exercise
(D) Rhabdomyolysis
(E) Corticosteroid therapy

445. A perivascular inflammatory infiltrate in skeletal muscle, as shown in the photomicrograph below, is likely to be seen in all the following EXCEPT

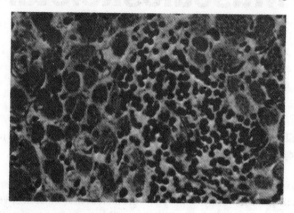

(A) hypersensitivity angiitis
(B) polymyositis
(C) polyarteritis nodosa
(D) cystic medial necrosis
(E) systemic sclerosis

446. A sex-linked recessive mode of inheritance exists in

(A) myotonic dystrophy
(B) limb-girdle dystrophy
(C) facioscapulohumeral dystrophy
(D) Duchenne's muscular dystrophy
(E) polymyositis

447. Osteogenesis imperfecta type I is characterized by

(A) a hereditary defect in osteoclastic function
(B) defective synthesis of type II collagen
(C) defective synthesis of osteoid matrix
(D) early death
(E) bone marrow aplasia

448. Characteristics or components of normal bone in the adult skeleton include all the following EXCEPT

(A) osteoblasts
(B) osteoid
(C) type I collagen
(D) lamellar bone
(E) woven bone

449. Diseases affecting the epiphyseal plate include all the following EXCEPT

(A) cretinism
(B) achondroplasia
(C) osteopetrosis
(D) scurvy
(E) Hurler's syndrome

450. The atypical rhabdomyoblasts illustrated in the photomicrograph below may be seen in all the following lesions EXCEPT

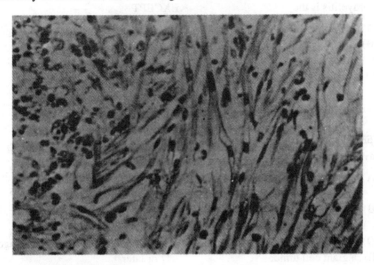

(A) sarcoma botryoides
(B) myositis ossificans
(C) mixed heterologous müllerian tumor of the uterus
(D) adult pleomorphic rhabdomyosarcoma
(E) embryonal rhabdomyosarcoma

---

451. Osteomalacia may best be characterized as

(A) failure of bone remodeling
(B) failure of bone mineralization
(C) failure of osteoid formation
(D) reactive bone formation
(E) reduction in amount of normally mineralized bone

452. Features of the normal process of fracture healing include

(A) pseudoarthrosis
(B) a sequestrum
(C) an involucrum
(D) a cloaca
(E) a cartilaginous callus

453. Which of the following statements about osteoid osteoma is true?

(A) It occurs predominantly in older adults
(B) Pain occurs predominantly at night
(C) It is associated occasionally with Gardner's syndrome
(D) It is frequently located in the spine
(E) Occasional malignant change occurs

454. The part of a long bone initially involved in hematogenous osteomyelitis is the

(A) metaphyseal region
(B) diaphysis
(C) epiphysis
(D) area around the entrance of the nutrient artery
(E) medullary cavity

455. The most common tumor that involves bone is

(A) a metastatic tumor from an extraosseous site
(B) osteogenic sarcoma
(C) multiple myeloma
(D) chondrosarcoma
(E) a giant cell tumor

456. Bilateral segmental osteonecrosis or avascular necrosis (AVN) of the femoral head is most often associated with

(A) systemic steroid therapy
(B) irradiation therapy
(C) sickle cell disease
(D) alcoholism
(E) fracture of the femoral neck

457. Osteosarcoma (osteogenic sarcoma) has an increased incidence in all the following conditions EXCEPT

(A) Paget's disease
(B) retinoblastoma
(C) fibrous dysplasia
(D) plasmacytoma
(E) osteochondromatosis

458. Characteristics of Ewing's sarcoma include all the following EXCEPT

(A) primary occurrence prior to age 20
(B) primary occurrence in the epiphysis of long bones
(C) onion-skin pattern on x-ray
(D) basophilic cells resembling lymphocytes
(E) PAS-positive intracytoplasmic glycogen

459. All the following statements about chondrosarcoma are true EXCEPT that

(A) it is most frequent in middle age or later
(B) the peripheral type can arise from enchondroma
(C) it is common in the pelvic bones
(D) histologic analysis is of prognostic significance
(E) it is the second most common malignant bone tumor

460. Tuberculous spondylitis (Pott's disease) is characterized by all the following EXCEPT

(A) involvement of thoracic and lumbar vertebrae
(B) hematogenous spread
(C) proliferative synovitis with pannus
(D) destruction of intervertebral disks
(E) formation of psoas abscess

461. All the following diseases may be associated with the grossly deformed joint depicted in the photograph below EXCEPT

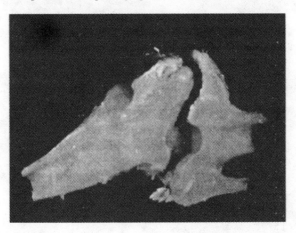

(A) leprosy
(B) psoriasis
(C) syringomyelia
(D) pernicious anemia
(E) diabetes mellitus

---

462. Which of the following fibroosseous bone disorders is most likely to be associated with skin lesions?

(A) Osteoid osteoma
(B) Albright's syndrome
(C) Nonossifying fibroma
(D) Polyostotic fibrous dysplasia
(E) Monostotic fibrous dysplasia

463. Secondary gout may be seen in association with all the following EXCEPT

(A) polycythemia
(B) psoriasis
(C) hemolytic anemias
(D) myeloproliferative diseases
(E) chondrocalcinosis

464. The lesion illustrated in the photomicrograph below is most likely

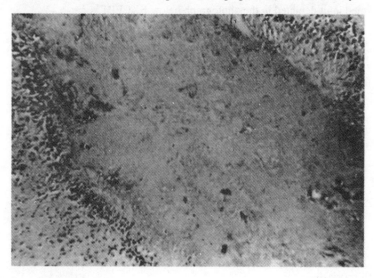

(A) a rheumatoid nodule
(B) myositis ossificans
(C) necrotizing panniculitis
(D) polymyositis
(E) fat necrosis

465. A 54-year-old man presents with chronic knee pain. Resection of the patella reveals chalky white deposits on the surface of intraarticular structures. Histologic sections reveal long, needle-shaped, negatively birefringent crystals. The photomicrograph below was taken under polarized light. These findings are most consistent with a diagnosis of

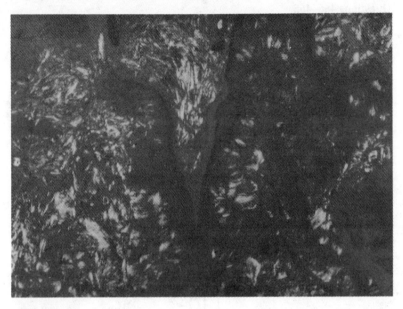

(A) osteoarthritis
(B) rheumatoid arthritis
(C) ochronosis
(D) gout
(E) pseudogout

DIRECTIONS: The group of questions below consists of lettered headings followed by a set of numbered items. For each numbered item select the **one** lettered heading with which it is **most** closely associated. Each lettered heading may be used **once, more than once, or not at all.**

Questions 466–468

For each bone lesion, select the lettered location and general configuration with which it is most likely to be associated in the diagram.

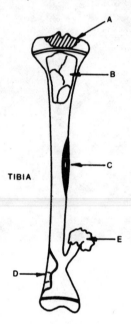

TIBIA

466. Giant cell tumor of bone (osteoclastoma)

467. Unicameral (solitary) bone cyst

468. Osteochondroma

Musculoskeletal System
Answers

440. The answer is E. (*Robbins, 5/e, pp 1275–1277. Rubin, 2/e, pp 1350–1352.*) Two functional types of muscle fibers are determined by the lower motor neuron innervating the muscle fiber. "Slow-twitch" (type 1, red) fibers are high in myoglobin (a red pigment), oxidative enzymes, and mitochondria; "fast-switch" (type 2, white) fibers are high in glycolytic enzymes (Embden-Meyerhof pathway), glycogen, and phosphorylase. ATPase stains type 2 fibers darkly and type 1 fibers almost not at all. Since human skeletal muscle is normally composed of a random mixture of both type 1 and type 2 fibers, ATPase staining normally has a "checkerboard" pattern. Atrophic muscle fibers are smaller and have an angulated appearance on cross-section. In normal muscle, less than 5 percent of the fibers have central nuclei. An increase in the percentage of central nuclei is a nonspecific abnormal finding. Hypercontraction bands are particularly frequent in Duchenne's muscular dystrophy. Ring fibers, in which the peripheral myofilament runs abnormally in a circumferential pattern, are particularly characteristic of myotonic dystrophy.

441. The answer is C. (*Henry, 18/e, pp 273–274. Rubin, 2/e, p 528.*) Creatine kinase (CK) is an enzyme found mainly in skeletal muscle, the myocardium, and the brain. Diseases that produce skeletal muscle destruction, such as all types of muscular dystrophy, polymyositis, viral myositis, and rhabdomyolysis, produce elevated levels of CK in the blood. Neurogenic muscle diseases, such as myasthenia gravis, multiple sclerosis, poliomyelitis, and parkinsonism, have normal levels of CK because there is no destruction of the muscle. Total CK activity is increased following a myocardial infarction and also following cerebrovascular diseases with cerebral ischemia. Serum CK levels have an inverse relationship with thyroid activity; that is, levels are increased in hypothyroid patients, but are low-normal to decreased in amount in patients with hyperthyroidism.

442. The answer is C. (*Robbins, 5/e, pp 1277–1278. Rubin, 2/e, pp 1359–1361, 1365–1368.*) Histologic features of muscle biopsy specimens may suggest certain muscle disorders. Denervation causes atrophy of the fibers, which become angulated. Another change seen in denervated muscle is the presence of distinctive three-zoned fibers called *target fibers*. Reinnervation is characterized by type-specific grouping of fibers, which is in contrast to the mixed, "checkerboard" pattern of type 1 and type 2 fibers seen in normal skeletal muscle. Variation in size and shape along with degenerative changes and intrafascicular fibrosis are features of muscular dystrophy. Eosinophils within muscle are found in association with parasitic infections, the most common of which is trichinosis. Lymphocytes and macrophages within muscle are seen in polymyositis.

443. The answer is A. *(Robbins, 5/e, pp 143–144, 1223–1227, 1242–1243, 1245.)* Paget's disease, osteitis deformans, is characterized by an uncoupling of osteoblastic and osteoclastic activity and is divided into three phases: an initial osteoclastic (osteolytic) resorptive stage, a mixed osteoblastic and osteoclastic activity stage, and a late sclerotic, burnt-out stage. Histologically, prominent osteoid seams separate irregular islands of bone into a mosaic ("jigsaw") pattern. The osteoclasts of Paget's disease are characteristically large with an increased number of hyperchromatic nuclei and viral inclusions. Because of the high bone turnover, the serum alkaline phosphatase level is markedly increased, and collagen breakdown products, such as hydroxyproline and hydroxylysine, are increased in amount in the serum and the urine. Gaucher's disease is characterized by the accumulation of glucocerebroside in macrophages, which then have an appearance described as "wrinkled tissue paper." These cells then accumulate in many organs, including the bone. Fibrous dysplasia histologically reveals a "Chinese-letters" effect of the bony trabeculae, which are surrounded by a cellular, fibrous stroma, with osteoblasts and osteoclasts decreased at the periphery of entrapped woven bone. Giant cell tumors of bone, usually occurring at the junction of the metaphysis and the epiphysis of a long bone, produce a multiloculated ("soap bubble") appearance on x-ray. They are composed of numerous osteoblastic giant cells found in a background of fibroblast-like neoplastic spindle cells. Brown tumors of bone are areas of fibrosis with hemosiderin-laden macrophages and many osteoclastic and foreign-body type giant cells. They occur in patients with primary hyperparathyroidism.

444. The answer is A. *(Robbins, 5/e, pp 213–214, 1292, 1289–1291. Rubin, 2/e, pp 1359–1361, 1364–1365, 1370.)* Myasthenia gravis is an acquired autoimmune disease with circulating antibodies to the acetylcholine receptors at the myoneural junction. These antibodies cause abnormal muscle fatigability, which typically involves the extraocular muscles and leads to ptosis and diplopia. Other muscles may also be involved, and this may cause many different symptoms, such as problems with swallowing. Two-thirds of patients with myasthenia gravis have thymic abnormalities; the most common is thymic hyperplasia. A minority of patients have a thymoma. Lack of lactate production during ischemic exercise is seen in metabolic diseases of muscle caused by a deficiency of myophosphorylase. Dermatomyositis is an auto-immune disease produced by complement-mediated cytotoxic antibodies against the microvasculature of skeletal muscle. Rhabdomyolysis is destruc-tion of skeletal muscle that releases myoglobin into the blood. This may cause myoglobinuria and acute renal failure. Rhabdomyolysis may follow an in-fluenza infection, heat stroke, or malignant hyperthermia. Corticosteroid ther-apy may cause muscle weakness and selective type 2 atrophy.

445. The answer is D. *(Robbins, 5/e, pp 210–214, 492–496, 502.)* Cystic medial necrosis is not inflammatory, but degenerative. Hypersensitivity angi-itis primarily affects small vessels; polyarteritis nodosa affects small to medium-sized arteries. In addition to interstitial inflammation (often perivas-cular), patients with polymyositis have histologic evidence of muscle fiber death. Perivascular inflammation is one of the early skeletal muscle changes in scleroderma (systemic sclerosis).

446. The answer is D. *(Anderson, 9/e, pp 2111–2112. Robbins, 5/e, pp 1285–1287.)* Classification of the muscular dystrophies is based on the mode of inheritance and clinical features. Inheritance of the Duchenne type is by an X-linked recessive trait, with the gene located on the short arm of the X chro-mosome, although spontaneous mutations are fairly common. Autosomal dominant inheritance characterizes both myotonic dystrophy and the fa-cioscapulohumeral type, while limb-girdle dystrophy is autosomal recessive. In Duchenne's muscular dystrophy, males are affected and symptoms begin before the age of 4. Pelvic-girdle muscles are affected with resultant difficulty in walking, and this is followed by shoulder-girdle weakness and eventual in-volvement of respiratory and cardiac muscles with death from respiratory failure before age 20. Histologic changes include rounded, atrophic fibers, hypertrophied fibers, degenerative and regenerative changes in adjacent my-ocytes, and necrotic fibers invaded by histiocytes. Elevation of serum creatine kinase is marked.

447. The answer is C. *(Robbins, 5/e, pp 1218–1219.)* Osteogenesis imper-fecta (OI), or brittle bone disease, constitues a group of disorders often inher-ited as autosomal dominant traits and caused by genetic mutations involving the synthesis of type I collagen, which comprises about 90 percent of the os-teoid, or bone matrix. Very early perinatal death and multiple fractures occur in OI type II, which is often autosomal recessive. The major variant of OI, type I, is compatible with survival; after the perinatal period fractures occur in addition to other signs of defective collagen synthesis such as thin, translu-cent, blue sclerae; laxity of joint ligaments; deafness from otosclerosis; and abnormal teeth. A hereditary defect in osteoclastic function with decreased bone resorption and bone overgrowth, which sometimes narrows or obliterates the marrow cavity, is characteristic of osteopetrosis, or marble bone disease.

448. The answer is E. *(Robbins, 5/e, pp 1213–1216. Rubin, 2/e, pp 1276–1279.)* Bone is composed of cells, a mineralized matrix, and an organic matrix. The normal cellular component of bone includes osteoblasts (protein-synthesizing, alkaline phosphatase–containing cells arranged in a line along the bone surface), osteocytes (an osteoblast embedded in bone matrix that has lost the capacity for protein synthesis), and osteoclasts (large, multinucleate, bone-resorbing cells with numerous lysosomes, found on the surface of bones in Howship's lacunae). The mineralized matrix consists of hydroxyapatite, which is composed mainly of calcium and phosphate. The organic matrix consists mainly of type I collagen, which is secreted by osteoblasts. Bone may be organized into woven bone or lamellar bone, each of which may be mineralized or unmineralized. The unmineralized bone is called *osteoid*. Lamellar bone has a parallel arrangement of type I collagen and few osteocytes; it is formed slowly and its presence is normal in the adult skeleton. Woven bone has an irregular arrangement of type I collagen fibers and numerous osteocytes; it is formed rapidly and is always pathologic if found in the adult skeleton. It is found in newly formed bone, such as early in fracture repair or bone-forming tumors.

449. The answer is C. *(Robbins, 5/e, pp 1222–1223. Rubin, 2/e, pp 1282–1287.)* The epiphyseal plate (growth plate), a layer of modified cartilage lying between the diaphysis and the epiphysis, consists of the following zones: reserve (resting) zone, proliferating zone, zone of hypertrophy, zone of calcification, and zone of ossification. Many disorders affect the epiphyseal plate. Cretinism (congenital hypothyroidism) results in mental retardation and dwarfism. The skeletal abnormalities result in defects in cartilage maturation of the epiphyseal plate. In achondroplasia, the most common inherited form of dwarfism, the zone of proliferating cartilage is either absent or greatly thinned. This in turn causes the epiphyseal plate to be thin. Vitamin C is essential for the normal synthesis and structure of collagen. In scurvy (vitamin C deficiency) there is a lack of osteoblastic synthesis of collagen (causing excess growth of chondrocytes at the epiphyseal plate) and fragility of the basement membrane of capillaries (causing periosteal hemorrhage). Many of the mucopolysaccharidoses (MPS) involve skeletal deformities. Hurler's syndrome (MPS IH) is associated with increased tissue stores and excretion of dermatan sulfate and heparan sulfate. These mucopolysaccharides also accumulate in the chondrocytes of the growth plate, resulting in dwarfism. *Gargoylism* describes the characteristic clinical appearance of these patients. Osteopetrosis (marble bone disease) is a rare inherited disease that involves osteoclasts with decreased functioning and lack of the usual ruffled borders.

This abnormality results in reduced bone resorption and bone overgrowth. Instead of affecting the epiphyseal plate, the long bones are widened in the metaphysis and diaphysis and have a characteristic "Erlenmeyer flask" appearance. Loss of the medullary cavity often results in anemia, and multiple fractures are frequent as the bones are structurally weak. The severe autosomal recessive form causes death in infancy, but the more common autosomal dominant adult form is relatively benign.

450. The answer is B. *(Robbins, 5/e, pp 1264, 1267–1268.)* Myositis ossificans is a benign condition characterized by fibrous repair of a skeletal muscle or subcutaneous fat, hematoma with secondary cartilage formation, ossification, and calcification. The other lesions mentioned are malignant neoplasms that may contain a variety of mesodermal tissues. The rhabdomyoblasts, if elongated, are called "tadpole," or "strap," cells.

451. The answer is B. *(Robbins, 5/e, pp 1219–1223, 1225–1227. Rubin, 2/e, pp 1300–1310.)* Osteomalacia (soft bones) is a disorder of adults characterized by inadequate mineralization of newly formed bone matrix and is most often associated with abnormalities of vitamin D metabolism (such as dietary deficiency or intestinal malabsorption of vitamin D), hypoparathyroidism, or chronic renal diseases. Rickets is a similar condition that occurs in children. Defective mineralization results in an increase in the thickness of the osteoid seams, such as seen in vitamin C deficiency (scurvy), and not in failure of osteoid formation. Osteopetrosis, marble bone, is a bone modeling abnormality related to hypofunction of the osteoclasts. Osteoporosis results from a reduction in the mass of bone, which still has the normal ratio of mineral to matrix. Reactive bone formation occurs in bone or soft tissue in response to such conditions as tumors, infections, or trauma.

452. The answer is E. *(Robbins, 5/e, pp 1227–1231. Rubin, 2/e, pp 1288–1290, 1294–1296.)* Normal fracture healing is characterized initially by an inflammatory phase, which lasts a few days. This is followed by a reparative phase, which lasts a few weeks and is associated with the formation of a cartilaginous callus. Finally there is a remodeling phase, which lasts for months to years. Osteomyelitis is inflammation of bone caused by an infectious organism rather than fracture healing. Organisms may be introduced into the bone by direct penetration or hematogenous spread. The initial focus of infection of the bone in hematogenous osteomyelitis is the metaphyseal area. The area of infection, or abscess, may extend into the cortex, destroying perforating arteries and causing necrosis of the cortex. The necrotic bone within the inflammation and debris is the sequestrum, and it may be surrounded by periosteal new bone formation, the involucrum. The abscess may drain through the bone, forming a draining sinus called the *cloaca*. An area of infection may be walled off and contained but still a chronic nidus of infection. This is called a *Brodie's abscess.*

453. The answer is B. *(Robbins, 5/e, pp 814, 1233–1234.)* Osteoid osteoma (OO) occurs predominantly in children or young adults in the second and third decades of life as a benign osteoblastic (bone-forming) lesion of small size, which by definition is less than 3 cm. In osteoid osteoma malignant change does not occur, unlike the closely related but larger osteoblastoma, in which there is occasional malignant change. OO is often located in the diaphyseal cortex of tibia or femur, unlike osteoblastoma, which occurs in the spine (vertebral arch) or medulla of long bones. Rarely, osteoma, another osteoblastic tumor, is associated with Gardner's syndrome, in which colonic polyposis and osteomas, epidermal cysts, and fibromatosis occur. Night pain, relieved by salicylates, is prominent with OO. OO consists of a very small, often radiolucent nidus of slender, mineralized osteoid trabeculae with intervening connective tissue; the entire lesion is enclosed by dense sclerotic bone. Treatment is complete excision of the nidus to prevent recurrence.

454. The answer is A. *(Rubin, 2/e, pp 1294–1296.)* Nutrient arteries to long bones divide to supply the metaphyses and diaphyses. In the metaphyses, the arteries become arterioles and finally form capillary loops adjacent to epiphyseal plates. This anatomic feature allows bacteria to settle in the region of the metaphysis and makes it the site initially involved in hematogenous osteomyelitis. As a consequence of vascular and osteoclastic resorption, the infected bone is replaced by fibrous connective tissue. Persistent chronic osteomyelitis is often associated with sequelae that include amyloidosis and the appearance of malignant tumors in old sinus tracts within the damaged bone.

455. The answer is A. *(Anderson, 9/e, pp 2055–2056. Robbins, 5/e, p 1246.)* Metastases account for the majority of bone tumors, followed in frequency by multiple myeloma and osteogenic sarcoma. Common carcinomas that metastasize to bone include lung, thyroid, breast, prostate, and renal cell carcinomas. Whereas most metastatic carcinomas to bone produce osteolytic radiologic lesions, prostate carcinoma tends to produce osteoblastic metastases. The serum calcium and alkaline phosphatase may be elevated in osseous metastases.

456. The answer is A. *(Anderson, 9/e, pp 163–164. Robbins, 5/e, pp 1229–1230.)* AVN of bone is a moderately frequent complication of high-dose systemic corticosteroid therapy—the usual cause of bilateral segmental infarction or AVN of the femoral head. Clinical features include sudden onset of severe pain and difficulty in walking. Within the femoral head a triangular yellow area of necrotic bone is found beneath the viable articular cartilage, and x-ray may show a crescent sign or space between cartilage and underlying infarct. Fracture of the subcapital femoral neck is frequently associated with unilateral AVN; the other conditions listed are much less frequently associated.

457. The answer is D. *(Robbins, 5/e, pp 1236–1244. Rubin, 2/e, pp 1318–1319.)* Osteosarcoma is the most common primary malignant bone tumor excluding multiple myeloma and lymphoma and is the most common bone cancer of children. In two-thirds of cases it is associated with mutations of the retinoblastoma (Rb) gene. Patients with retinoblastoma are at an increased risk for developing osteogenic sarcoma. In older patients, there is an association with multifocal Paget's disease of bone, radiation exposure (as in painters of radium watch dials), fibrous dysplasia, osteochondromatosis, and chondromatosis. Osteosarcomas usually arise in the metaphyses of long bones of the extremities, although they may involve any bone. They are composed of malignant osteoblasts and show marked variation histologically depending on the amount of type I collagen, osteoid, and spicules of woven bone produced. Osteosarcomas produce a characteristic sunburst x-ray pattern due to calcified perpendicular striae of reactive periosteum adjacent to the tumor. They may also show periosteal elevation at an acute angle (Codman's triangle) or penetrate cortical bone with extension into the adjacent soft tissue. These tumors metastasize hematogenously and usually spread to the lungs early in the course of the disease. With surgery, radiation, and chemotherapy the 5-year survival is now about 60 percent. Plasmacytoma is not associated with an increased incidence of osteogenic sarcoma.

458. The answer is B. *(Robbins, 5/e, p 1244. Rubin, 2/e, p 1322.)* Ewing's sarcoma is an uncommon tumor primarily affecting patients younger than 20 years of age. It arises in the medullary cavity and is usually located in the diaphysis or metaphysis of the long bones, not the epiphysis. Most cases have a reciprocal translocation between chromosomes 11 and 22. In about half of the cases of Ewing's sarcoma, reactive new bone formation may cause concentric "onion-skin" layering. Histologically the tumor is composed of small, uniform, round cells similar in appearance to lymphocytes. Occasionally the tumor cells form rosettes around central blood vessels (Homer-Wright pseudorosettes), indicating neural differentiation. PAS staining of glycogen-positive, diastase-sensitive cytoplasmic granules within the tumor cells of Ewing's sarcoma differentiates this lesion from lymphoma and neuroblastoma. With a combination of chemotherapy, radiation, and surgery, the 5-year survival is now 75 percent.

459. The answer is E. *(Robbins, 5/e, pp 1240–1241.)* Chondrosarcoma shows a peak incidence in the sixth and seventh decades. Most chondrosarcomas (85 percent) arise de novo, but the peripheral type, unlike the central type, may arise in benign tumors of cartilage, especially if they are multiple. Frequent sites of origin include pelvic bones (50 percent), humerus, femur, ribs, and spine. Although a fairly common form of bone cancer, chondrosarcoma is preceded in frequency by metastatic carcinoma, multiple myeloma, and osteosarcoma. Histologic grading is most important in prognosis since grade I and grade II lesions present very good 5-year survival rates following surgery, unlike grade III, poorly differentiated tumors, which invade quickly and metastasize to lungs.

460. The answer is C. *(Robbins, 5/e, pp 1231–1232, 1249–1250.)* Pott's disease of the spine is caused by tuberculous infection of the lower thoracic and lumbar vertebrae. Destruction of the intervertebral disks and adjacent vertebral bodies causes them to collapse, and these compression fractures may result in angular kyphosis or scoliosis. Caseous material may extend from the vertebrae into paravertebral muscles and along the psoas muscle sheath to form a psoas abscess in the inguinal regions. Tuberculous osteomyelitis occurs most often in the long bones and spine and via hematogenous spread from a primary site elsewhere. Chronic proliferative synovitis with pannus formation is characteristic of rheumatoid arthritis and Lyme arthritis. In Lyme arthritis there is also hyperplastic "onion-skin" arteriolar thickening (similar to that in syphilis).

461. The answer is B. *(Anderson, 9/e, pp 2068, 2158. Isselbacher, 13/e, pp 557, 1705.)* The photograph displays a grossly deformed knee joint, an example of neurogenic arthropathy (Charcot's joint). This is a rapidly destructive, often monarticular form of osteoarthritis. Destruction of the joint surface, subluxation or dislocation, and loose bodies are prominent, and the scarred, chronically inflamed synovium contains striking bone and cartilage detritus. The underlying neurologic lesion with its resultant loss of local proprioception and sensory nerve paths may occur in tabes dorsalis, syringomyelia, leprosy, diabetes, spina bifida, or chronic alcoholism. The rare association of arthritis and psoriasis characteristically affects the distal interphalangeal joints of hands and feet in asymmetric fashion.

462. The answer is B. *(Robbins, 5/e, pp 1241–1244. Rubin, 2/e, p 1314.)* Fibroosseous lesions of bone classically include fibrous dysplasia (FD), nonossifying fibroma (fibrous cortical defect), and osteoid osteoma. Histologically, FD shows a characteristic "Chinese-lettering" effect of the bony trabeculae, which are surrounded by a cellular, fibrous stroma, with osteoblasts and osteoclasts conspicuously decreased at the periphery of the entrapped woven bone. Histologically, nonossifying fibroma shows characteristic foam cell histiocytes within the lesions of the metaphysis. Osteoid osteomas are found within the diaphysis of long bones and contain osteoid trabeculae in a cellular, fibrous matrix, but unlike FD, this disease demonstrates (singular) peripheral trabecular osteoblasts. FD produces radiolucent bone lesions involving long bones and thorax, skull, and facial bones. *Monostotic FD* refers to single-bone involvement, *polyostotic FD* refers to involvement of multiple lesions or bones, and *Albright's syndrome* refers to polyostotic bone lesions, endocrinopathy (hyperthyroidism, thyrotoxicosis, hyperpituitarism, Cushing's syndrome), precocious puberty in females, and café-au-lait spots on the skin. The pigmented, macular café-au-lait spots are usually more irregular ("coast of Maine") in outline than the forms seen in neurofibromatosis. Monostotic FD is very rarely associated with the skin lesions.

463. The answer is E. *(Robbins, 5/e, pp 1255–1258.)* Diseases that lead to continued tissue synthesis and breakdown may produce hyperuricemia and clinical gout because of the resulting increase in nucleic acid turnover. This form of secondary gout may be seen in polycythemia vera, myeloid metaplasia, chronic leukemia, extensive psoriasis, and sarcoidosis. Cytotoxic drugs used in the chemotherapy of cancer may augment hyperuricemia. Decreased renal excretion of uric acid may also lead to secondary gout. Overproduction of uric acid may result from inborn errors of metabolism, as in the Lesch-Nyhan syndrome (deficiency of the enzyme hypoxanthine-guanine phosphoribosyltransferase (HGPRT). Chondrocalcinosis is pseudogout.

464. The answer is A. *(Anderson, 9/e, pp 2079, 2082–2083. Robbins, 5/e, pp 1249–1253.)* Rheumatoid arthritis frequently affects the small joints of the hands and feet. The larger joints are involved later. Subcutaneous nodules, with a necrotic focus surrounded by palisades of proliferating cells, are seen in some cases. In the joints, the synovial membrane is thickened by a granulation tissue pannus that is infiltrated by many inflammatory cells. Nodular collections of lymphocytes resembling follicles are characteristically seen. The thickened synovial membrane may develop villous projections, and the joint cartilage is attacked and destroyed.

465. The answer is D. *(Robbins, 5/e, pp 25–26, 1247–1253, 1255–1259.)* Gout is associated with increased serum levels of uric acid, even though less than 15 percent of all persons with elevated serum levels of uric acid develop symptoms of gout. Gout may be classified as primary or secondary. Secondary gout may result from increased production of uric acid or from decreased excretion of uric acid. Primary (idiopathic) gout usually results from impaired excretion of uric acid by the kidneys. Most patients present with pain and redness of the first metatarsophalangeal joint, the "great toe."

Sodium urate crystals—needle-shaped, negatively birefringent crystals—precipitate to form chalky white deposits. Urate crystals may precipitate in extracellular soft tissue, such as the helix of the ear, forming masses called tophi. Pseudogout is caused by deposition of calcium pyrophosphate dihydrate (CPPD) in synovial membranes, which also forms chalky white areas on cartilaginous surfaces. CPPD crystals are not needle-shaped like urate crystals, but are short, stubby, and rhomboid; they are also birefringent. The degenerative joint disease osteoarthritis is the single most common form of joint disease. It is a "wear and tear" disorder that destroys the articular cartilage, resulting in smooth (eburnated, "ivory-like") subchondral bone. Rheumatoid arthritis, a systemic disease frequently affecting the small joints of the hands and feet, is associated with rheumatoid factor. Rheumatoid factors are antibodies, usually IgM, which are directed against the Fc fragment of IgG. In the joints, the synovial membrane is thickened by a granulation tissue, a pannus, that consists of many inflammatory cells, mainly lymphocytes and plasma cells. Ochronosis, caused by a defect in homogentisic acid oxidase, is associated with deposition of dark pigment in the cartilage of joints and degeneration of the joints.

466–468. The answers are 466-A, 467-B, 468-E. *(Anderson, 9/e, pp 2021–2022, 2043–2045. Robbins, 5/e, pp 1237–1238, 1245–1246. Rubin, 2/e, pp 1315–1316.)* Osteoclastoma, the giant cell tumor of bone, usually produces a lytic lesion involving the epiphysis of long bones. The proximal tibia is a common site. There are many pitfalls involved in making a diagnosis of giant cell tumor of bone. The main problem involves the difficulty of distinguishing the bone destruction that is a true neoplasm from bone destruction that is the result of various types of osteoclastic-osteoblastic activity. Direct communication with the radiologist and, preferably, the orthopedic surgeon is, therefore, nearly mandatory for the pathologist when making a diagnosis.

Unicameral, or solitary, cysts are loculated, lytic lesions of bone that characteristically abut on the epiphyseal plate in older children and produce cortical irregularities. Regions involved in the benign lesion are prone to fracture.

Osteochondromas are cauliflower-like lesions that contain a core of cortical and medullary bone and a cartilage cap that decreases in width as age increases. They usually protrude from the metaphyses of long bones and may be multiple.

Nonossifying fibromas of bone—usually well-demarcated, eccentric, lytic metaphyseal lesions—most commonly occur in the tibia and femur. They are histologically identical to fibrous cortical defects and consist of a fibroblastic growth without concomitant bone formation.

Skin and Breast

DIRECTIONS: Each question below contains five suggested responses. Select the **one best** response to each question.

469. The clinical photograph below suggests that the patient

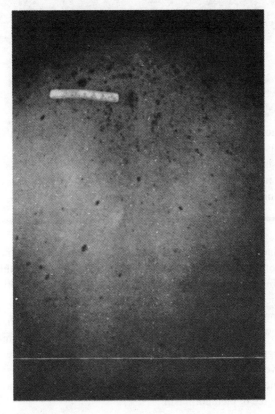

(A) has Leser-Trelat sign
(B) has multiple basal cell nevus syndrome
(C) is at risk for developing malignant melanoma
(D) has leopard syndrome
(E) has Torres's syndrome

470. Which of the following pairs of disorders would most appropriately be considered in the differential diagnosis for the lesion seen in the photomicrograph below?

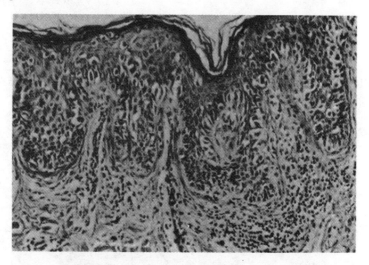

(A) Superficial spreading malignant melanoma in situ and Paget's disease
(B) Mycosis fungoides and metastatic carcinoma
(C) Psoriasis and lichen planus
(D) Lupus erythematosus and lupus vulgaris
(E) Leukemia and lymphoma

471. The incidence of malignant melanoma of the skin appears to be increasing in the United States. Which of the following is most significant in predicting the clinical behavior following diagnosis?

(A) The degree of pigmentation
(B) The level and depth
(C) The amount of inflammation
(D) The degree of pleomorphism
(E) The state of nutrition

472. Diseases developing from cells found normally within the epidermis include all the following EXCEPT

(A) squamous cell carcinoma
(B) Merkel cell carcinoma
(C) melanoma
(D) Letterer-Siwe disease
(E) urticaria pigmentosa

473. Malignant or premalignant lesions of the skin include

(A) acrochordon
(B) senile (actinic) keratosis
(C) keratoacanthoma
(D) dermatofibroma
(E) dermoid cyst

474. An adult patient develops crops of bullae and vesicles in the mouth and later on the skin of the trunk. A skin biopsy is inconclusive but shows a suprabasal acantholysis of the overlying epidermis. Direct immunofluorescence of the skin can be used to identify all the following EXCEPT

(A) bullous pemphigoid
(B) pemphigus vulgaris
(C) dermatitis herpetiformis
(D) erythema multiforme
(E) discoid lupus erythematosus (DLE)

475. Mycosis fungoides is correctly characterized by which of the following statements?

(A) It is more common in females
(B) It represents cutaneous spread of a primary nodal lymphoma
(C) It is characterized histologically by microabscesses of Munro
(D) It is a cutaneous lymphoma of CD4+ T-cell lineage
(E) It is a cutaneous lymphoma of CD8+ T-cell lineage

476. True statements concerning basal cell carcinoma of the skin include all the following EXCEPT

(A) it is locally destructive but rarely metastasizes
(B) histologically it typically shows large cells with abundant, glassy, eosinophilic cytoplasm
(C) peripheral palisading is a common histologic feature
(D) clinical appearance is a pearly papule with raised margins and a central ulcer
(E) recognized variants include morphea-like, superficial, and pigmented

477. Lobular panniculitis with vasculitis is seen in

(A) erythema nodosum
(B) erythema multiforme
(C) erythema induratum
(D) Weber-Christian disease
(E) pseudoxanthoma elasticum

478. All the following are the result of melanocytic hyperplasia EXCEPT

(A) freckle
(B) lentigo
(C) junctional nevus
(D) blue nevus
(E) Spitz tumor

479. True statements about the condition seen in the photomicrograph below include all the following EXCEPT

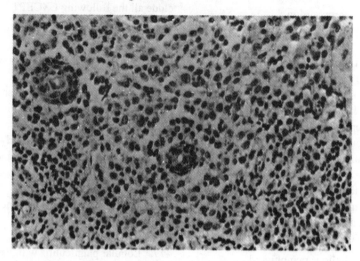

(A) it is often misdiagnosed clinically as seborrheic dermatitis
(B) it may have associated otitis media
(C) it may involve multiple viscera
(D) diabetes mellitus is fairly commonly associated
(E) Birbeck granules can be observed in the cells

---

480. A 37-year-old woman presents with a lump in the upper outer quadrant of the left breast, which shows a wide spectrum of benign breast disease on pathologic examination. Which of the following is considered to indicate the greatest risk for subsequent carcinoma of the breast?

(A) Intraductal papillomatosis
(B) Sclerosing adenosis
(C) Focal papillomatosis
(D) Marked apocrine metaplasia
(E) Epithelial hyperplasia of the ducts

481. A 23-year-old woman presents with a rubbery, freely movable 2-cm mass in the upper outer quadrant of the left breast. A biopsy of this lesion would most likely histologically reveal

(A) large numbers of neutrophils
(B) large numbers of plasma cells
(C) duct ectasia with inspissation of breast secretions
(D) necrotic fat surrounded by lipid-laden macrophages
(E) a mixture of fibrous tissue and ducts

482. The differential diagnosis of the lesion with dense lymphocytic infiltration depicted below could include all the following EXCEPT

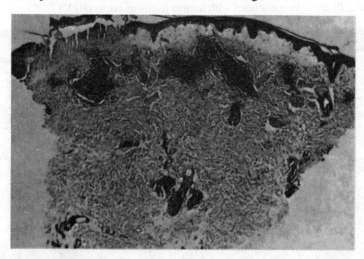

(A) lupus erythematosus
(B) urticaria pigmentosa
(C) polymorphous light eruption
(D) pseudolymphoma
(E) malignant lymphoma

---

483. A papillary lesion is seen in a biopsy from a 32-year-old woman who presented with sanguineous discharge from the nipple. All the following would be useful in differentiating benign intraductal papilloma from papillary adenocarcinoma EXCEPT

(A) a cribriform pattern
(B) knowledge of the presence or absence of cell uniformity
(C) fibrovascular cores
(D) the age of the patient
(E) two cell types (epithelial and myoepithelial)

484. A menopausal woman is given a diagnosis of lobular carcinoma of the breast. True statements regarding this lesion include all the following EXCEPT

(A) it represents about 10 percent of breast carcinomas
(B) epidermal infiltration is characteristic
(C) biopsies of the contralateral breast are indicated
(D) it tends to be multifocal
(E) a single file pattern of infiltration is characteristic

485. The photomicrograph below is from a small, papillary lesion found on the dorsal surface of the left hand of an 18-year-old woman. This lesion is most likely to be associated with human papillomavirus (HPV)

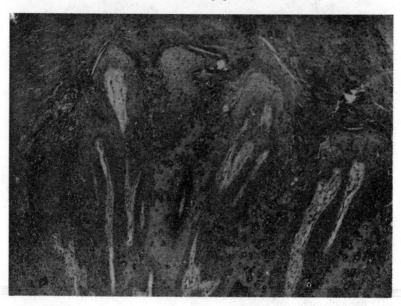

(A) types 1 or 3
(B) types 2 or 4
(C) types 5 or 8
(D) types 6 or 11
(E) types 16 or 18

486. Which of the following diseases of the skin is characterized by homogeneous intracytoplasmic inclusions within the epidermal cells of the stratum granulosum?

(A) Molluscum contagiosum
(B) Impetigo
(C) Tinea
(D) Erythema migrans
(E) Pediculosis

487. Clinical risk factors for development of carcinoma of the female breast include all the following EXCEPT

(A) early menopause
(B) nulliparity
(C) history of endometrial cancer
(D) early menarche
(E) obesity

488. A 37-year-old woman presents with a recurrent swelling in her left upper eyelid. The lesion is biopsied by an ophthalmologist, and a section from that specimen, seen in the photomicrograph below, is characteristic of a

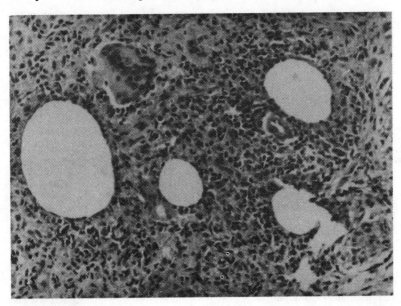

(A) chalazion
(B) hordeolum
(C) xanthelasma
(D) hydrocystoma
(E) sebaceous carcinoma

---

489. Which of the following statements most accurately describes inflammatory breast cancer?

(A) Inflammation improves the prognosis
(B) Inflammation is increased in Paget's disease
(C) Acute inflammatory cells are present
(D) Chronic inflammatory cells are present
(E) Lymphatic permeation is present

490. The most important factor related to the prognosis of breast cancer is

(A) the presence of activated oncogenes
(B) the histologic type and grade
(C) the size of the tumor
(D) the status of axillary lymph nodes
(E) the presence of estrogen receptors

491. An excisional biopsy of the nipple area, taken from a 46-year-old woman, is shown below. The patient complained of discharge from the nipple for approximately 4 months. The most likely diagnosis is

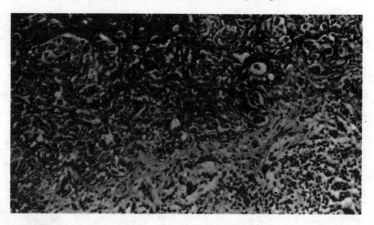

(A) fibroadenoma
(B) epidermoid carcinoma
(C) eczematous inflammation
(D) Paget's disease of the breast
(E) mammary fibromatosis

492. A number of malignant tumors of the breast have been known in some instances to have a deceptively bland histologic appearance and hence have at times been misdiagnosed as benign by the pathologist. These potentially deceptive tumors include all the following EXCEPT

(A) duct carcinoma
(B) tubular carcinoma
(C) angiosarcoma
(D) papillary carcinoma
(E) metastasizing mucinous carcinoma

493. All the following factors have shown an association with gynecomastia EXCEPT

(A) Leydig cell tumors
(B) seminomas
(C) Sertoli cell tumors
(D) alcoholic cirrhosis
(E) digitalis therapy

494. A 16-year-old girl undergoes biopsy of a breast lump that shows the changes in the photomicrograph below. What is the most appropriate course of action?

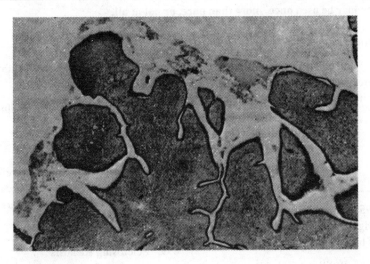

(A) Radiotherapy
(B) Local excision
(C) Radical mastectomy
(D) Modified radical mastectomy
(E) No further therapy

DIRECTIONS: Each group of questions below consists of lettered headings followed by a set of numbered items. For each numbered item select the **one** lettered heading with which it is **most** closely associated. Each lettered heading may be used **once, more than once, or not at all.**

Questions 495–497

Match the characteristic features with the appropriate acanthotic skin disease.

(A) Psoriasis
(B) Lichen planus
(C) Verruca vulgaris
(D) Pemphigus vulgaris
(E) Acanthosis nigricans

495. Elongated, saw-toothed rete ridges and liquefaction degeneration of basal layer

496. Papillary, folded hyperkeratosis and melanin pigmentation of basal layer

497. Parakeratosis and elongation of clubbed rete ridges and dermal papillae

Questions 498–500

Match each breast disease with the appropriate description.

(A) Is characteristically painful
(B) May have mesenchymal differentiation
(C) Is frequently bilateral
(D) Never predisposes to carcinoma
(E) Produces scirrhous tumors

498. Ductal carcinoma

499. Sclerosing adenosis

500. Cystosarcoma phylloides

Skin and Breast

Answers

469. The answer is C. *(Robbins, 5/e, pp 1177–1178, 1181–1182. Rubin, 2/e, pp 1219–1220.)* The clinical photograph depicts the presence of the dysplastic nevus syndrome, first described by Dr. Wallace Clark and his coworkers Drs. Mark Greene, David Elder, and E. Bondi in Philadelphia during the mid 1970s. This valuable finding elucidated the presence of abnormal nevi that are at least a marker for the development of malignant melanoma. These nevi, while not malignant, have atypical features compared with those of normal nevi, such as irregular borders, a pink base, and irregular pigmentation. The Leser-Trelat sign refers to the development of multiple seborrheic keratoses over a short period of time in older patients who have visceral malignancy, while the basal cell nevus syndrome is dominantly inherited with the association of numerous basal cell carcinomas forming throughout life, bifid ribs, keratocysts of the mandible, unusual facies, and abnormalities of the central nervous system and reproductive system. A familial occurrence of dysplastic nevus syndrome with basal cell nevus syndrome was elucidated at the 1985 meeting of the International Academy of Pathologists by Elliot Foucar. The leopard syndrome refers to multiple flat lentigines that are not premalignant for melanoma, in addition to cardiac abnormalities and ocular hypertelorism. Recent studies have shown that the dysplastic nevus syndrome is not only familial, but may be sporadic in about 6 percent of the general population. The risk of developing melanoma in the dysplastic nevus familial situation is greatly increased over that in the general population. It has been stated that patients with dysplastic nevi belonging to a kindred with dysplastic nevus and familial malignant melanoma have a 100-fold risk of developing malignant melanoma over their entire lifetime.

470. The answer is A. *(Robbins, 5/e, pp 1105, 1179–1181, 1190–1192, 1197–1200.)* The photomicrograph was taken from a patient with superficial spreading malignant melanoma in situ; it shows individual cells resembling Paget's disease invading the upper regions of the epidermis. The basement membrane zone is intact and there are lymphocytes in the underlying dermis. Cells with clear cytoplasm and malignant-appearing nuclei such as shown here resemble those of Paget's disease, from which they must be distinguished. Some cells of mycosis fungoides will resemble this, but they occur in nest formations called Pautrier's abscesses. Metastatic carcinoma can produce lesions that resemble malignant melanoma, but these are problems relating to the dermis. Leukemia-lymphoma infiltrates mainly involve the dermis, although the epidermis may become ulcerated and atrophic. Lupus erythematosus and lichen planus produce subepidermal lymphocytic infiltrates with no involvement of the epidermis itself. Psoriasis produces parakeratosis and elongtated rete ridges but no abnormal cells in the epidermis.

471. The answer is B. *(Robbins, 5/e, pp 1179–1181. Rubin, 2/e, pp 1218–1228.)* Although malignant melanoma of the skin is not as common as squamous and basal cell carcinoma, it is an exceedingly important and somewhat mysterious tumor owing to its often devastating clinical course and occasionally unpredictable behavior. There appear to be strong immune factors that presumably account for some well-documented remissions, lengthy survival after distant metastasis, and rapid growth in renal transplant patients. However, most patients with this form of cancer pursue a course characterized by eventual distant and visceral metastasis, especially if the histologic type is either nodular or superficial spreading. The subtype called *lentigo maligna melanoma,* found in the sun-exposed skin of elderly patients, generally has a much more favorable outlook. The most important predictors of outcome are the level of penetration into the subepidermis and reticular dermis (Clark levels I through V: I, in situ, V, invasion of subcutaneous fat) and the actual depth of invasion, measured in millimeters with an ocular micrometer (Breslow depth). The survival at 5 years is 90 percent if the tumor is Clark I or II and 0.76 mm or less in depth, but survival falls to 40 to 48 percent if the tumor is level III or IV and greater than 1.9 mm in depth. While some melanoma cells may show cytologic pleomorphism, many aggressive melanomas exhibit uniformity and blandness. Recent work has shown that melanomas arising in the region of the shoulder, upper trunk, and back in men behave in an aggressive fashion.

472. The answer is E. *(Robbins, 5/e, pp 1173, 1186–1188. Rubin, 2/e, pp 1179–1181, 1185.)* The skin is made up of the epidermis and the dermis. The epidermis is composed of stratified keratinocytes, which produce keratin, tonofibrils, and keratohyaline bodies. The epidermal keratinocytes may give rise to squamous cell carcinomas. Several cell types normally immigrate into the epidermis. Melanocytes are dendritic cells that originate in the neural crest, migrate into the basal layer of the epidermis, and contain melanosomes. They may give rise to malignant melanomas. Langerhans cells are dendritic cells that process antigens, contain distinctive organelles (the racket-shaped Birbeck granules), and may give rise to one of the forms of Langerhans cell histiocytosis (histiocytosis X), such as Letterer-Siwe disease. Merkel cells, attached to keratinocytes by desmosomes, have distinctive membrane-bound, dense-core granules and may give rise to Merkel cell carcinoma. Mast cells are normally found about venules within the dermis, not the epidermis. They may proliferate, causing the disease urticaria pigmentosa.

473. The answer is B. *(Robbins, 5/e, pp 1182–1186, 1188–1189.)* Fibrous histiocytoma (dermatofibroma, sclerosing hemangioma) is a benign dermal tumor of fibroblasts and histiocytes, proliferating in cartwheel or storiform pattern, in which small blood vessels may form a prominent component. Senile (actinic, solar) keratosis is a premalignant skin lesion with focal atypia of keratinocytes of the lower layers of the epidermis. There is often a history of chronic exposure to the sun, and there is a high incidence in the southern United States. Other precancerous skin lesions include erythroplasia of Queyrat and Bowen's disease. Keratoacanthoma, a benign tumor, may resemble squamous cell carcinoma both clinically and histologically, but penetration of the dermis never extends deeper than adjacent hair follicles. The lesion is cup-shaped with central keratin; biopsy or excision excludes squamous carcinoma. An achrochordon (skin tag) is a benign fibroepithelial polyp of the skin. The dermoid cyst is similar to the benign epidermal inclusion cyst except that it also has dermal appendage structures attached to the wall of the cyst.

474. The answer is D. *(Robbins, 5/e, pp 1199–1205. Rubin, 2/e, pp 1190–1205.)* Patients of either sex in the fourth to sixth decade who develop oral vesicles followed by disseminated bullae are likely to have pemphigus vulgaris, one of the blistering (bullous) dermatoses. The differfential diagnosis in this setting is widespread and can include various forms of erythema multiforme (or Stevens-Johnson syndrome in the young) and bullous pemphigoid, as well as pemphigus vulgaris. Common to most bullous dermatoses is the presence of epidermal cell separation, which produces spaces and clefts (acantholysis) that are visible in ordinary tissue sections and specific to location within the epidermis. The bullae may be subcorneal, intraepidermal, suprabasal, or subepidermal, and multiple diseases can be grouped according to acantholysis location. To categorize the type of disease further, direct immunofluorescence testing can be done on a fresh skin lesion, using antibodies to immunoglobulins, fibrin, and complement. Pemphigus vulgaris shows a characteristic "basket-weave" pattern in the epidermis to IgG, IgA is found at the tips of the dermal papillae in dermatitis herpetiformis, and linear bands of IgG and complement are found in the subepidermal zones in bullous pemphigoid, whereas erythema multiforme has no immunofluorescent pattern. In DLE, direct immunofluorescence shows a granular band of immunoglobulin and complement at the dermoepidermal junction (lupus band test), and this may be present in "normal" skin in patients with systemic lupus erythematosus.

475. The answer is D. *(Robbins, 5/e, pp 1109–1192.)* Mycosis fungoides is part of the spectrum of malignant T-cell lymphomas, mostly of the CD4+ T-cell subset, with a predilection for the skin. It is more common in males and the incidence increases with age. It arises primarily in the skin but more than 70 percent of patients have extracutaneous spread with lymph nodes, spleen, liver, and lungs most often involved. Clinically it presents as cutaneous patches, plaques, or nodules and is often misdiagnosed as psoriasis or other dermatitides. Histologically there is a bandlike infiltrate in the upper dermis of atypical lymphocytes with markedly convoluted nuclei—the Sézary-Lutzner cells. These show epidermotropism and form characteristic intraepidermal clusters known as *Pautrier's microabscesses*. In some cases there is generalized erythroderma and Sézary-Lutzner cells in the peripheral blood. This is known as the Sézary syndrome.

476. The answer is B. *(Robbins, 5/e, p 1187. Rubin, 2/e, pp 1230–1232.)* Basal cell carcinoma, arising from the pluripotential cells in the basal layer of the epidermis, is the most common tumor in patients with pale skin. This carcinoma is locally invasive and may be quite destructive. Metastasis, however, is quite rare. The classic clinical appearance is a pearly papule with raised margins and a central ulcer. Variants, which are not infrequent, include the superficial type (which may be multifocal), the morphea-like type (which has marked fibrosis and is difficult to eradicate locally), and the pigmented type (which may be mistaken clinically for malignant melanoma). Histologically the cells are deeply basophilic with palisading at the periphery of groups of tumor cells and peritumoral clefting. Abundant eosinophilic cytoplasm may be seen in squamous cell carcinomas, not basal cell carcinoma.

477. The answer is C. *(Robbins, 5/e, pp 1195–1196. Rubin, 2/e, pp 1202–1204, 1213–1215.)* Inflammation of the subcutaneous adipose tissue, panniculitis, may affect the connective tissue septa (septal panniculitis) or the fat lobule (lobular penniculitis). Erythema nodosum is a self-limited disease triggered by several agents, including drugs and microorganisms. It consists of inflammation of the fibrous septa without vasculitis. Weber-Christian disease is characterized by recurring groups of tender nodules within the subcutaneous fat and inflammatory cells within the lobules with necrosis of adipocytes. There is no vasculitis. Erythema induratum is a chronic disease found primarily on the legs of women. It is associated with vasculitis and is considered to be a vascular hypersensitivity reaction. There is chronic inflammation in the subcutaneous lobules with tuberculoid granulomas and fat necrosis. Erythema multiforme is an acute, self-limited disorder that usually occurs as a reaction to a drug or infectious agent. Histologic examination reveals lymphocytic infiltration, with possible subepidermal bullae, and epidermal necrosis. Pseudoxanthoma elasticum is a hereditary disorder characterized by fragmented and thickened elastic fibers in the dermis and thickened, yellow-orange skin in the axillary folds and inguinal regions.

478. The answer is A. *(Robbins, 5/e, pp 1176–1181. Rubin, 2/e, pp 1218–1228.)* Melanocytic hyperplasia, which causes hyperpigmentation of the skin, can be classified into several types of lesions. A lentigo consists of melanocytic hyperplasia in the basal layers of the epidermis along with elongation and thinning of the rete ridges. Two types of lentigines are lentigo simplex and lentigo senilis ("liver spots"). Increased numbers of melanocytes may form clusters located either at the tips of the rete ridges in the epidermis (junctional nevus), within the dermis (intradermal nevus), or both at the tips of the rete ridges and within the dermis (compound nevus). A blue nevus is composed of highly dendritic melanocytes that penetrate more deeply into the dermis. This deep location gives the lesion its characteristic blue color. The Spitz tumor (epithelioid cell nevus) is a benign lesion composed of groups of epithelioid and spindle melanocytes found in children and young adults. It may be mistaken histologically for a malignant melanoma. A freckle (ephelis) is a pigmented lesion caused by increased melanin pigmentation within keratinocytes of the basal layer of the epidermis. There is no increase in the number of melanocytes. These lesions fade with the lack of sun exposure.

479. The answer is D. *(Robbins, 5/e, pp 666–667, 1190.)* The photomicrograph demonstrates the presence of Langerhans cells in an infiltrated fashion into the upper dermis and shows the reniform nuclei and crowding characteristic of the disorder previously referred to as a form of *histiocytosis X*. These are now known to be disorders of Langerhans cells, which have surface membrane FC receptors and react with antibodies to thymocyte differentiation antigens (CD1) and ultrastructural granules referred to as *Birbeck granules,* which have the appearance of tennis rackets when seen by electron microscopy. The Letterer-Siwe form arises in children, often in infants, and presents with cutaneous lesions that resemble seborrheic dermatitis (or cradle cap). Often these patients present with fever and otitis media or mastoiditis, which call attention to the disorder. If the disease disseminates it may involve organs of the mononuclear phagocyte system, including the spleen, liver, lymph nodes, bone marrow, and lungs. On x-ray, lesions are reflected by cystic radiolucent areas that can be seen in the skull, pelvis, and long bones. Patients often have anemia and thrombocytopenia, which can contribute to a terminal outcome owing to infections. Many infants died from the disorder in years past, but with the use of chemotherapy and improvement of underlying hypoimmunity, there has been a reversal of the death rate. Diabetes insipidus, not diabetes mellitus, is a fairly common accompaniment of multifocal Langerhans cell histiocytosis.

480. The answer is E. *(Robbins, 5/e, pp 1093–1097.)* The spectrum of benign breast disease includes fibrocystic disease, which is probably a misnomer; adenosis, both slcerosing and microglandular; intraductal papillomas and papillomatosis; apocrine metaplasia; fibrous stromal hyperplasia; and hyperplasia of the epithelial cells lining the ducts and ductules of the breasts. At one time or another each of the above was considered to be a forerunner of carcinoma; however, with extensive studies in the literature, none of these has been shown to necessarily correlate with a greater risk of developing carcinoma with the exception of epithelial hyperplasia, particularly when atypical. With any of the features, but especially epithelial hyperplasia, adding a positive family history of breast cancer in a sibling, mother, or maternal aunt markedly increases the risk for developing carcinoma of the breast in the given patient. Owing to the advances and technology of xeromammography, there has been an increased interest in calcifications, which are markers for carcinoma of the breast. These calcifications, however, do not necessarily occur within the cancerous ducts themselves and can be found frequently in either adenosis adjacent to the carcinoma or even in normal breast lobules in the region. Stipple calcification as seen by xeromammography is regarded by some workers as an indication for a biopsy of the region.

481. The answer is E. *(Robbins, 5/e, pp 1091–1093, 1097–1098. Rubin, 2/e, pp 978, 982.)* The most common benign neoplasm of the breast is the fibroadenoma. It typically occurs in the upper outer quadrant of the breast in women between the ages of 20 and 35. These lesions originate from the terminal duct lobular unit and histologically reveal a mixture of fibrous connective tissue and ducts. Clinically, fibroadenomas are rubbery, freely movable, oval nodules that usually measure 2 to 4 cm in diameter. Numerous neutrophils are seen in acute bacterial infection of the breast (acute mastitis), which is usually seen in the postpartum lactating or involuting breast. Dilatation of the breast ducts (ectasia) with inspissation of breast secretions is characteristic of mammary duct ectasia. It is common in elderly women. If large numbers of plasma cells are also present, the lesion is called *plasma cell mastitis*. Fat necrosis of the breast, associated with traumatic injury, is characterized by necrotic fat surrounded by lipid-laden macrophages and a neutrophilic infiltration.

482. The answer is B. *(Anderson, 9/e, pp 1769–1771, 1775–1776, 1827. Lever, 7/e, p 497.)* Dense lymphocytic infiltration of the skin carries with it a differential diagnosis that includes the five L's: lupus, light, lymphoma, pseudolymphoma, and lymphotic infiltration of the skin (Jessner). All are characterized by lymphoid hyperplasia of the dermis. Leukemic lymphomas are diagnosed by atypical sheets of lymphoblastic cells with mitoses; lupus erythematosus is characterized by lymphoid infiltration around the follicles and vessels of the dermis. Light eruptions are characterized by a lymphocytic perivascular inflammation of the skin of the face. A difficult differential diagnosis includes lymphocytic infiltration of the skin (Jessner), which often has an increase in dermal mucopolysaccharides that can be demonstrated by alcian blue stains. In urticaria pigmentosa, a localized cutaneous form of mastocytosis that affects mainly children, there is infiltration of mast cells in the upper and middle dermis.

483. The answer is D. *(Anderson, 9/e, pp 1731–1732, 1737–1739.)* The histologic distinction between benign, cystic intraductal papillomas of the breast and papillary adenocarcinomas is based on multiple criteria. The age of the patient is not of immense importance, since papillomas occur in both younger and older women. Benign papillomas are structured with a complex arrangement of papillary fronds of fibrovascular stalks, covered by one or (usually) two types of cells (epithelial and myoepithelial). Papillary carcinomas are usually of one monotonous cell type and have either no fibrovascular stalks or only a few of them. Papillary carcinomas show a uniform growth of cells with similar appearance with enclosed tubular spaces; the whole arrangement bridges across the entire lumen at times or simply lines the outer rim of the duct (cribriforming). Peripheral invasion of the stroma, if present at all, makes the diagnosis of carcinoma rather certain. There are lesions in which the differentiation is exceedingly difficult, even in the hands of renowned surgical pathologists. Many competent pathologists understandably prefer to defer the diagnosis on all papillary lesions of the breast on frozen section until well-fixed and optimally prepared permanent sections are available.

484. The answer is B. *(Robbins, 5/e, pp 1105–1106.)* Lobular carcinoma composes up to 10 percent of all histologic types of breast cancer, with duct carcinoma being the most common (70 to 75 percent of the total). It presumably arises from the terminal duct epithelium of the lobule, and it carries a high propensity to multifocality and bilateral breast involvement. There is evidence that this form of breast cancer gives rise to multiple, separate primaries within both breasts. For this reason, breast therapists currently advocate biopsies of the contralateral breast when the tumor is diagnosed. The lobular architectural spectrum begins with lobular hyperplasia and may then progress to lobular neoplasia, atypical lobular neoplasia (lobular carcinoma in situ), and, finally, infiltrating lobular carcinoma. Histologically, the tumor cells infiltrate in a characteristic single file pattern. Invasion of the epidermis by malignant cells is characteristic of Paget's disease.

485. The answer is B. *(Silverberg, 2/e, p 195. Robbins, 5/3, pp 1205–1206. Rubin, 2/e, pp 1228–1229.)* Verrucae (warts) are cutaneous lesions caused by human papillomaviruses (HPV) that belong to the DNA-containing papovavirus group. Verrucae are classified according to their location and morphology. Verruca vulgaris, the most common type of wart, may occur anywhere on the body, but most commonly, it is located on the dorsal surface of the hands. The photomicrograph reveals characteristic features of verrucae vulgaris including hyperkeratosis, papillary hyperplasia of the epidermis, and numerous, large, keratohyaline granules within the epidermal cells. Verrucae vulgaris have been associated with several types of HPV, including types 2 and 4. Plantar warts, hyperkeratotic lesions on the soles similar to a callus, are associated with HPV type 1, while verruca plana, typically found on the face, is associated with HPV type 3. Venereal warts, also called *condyloma acuminata,* are associated with HPV types 6 and 11. Carcinoma may develop in condyloma acuminata, in which case HPV types 16 and 18 are more frequently identified. Bowenoid papulosis, multiple hyperpigmented papules on the genitalia, are associated with HPV types 16 and 18. Epidermodysplasia verruciformis is an autosomal recessive disease associated with impaired cell-mediated immunity and the widespread development of multiple flat warts. These lesions have been associated with HPV types 5 or 8. Some of these lesions may develop into squamous cell carcinomas.

486. The answer is A. *(Robbins, 5/e, pp 1206–1209.)* Intracytoplasmic inclusions are characteristic of viral diseases. Of all the skin diseases listed, only molluscum contagiosum is caused by a virus. It is caused by a poxvirus, which has a characteristic brick-shape appearance with a dumbbell-shaped DNA core. Molluscum is a self-limited pruritic disease of the skin that typically occurs on the trunk or the anogenital region. Impetigo is a common bacterial infection of the skin caused by either coagulase-positive staphylococci or group A beta-hemolytic streptococci. Tinea is caused by superficial fungal infection of the skin, and different types include tinea capitis, tinea corporis, tinea pedis (athlete's foot), and tinea versicolor, which is caused by *Malassezia furfur.* Erythema migrans describes a characteristic expanding erythematous lesion that may be caused by either the bite of the brown recluse spider or by *Ixodes dammini,* the vector for the spirochete that causes Lyme disease. Pediculosis is a pruritic infection that may be caused by the head louse, the crab louse, or the body louse.

487. The answer is A. *(Robbins, 5/e, pp 1100–1101. Rubin, 2/e, pp 982–984.)* Long and continuous exposure to endogenous estrogens increases the risk of developing breast carcinoma. Therefore, late menopause (after age 50), early menarche (especially before age 13), and nulliparity are all risk factors. Endometrial adenocarcinoma and occasional ovarian cancers are also associated with continuous estrogen stimulation with a resultant higher risk of the development of breast cancer in the same patient. Other factors include obesity—estrogen metabolism is altered in obese women and synthesis of estrone increased. Family history is significant, especially if mother and sister had premenopausal breast cancer, in which case there is an increased risk of 50 times that of controls. A past history of breast cancer, especially of lobular type, means greater risk of contralateral breast carcinoma. Hormonal and genetic factors and obesity are probably the major risk factors.

488. The answer is A. *(Silverberg, 2/e, pp 2047–2050. Rubin, 2/e, p 1458.)* Many lesions of the eyelid are submitted for pathologic examination. One of the most common eyelid lesions is the chalazion, a chronic inflammatory reaction to lipid released into the tissue from the eyelid's sebaceous glands of Meibom or Zeis. Characteristic histologic features of this lesion include a chronic inflammatory reaction with giant cells that surround empty spaces where the lipid vacuoles from the sebaceous glands had been located. Because the major clinical disorder to be differentiated from chalazia is a sebaceous carcinoma, ophthalmologists biopsy recurrent lesions suspected of being chalazia to rule this out. Hordeolums (styes) are acute staphylococcal infections of the eyelash follicles (external hordeolum) or the Meibomian glands (internal hordeolum). Xanthelasma, yellow plaques on the skin, histologically reveal aggregates of foamy macrophages within the dermis. Hydrocystomas are one type of cyst that may affect the eyelid and may be lined by apocrine or eccrine cells.

489. The answer is E. *(Robbins, 5/e, p 1106.)* Inflammatory breast carcinoma is often misunderstood because of the qualifying adjective "inflammatory." The term does not refer to the presence of inflammatory cells, abscess, or any special histologic type of breast carcinoma; rather, it refers to more of a clinical phenomenon, in that the breast is swollen, erythematous, and indurated and demonstrates a marked increase in warmth. These changes are caused by widespread lymphatic and vascular permeation within the breast itself and in the deep dermis of the overlying skin by breast carcinoma cells.

The clinical induration and erythema are presumably related to lymphatic-vascular blockage by tumor cells; if present, these findings mean a worse prognosis for the patient.

490. The answer is D. *(Robbins, 5/e, pp 1099, 1107–1108.)* Carcinoma of the breast still causes about 20 percent of female cancer deaths and is the leading cause of death worldwide in women over 40 years of age. It is difficult to predict survival rate, but the status of the axillary nodes is of major importance since negative nodes suggest 70 to 80 percent 10-year survival. There is a significant decrease in 5-year survival if one to three nodes are positive (only 50 percent), and four or more positive nodes at the time of diagnosis usually mean about 20 percent disease-free survival. Obviously, a large size of involved nodes, invasion of the capsule, and fixation to adjacent tissue adversely affect survival. The histologic type and grade of tumor and its size are important also, but nodal involvement (number and size) is the outstanding factor in prognosis. Unfortunately, more than 20 percent of patients with negative lymph nodes do have recurrences and die within 10 years. Although they are of lesser prognostic importance in breast cancers, high levels of estrogen receptors have a better prognosis than lower levels or none, although the best response to endocrine (antiestrogen) ablation therapy is noted with tumors containing both estrogen and progesterone receptors. Amplified or activated tumor oncogenes, particularly c-*erb* B2, may be associated with an aggressive tumor and poor prognosis.

491. The answer is D. *(Robbins, 5/e, p 1105. Rubin, 2/e, pp 986–987.)* The biopsy shows infiltration of the nipple by large cells with clear cytoplasm, which is diagnostic of Paget's disease. These cells are usually found both singly and in small clusters in the epidermis. Paget's disease is always associated with (in fact begins with) an underlying intraductal carcinoma that extends to infiltrate the skin of nipple and areola. Paget cells may resemble the cells of superficial spreading melanoma, but they are PAS-positive diastase-resistant (mucopolysaccharide- or mucin-positive), unlike melanoma cells. Eczematous dermatitis of the nipples is a major differential diagnosis but is usually bilateral and responds rapidly to topical steroids. Paget's disease should be suspected if "eczema" persists more than 3 weeks with topical therapy. Paget's disease occurs mainly in middle-aged women but is unusual. In Paget's disease of the vulvar-anal-perineal region, there is very rarely underlying carcinoma. Mammary fibromatosis is a rare, benign, spindle cell lesion affecting women in the third decade. Clinically, it may mimic cancer with retraction or dimpling of skin. It should be treated by local excision with wide margins since there is risk of local recurrence.

492. The answer is A. *(Anderson, 9/e, pp 1741–1745, 1748.)* The most notorious malignant tumor of the breast, presenting a deceptively innocuous histologic and cytologic appearance, is angiosarcoma, with its almost unrecognizable anastomosing clear channels lined by flattened and barely visible endothelial cells. If this combination is seen within unequivocal breast lobules and ducts, the pathologist must suspect angiosarcoma. Well-differentiated adenocarcinoma of the breast (tubular carcinoma) demonstrates a tumor that is rather benign in appearance, with small ducts lined by single and innocuous-appearing epithelial cells. Whereas the primary site of mucinous carcinoma of the breasts (colloid carcinoma), with its "cysts" filled with extracellular mucin and signet-ring cells, presents no problem in diagnosis, biopsies of metastatic lesions will not infrequently show sheets of bland granular cells with pinpoint nuclei resembling granular cell tumor of the skin, a benign lesion. Early intraductal papillary carcinomas have been misdiagnosed at times as benign intraductal papillomas, and the reverse error has also occurred. Infiltrating duct (scirrhous) carcinoma presents no diagnostic problem in either frozen or permanent section analysis for the pathologist.

493. The answer is B. *(Robbins, 5/e, pp 1109–1110.)* Gynecomastia is enlargement of the male breast with marked hyperplasia of duct epithelium and proliferation of periductal connective tissue. No lobular or acinar tissue exists. Gynecomastia often occurs in response to hyperestrinism and may be found with functioning testicular tumors such as Leydig (interstitial) cell or, rarely, Sertoli cell tumors. The major cause of hyperestrinism in the male is cirrhosis because of deficient breakdown of estrogenic substances by the damaged liver. Digitalis therapy occasionally causes gynecomastia, and Klinefelter's syndrome frequently does so because very reduced circulating androgen results in relative hyperestrinism.

494. The answer is B. *(Anderson, 9/e, pp 1730–1731. Robbins, 5/e, pp 1098–1099.)* The lesion depicted in the photomicrograph is that of a cellular fibroadenoma, a basically benign neoplasm of the breast. Mueller initially described cystosarcoma phylloides in 1838 and named it for the resemblance of the lesion to leaves. In older women if the stroma is hypercellular with mitoses and peripheral infiltrative borders, it has the capacity to metastasize. In the adolescent female, cellular stroma of spindle cells with occasional mitoses, such as in this example, may not behave in a malignant fashion as in older women. Because most lesions like these behave in a benign fashion, conservative but total excision with a small rim of normal tissue surrounding the lesion is all that is necessary in the adolescent.

495–497. The answers are 495-B, 496-E, 497-A. *(Anderson, 9/e, pp 1757, 1759–1760, 1762–1763, 1772–1774, 1794–1795. Robbins, 5/e, pp 1197–1199, 1205–1206.)* Acanthosis, or thickening of the epidermis, through hyperplasia of the malpighian layer often occurs with hyperkeratosis, but not always. Although four of the listed lesions are acanthotic, pemphigus vulgaris is acantholytic with loss of intercellular bridges (desmosomes). This type of intraepidermal vesiculation is seen in the bullae of pemphigus vulgaris; cleavage is just above the basal layer. Biopsy and immunofluorescence are necessary for diagnosis of pemphigus.

Psoriasis occurs in up to 2 percent of the population in Western countries. It is a hereditary skin disease with silver-white, scaling plaques often in sites of repeated trauma. Removal of scale results in minute drops of blood (Auspitz sign). Abnormalities of the nails are found in 25 percent of patients, especially in those with arthritis, and include pitting and yellow-brown "oil spots" under the nail. Histologically, there is marked epidermal thickening and thinning with elongation of rete ridges, parakeratotic hyperkeratosis (nuclei retained in the stratum corneum), and increased mitosis of keratinocytes and other cells above the basal layer. Polymorphonuclear neutrophils (PMNs) form the microabscesses of Munro in the stratum corneum of the epidermis.

Lichen planus is an acute or chronic inflammation of the skin and mucous membranes characterized by flat-topped, pruritic, purple papules on the skin and white oral papules. Histologically, lesions show acanthosis with elongated, saw-toothed rete ridges and liquefaction degeneration of the basal layer, often with necrotic basal cells in the papillary dermis, which form colloid or Civatte bodies. There is usually a bandlike lymphocytic infiltrate along the dermoepidermal junction.

Verruca vulgaris, the common wart, is one of the human papillomavirus (HPV 1, 2, 3, 4) infections of the papovavirus group. It may occur anywhere but most commonly appears on the hands and fingers of schoolchildren as firm 1- to 10-mm papules. Histologically, the lesion shows a papillary acanthosis and cells of the stratum granulosum often display perinuclear vacuoles (koilocytosis). Intranuclear viral particles are seen by EM. A characteristic finding is of "reddish-brown" dots (thrombosed capillary loops) seen with a hand lens on the surface.

Acanthosis nigricans occurs most typically in flexures (axilla, groin, anogenital region) and is usually associated with other benign or malignant conditions. The juvenile type is autosomal dominant with variable penetrance and occurs usually in association with obesity or endocrine disorders. The adult type (about 20 percent of all cases) often occurs with occult adenocarcinoma (usually gastric) but has occurred with oral contraceptive use. Folding of a hyperkeratotic epidermis with basal layer darkened with melanin is characteristic of acanthosis nigricans.

498–500. The answers are 498-E, 499-D, 500-B. *(Robbins, 5/e, pp 1095, 1098–1109.)* Diseases of the breast that are often painful include galactocele, duct ectasia, and fibrocystic disease. Infiltrating ductal carcinoma rarely causes pain but is likely to produce scirrhous tumors causing a firm or hard mass.

Cystosarcoma phylloides may be either benign or malignant and has a cellular myxoid stroma in which osteoid or chondroid foci may appear. It forms a large, lobulated, and cystic lesion and malignant change is accompanied by rapid increase in size. Metastases occur only in about 15 percent of cases.

Sclerosing adenosis is benign, does not predispose to carcinoma, is often unilateral, and arises in the upper outer quadrant. It displays clinical and histologic features difficult to distinguish from carcinoma.

None of these three lesions tends to be bilateral—unlike both lobular carcinoma and fibrocystic disease.

Bibliography

Adams RD, Victor M: *Principles of Neurology,* 5/e. New York, McGraw-Hill, 1993.

Anderson WA, Kissane JM (eds): *Pathology,* 9/e. St. Louis, Mosby, 1989.

Brawer MK: Prostatic intraepithelial neoplasia: A premalignant lesion. *Hum Pathol* 23:242–248, 1992.

Duchin JS, et al: Hantavirus pulmonary syndrome: A clinical description of 17 patients with a newly recognized disease. *N Engl J Med* 330:949–955, 1994.

Fawcett DW: *A Textbook of Histology,* 12/e. New York, Chapman & Hall, 1994.

Henry JB, et al (eds): *Clinical Diagnosis and Management by Laboratory Methods,* 18/e. Philadelphia, Saunders, 1991.

Isselbacher KJ, et al (eds): *Harrison's Principles of Internal Medicine,* 13/e. New York, McGraw-Hill, 1994.

Joklik WK, et al (eds): *Zinsser Microbiology,* 20/e. Norwalk, CT, Appleton & Lange, 1992.

Lee GR, et al (eds): *Wintrobe's Clinical Hematology,* 9/e. Philadelphia, Lea & Febiger, 1993.

Lever WF, Schaumberg-Lever G: *Histopathology of the Skin,* 7/e. Philadelphia, Lippincott, 1990.

Robbins SL, Cotran RS: *Pathologic Basis of Disease,* 5/e. Philadelphia, Saunders, 1994.

Rubin E, Farber JL: *Pathology,* 2/e. Philadelphia, Lippincott, 1994.

Silverberg SG (ed): *Principles and Practice of Surgical Pathology,* 2/e. New York, Churchill Livingstone, 1990.